CN01263827

Diagnosis and Management of

Breast Disease

Diagnosis and Management of

Breast Disease

Richard E. Blackwell, PhD, MD
Professor of Obstetrics and Gynecology
Director, Division of Reproductive Biology and Endocrinology
University of Alabama at Birmingham
Birmingham, Alabama

James C. Grotting, MD, FACS
Clinical Professor of Plastic Surgery
University of Alabama at Birmingham
Birmingham, Alabama

b

**Blackwell
Science**

Blackwell Science

Editorial offices:

238 Main Street, Cambridge,
  Massachusetts 02142, USA
Osney Mead, Oxford OX2 0El, England
25 John Street, London WC1N 2BL, England
23 Ainslie Place, Edinburgh EH3 6AJ, Scotland
54 University Street, Carlton, Victoria 3053,
  Australia
Arnette Blackwell SA, 224 Boulevard Saint
  Germain, 75007 Paris, France
Blackwell Wissenschafts-Verlag GmbH
  Kurfürstendamm 57, 10707 Berlin, Germany
Zehetnergasse 6, A-1140 Vienna, Austria

Distributors:

USA
Blackwell Science, Inc.
238 Main Street
Cambridge, Massachusetts 02142
(Telephone orders: 800–215–1000
  or 617–876–7000; Fax orders: 617–492–5263)

Canada
Copp Clark, Ltd.
2775 Matheson Blvd. East
Mississauga, Ontario
Canada, L4W 4P7
(Telephone orders: 800–263–4374
  or 905–238–6074; Fax orders: 03–9349–3016)

Australia
Blackwell Science Pty., Ltd.
54 University Street
Carlton, Victoria 3053
(Telephone orders: 03–347–0300)

Outside North America and Australia
Blackwell Science, Ltd.
c/o Marston Book Services, Ltd.
P.O. Box 2691
Abingdon
Oxon OX14 4YN
(Telephone orders: 44–1865–791155)

Acquisitions: Joy Ferris Denomme
Development: Debra Lance
Production: Heather Garrison
Manufacturing: Lisa Flanagan
Typeset by Huron Valley Graphics
Printed and bound by Edwards Brothers

© 1996 by Richard E. Blackwell and James C.
  Grotting
Printed in the United States of America

96 97 98 99 5 4 3 2 1

Library of Congress Cataloging-in-Publication
Data
Diagnosis and management of breast disease /
[edited by] Richard E.
  Blackwell, James C. Grotting.
      p.   cm.
    Includes bibliographical references
and index.
    ISBN 0–86542–405–5 (alk. paper)
    1. Breast—Cancer. 2. Breast—
Diseases. I. B lackwell, Richard
  E. II. Grotting, James C.
    [DNLM: 1. Breast Diseases—
diagnosis. 2. Breast Diseases—
  therapy.   WP 840 D5361 1996]
RC280.B8D438   1996
616.99'449—dc20
DNLM/ DLC
for Library of Congress   96–5096
                                          CIP

To Dr. Charles E. Flowers, Jr. and Dr. Hugh M. Shingleton. Their teaching, research, and clinical practice have had a major impact in improving the health care of women and in educating a generation of obstetricians/gynecologists.

R. E. B.

To my wife Ann, my sons Jimmy and Ben, and to our patients who have been faced with the spectrum of alterations to the breast form and function due to the disorders described herein.

J. C. G.

Contents

Contributors

Wanda K. Bernreuter, MD
Associate Professor of Diagnostic Radiology
University of Alabama at Birmingham
Birmingham, Alabama

Richard E. Blackwell, PhD, MD
Professor of Obstetrics and Gynecology
Director, Division of Reproductive Biology and Endocrinology
University of Alabama at Birmingham
Birmingham, Alabama

John T. Carpenter, Jr., MD
Professor of Medicine
University of Alabama at Birmingham
Birmingham, Alabama

David Ralph Crowe, MD
Associate Professor of Pathology
University of Alabama at Birmingham
Birmingham, Alabama

Gary W. DeVane, MD
Center for Infertility and Reproductive Medicine
Orlando, Florida

Peter H. Grossman, MD
Department of Surgery and Burn Care
Sherman Oaks Hospital
Sherman Oaks, California

James C. Grotting, MD, FACS
Clinical Professor of Plastic Surgery
University of Alabama at Birmingham
Birmingham, Alabama

Brian J. Hasegawa, MD, FRCS(C)
Attending Surgeon
Department of Plastic Surgery
Stratford General Hospital
Stratford, Ontario
Canada

Richard L.S. Jennelle, MD
Assistant Professor of Radiation Oncology
University of Alabama at Birmingham
Birmingham, Alabama

Philip J. Kenney, MD
Professor of Radiology
University of Alabama at Birmingham
Birmingham, Alabama

Olubunmi T. Lampejo, MD
Assistant Professor of Pathology
University of Alabama at Birmingham
Birmingham, Alabama

Norman S. Levine, MD
Professor and Chairman, Section of Plastic Surgery
University of Oklahoma Health Sciences Center
Oklahoma City, Oklahoma

Nancy S. Pile, MD
Assistant Professor of Radiology
Mammography and Musculoskeletal Sections
University of Alabama at Birmingham
Birmingham, Alabama

Eli Reshef, MD
Assistant Professor of Reproductive Endocrinology
Department of Obstetrics and Gynecology
University of Oklahoma Health Sciences Center
Oklahoma City, Oklahoma

Eva Rubin, MD
Professor of Radiology
University of Alabama at Birmingham
Birmingham, Alabama

Merle M. Salter, MD, FACR
Clinical Professor of Radiation Oncology
University of Alabama at Birmingham
Birmingham, Alabama

Joseph S. Sanfilippo, MD
Professor of Obstetrics and Gynecology
Director of Reproductive Endocrinology
University of Louisville School of Medicine
Louisville, Kentucky

Charles R. Shumate, MD, FACS
Surgical Oncologist
Surgical Associates, P.C.
Birmingham, Alabama

Preface

Throughout history, the breast has assumed a prominent role in art and literature. It has been identified as an object of beauty and sexuality, and as such its role goes far beyond its primary function of lactation. Because of the importance attached by society to the breast, any pathology of the organ is viewed by the patient with alarm. With the exception of carcinoma, disorders of the breast are not life-threatening; however, any deviation from normal size and appearance must be thoroughly evaluated. It is the purpose of this text to furnish the primary care physician with a working guide to the diagnosis and management of breast disease. Emphasis has been placed on the epidemiology of breast disease, breast pathophysiology, appropriate diagnostic steps, point of referral, and treatment and outcome that both the patient and physician may expect.

We would like to give special thanks to Murrill Lynch, Dr. Blackwell's Administrative Associate and to Judy Hunt, Dr. Grotting's Administrative Assistant.

Richard E. Blackwell, PhD, MD
James C. Grotting, MD, FACS

Introduction

Richard E. Blackwell

COMPARATIVE ANATOMY OF LACTATION

As the result of selective pressures, certain apocrine sweat glands evolved into milk-producing organs in different species. Milk products vary widely among the different species, and undoubtedly the variation is related to nutritional requirements and environmental restrictions placed on the female. The mammary gland is unique among the animal kingdom in that only 4200 species of mammals possess this organ. The majority of these mammals (95%) belong to the subclass Eutheria. The only other mammals possessing mammary glands belong to the subclass Monotremata, which includes primitive egg-laying mammals, such as the duckbill platypus, and the subclass Metatheria, which contains the single-order Marsupialia (kangaroo) (1).

HISTORIC OVERVIEW

A commentary regarding the treatment of diseases of the breast is mentioned in the oldest recorded medical history from Egypt, the Edwin Smith papyrus. This manuscript dates back to about 1600 BC and contains 48 cases; the forty-fifth case was dedicated to the description of the treatment of breast cancer. Diseases such as this were treated with little success because Egyptian and Babylonian physicians suffered severe penalties for therapeutic failure. Greek culture was more forgiving, and Hippocrates' aphorism made many references to the relationship of the breast to pregnancy (e.g., when the pregnant uterus contains twins, if one breast becomes flaccid, one of the twins is expelled: if the right breast became flaccid, the male was expelled; but if it was the left breast, the female was expelled), menstrual function (a woman who is neither pregnant nor has lately delivered who has milk in her breast labors under obstructed menstruation), and mood lability (blood originating from the breasts of females denotes an attack of mania).

The first clinical description of breast cancer was written in Latin by Celsus in approximately the first century AD. He was the first to stage breast cancer but did not recommend treatment for stages II, III, or IV. Likewise, Galen, in approximately AD 200, accurately described cancer of the breast and recommended removal of black bile by purging and bleeding as a treatment. The concept of four humors was carried through the Middle Ages, although diseases of the breast were frequently treated with amputation and cautery. These techniques were refined during the Renaissance by Fabre in the late 1500s, who recommended compression of the breast before amputation, whereas Schultes recommended traction with heavy ligatures followed by amputation and cautery.

During the late eighteenth and nineteenth centuries, controversy existed as to the origin of milk. Many of the original drawings by Leonardo da Vinci showed the uterus and the mammary glands connected by a system of ducts. Such an idea may have arisen because of the observation that uterine cramping often is associated with nursing. Haller, in 1765, was the first to conclude that milk was derived from blood. This idea became firmly entrenched by the nineteenth century: "The secretion of milk would appear to illustrate, even more fully and clearly than do other glands, the truth on which we have so often insisted, that a secretion is eminently the result of the metabolic activity of the secretory cell. The blood is the ultimate source of milk, but it becomes milk only through the activity of the cell, and that activity consists largely in a metabolic manufacture by the cell and in the cell of the common things brought by the blood into the special things present in the milk."

The relationship of blood and milk production was further investigated by Sir Ashley Cooper, the English surgeon, who in 1845 described the lobular-alveolar anatomy of the breast, its blood supply, and innervation. He first described the early physiologic occurrence in milk letdown and lactogenesis. In the 1930s, Peterson showed by means of pressure monitors the separation of milk secretion and ejection (2). In 1928, Riddle, Bates, and Dykshorn extracted prolactin and showed it to be separate from other known pituitary hormones (3).

In the 1940s, Meites and Turner proposed that, in pregnancy, estrogen and progesterone promote full mammary growth and progesterones inhibit estrogen stimulation and prolactin secretion, and that at parturition an increase in circulating prolactin and cortisol is accompanied by a fall in estrogen and progesterone, which brings about the onset of lactation (4). Although incorrect in some aspects, the Turner-Meites hypothesis has remained intact for more than 40 years. Their observations were challenged by Clifton and Furth, who implanted pituitary mammotropic tumors which secreted prolactin, growth hormone, and corticotropin in the adrenalectomized rats (5). Mammary growth occurred in the absence of steroid hormones. Testing their own hypothesis, Chen and Meites also showed that estrogen stimulated the secretion of prolactin (6). While partially inhibiting the response, progesterone suppressed prolactin secretion below baseline levels. Finally, Kuhn proposed that elevated prolactin levels during pregnancy prevented the secretion of milk and that the withdrawal of this hormone after parturition is partially responsible for lactogenesis (7). Thus, a concept of multiple-hormone control of lactation evolved.

Knowledge of the anatomy and surgery of the breast proceeded at a similar pace. Camper, in the mid-1700s, described the internal mammary lymph nodes. Dran and Petit, in France, determined that breast cancer spread by metastasis, and they advocated the removal of the breast, underlying pectoral muscles, and axillary lymph nodes (8). The introduction of anesthesia by Morton and Crawford Long and the concept of antisepsis by Joseph Lister allowed surgery of the breast to undergo expediential growth. However, progress did not occur without setback. James Paget, in 1856, reported an operative mortality rate of 10% in 235 patients, with a 100% recurrence in 8 years (9). Samuel D. Gross, in the United Sates, performed simple mastectomy and removed lymph nodes only if they were grossly involved. His son, Samuel W. Gross, however, removed the entire breast, the skin covering the mammary fat, fascia of the pectoralis muscle, and lymph nodes. William Stewart Halsted, in the early 1900s, introduced the contemporary radical mastectomy (10). He recommended the removal of tissue in one piece, including the skin, and en bloc resection of the pectoralis major. His successor, Thomas Cullen, working with William Henry Welch at Johns Hopkins University, was the first to use frozen sections in the diagnosis of breast lesions in 1891 (11). Five years later, Grubbe first irradiated a breast cancer patient, and by 1898 Ehrlich had isolated the first alkylating agents that would serve as early chemotherapies (12).

References

1. Mepham T. Physiological aspects of lactation. In: McPhan T, ed. Biochemistry of lactation. New York: Elsevier, 1983:3.
2. Peterson LV. Lactation. Physiol Rev 1944;24:340.

4   Introduction

3. Riddle O, Bates R, Dykshorn S. The preparation, identification and assay of prolactin-A hormone of the anterior pituitary. Am J Physiol 1933; 105:191.

4. Meites J, Turner C. Studies concerning the mechanism controlling the initiation of lactation at parturition II: why lactation is not initiated during pregnancy. Endocrinology 1942;30:719.

5. Clifton K, Further J. Ducto-alveolar growth in mammary glands of adreno-gonadectomized male rats bearing mammotropic pituitary tumors. Endocrinology 1960;66:893.

6. Chen C, Meites J. Effects of estrogen and progesterone on serum and pituitary levels in ovariectomized rats. Endocrinology 1970;86:503.

7. Kuhn N. Progesterone withdrawal as the lactogenic trigger in the rat. J Endocrinol 1969;44:39.

8. le Dran F. Memoire avec une precis de plusiers observations sur le cancer. Mem Acad Roy Chir, Paris 1757;3:1–546.

9. Paget J. On the average duration of life in patients with scirrhosus cancer of the breast. Lancet 1856;1:62–63.

10. Halsted WS. The results of radical operations for cure of cancer of the breast. Am Surg 1907;46:1–19.

11. Cullen TS. A rapid method of making permanent specimens from frozen sections by the use of formalin. Bull J Hopkins Hosp 1895;6:67–73.

12. Page DL, Simpson JF. Benign, high-risk, and premalignant lesions of the mamma. In: Bland KI, Copeland EM, III, eds. The breast: comprehensive management of benign and malignant diseases. Philadelphia: WB Saunders, 1991:113–134.

Breast Anatomy, Physiology, Screening, and Self-Assessment

Richard E. Blackwell

The mammary gland lies on the pectoralis fascia and the musculature of the chest wall over the upper anterior rib cage. It is surrounded by layers of fat and is encased in skin. The tissue often extends into the axilla, which forms a tail of Spence. The mammary gland consists of approximately 12 to 20 glandular lobes that are connected by a ductal system. The ducts are surrounded by connective and periductal tissue, which is under hormonal control. The lactiferous ducts enlarge as they approach the nipple and are surrounded by pigmented areola. The ducts contain contractile smooth muscle fibers. The ductal tissue is lined by epithelial cells and fibrous septum, which runs from the lobules into the superficial fascia. Cooper's ligaments (suspensory ligaments) allow for mobility of the breast (Fig. 1.1). The major blood supply of the breast comes from the lateral thoracic and internal thoracic arteries, although components have been identified from the anterior intercostal vessels. The breast is innervated chiefly by the intercostal nerves carrying both sensory and autonomic fibers. The areola and nipple are innervated by the inferior ramus of the fourth intercostal nerve. Seventy-five percent of the lymphatic drainage involves axillary pathways, although the pectoral and apical lymph nodes are also involved, as are the parasternal nodes.

EMBRYOLOGY OF THE MAMMARY GLAND

The mammary gland is derived from ectoderm, and it can be identified 6 weeks after fertilization. At this point in gestation, the ectoder-

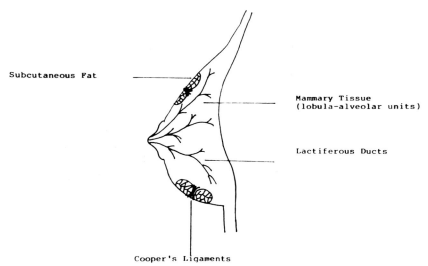

Subcutaneous Fat

Mammary Tissue
(lobula-alveolar units)

Lactiferous Ducts

Cooper's Ligaments

Figure 1.1.   *Gross anatomy of the breast.*

mal ridge forms from an ectodermal pit and begins to penetrate the mesenchyme, producing the mammary primordium. At 20 weeks gestation, 16 to 24 primitive lactiferous ducts invade the mesoderm. These ectodermal projections continue to branch and grow deeper into the tissue. Canalization occurs near term. It should be noted that, although the central lactiferous duct is present at birth, differentiation of the gland does not occur until it receives the appropriate hormonal signals.

Although mammary tissue remains unresponsive until pregnancy, it will respond to systemic hormone administration during fetal life. In the third trimester when fetal prolactin levels increase, terminal differentiation of ductal cells occurs. After birth, these cells revert to a more primitive state (1). The gland remains quiescent until puberty with the establishment of ovulatory menstrual cycles. At this juncture, breast development proceeds according to the descriptions of Marshall and Tanner. Although the hormonal regulations of mammogenesis is unclear, estrogen given in vitro appears to bring about ductal proliferation (2). In vitro, estrogens have not been shown to promote mammary growth. It has been suggested that various epidermal growth factors may be involved in the process (3). When progesterone is administered in vivo, lobular-aveolar development occurs (4). However, the administration of both estrogen and progesterone to hypophysectomized animals failed to promote mammogenesis (5). This strongly suggests that other hormones play a central role in mammogenesis. For instance, if the pituitary and adrenal glands are removed from oophorectomized rats, the addition of estrogen plus corticoids and growth hormone restores duct growth (6). This is comparable to the events that are seen at puberty.

Before pregnancy, breast lobules consist of ducts lined with epithelium that are embedded in connective tissue. The majority of tissues in the gland are of the connective and adipose type. There is scant contribution from glandular parenchyma, and a few sacculations arise from the ducts. The entire gland consists of the lactiferous system, the breasts undergo cyclic changes associated with normal ovulation, and the premenstrual breast engorgement noted by most women is secondary to tissue edema and hyperemia (7).

After conception, the mammary gland undergoes remarkable augmentation. Because the lobular-alveolar elements differentiate during the first trimester, it is possible to induce mammary development either with placental lactogen or prolactin in the absence of steroid hormones, as demonstrated both in vitro and in vivo (8). Although placental lactogen and prolactin increase throughout pregnancy, the data suggest that either of these hormones is capable of stimulating mammogenesis. The role of estrogen in mammogenesis is secondary because lactation has been reported in pregnancies with placental sulfatase enzyme deficiencies (9). Progesterone, while stimulating lobular-alveolar development, appears to antagonize the terminal effects induced by prolactin at least in vitro. Cortisol, while potentiating the action of prolactin on mammary differentiation, is unnecessary for either ductal or alveolar proliferation (10). A strong case can be made for the involvement of both insulin and other growth factors in stimulating mammogenesis. For instance, insulin is required for the survival of postnatal mammary tissue in vitro (11). It is possible that insulin-like molecules such as the somatomedins may be involved in the process. However, studies have suggested that epidermal growth factor may be involved in mammogenesis and, together with a group of corticoids, facilitate the accumulation of type IV collagen and component of the basal lamina, in which epithelial cells are supported.

BIOLOGY OF PROLACTIN PRODUCTION AND FUNCTION

Prolactin is unique among the pituitary hormones, and its secretion is inhibited rather than stimulated (Table 1.1). Dopamine, produced in the median eminence of the hypothalamus and secreted into the hypothalamic portal vessels, appears to be the principal inhibitor of both the synthesis and secretion of prolactin by the lactotrophs (12). Dopamine accounts for 70% of prolactin-inhibiting activity secreted into the hypothalamic portal system of the rat (13). When the infusion of exogenous dopamine is decreased in the primate, large increases in prolactin concomitantly occur (14). Dopamine acts on the lactotrophs by binding to high-affinity receptors on the plasma membranes and apparently acts through a cyclic adenosine monophosphate-calcium–dependent mechanism, leading to the inhibition of adenylate cyclase (15). Gamma-aminobutyric acid (GABA) is also an inhibitor of prolactin

Table 1.1.   Regulation of presecretion

Inhibitory	Stimulators
Dopamine	Vasoactive intestinal peptide (autocrine)
γ-aminobutyric acid	Thyrotropin-releasing hormone
TGF-β	Angiotensin II
	Serotonin
	Histamine
	Substance P
	Neurotensin
	GnRH (paracrine)
	GnRH-associated peptide
	TGF-α

TGF = transforming growth factor; GnRH = gonadotropin-releasing hormone.

secretion. Receptors for GABA have been isolated on lactotroph membranes. Compared to dopamine, however, the effect of GABA in inhibiting prolactin release is small (16).

A number of substances stimulate the release of prolactin. These include vasoactive intestinal peptide (VIP), thyrotropin-releasing hormone (TRH), angiotensin II, serotonin, and histamine. VIP is widely distributed throughout the central nervous system and is present in hypothalamic portal blood (17). It is probably produced by the pituitary gland as well as the gastrointestinal tract. VIP serves as an intrahypophysial regulator of prolactin secretion through an autocrine mechanism. TRH likewise induces a synthesis and secretion of prolactin and of thyroid-stimulating hormone (TSH). The physiologic release of these hormones is discordant at times. For example, the release of prolactin that occurs with suckling is not accompanied by the release of TSH. Angiotensin II has also been shown to stimulate prolactin secretion in vivo and in vitro, and receptors for this compound are found on the lactotroph membrane (18). Likewise, it is distributed throughout the brain. Serotonin can also stimulate a significant release in prolactin secretion, and the administration of serotonin antagonist cyproheptadine blocks the response. Histamine-like neurotransmitters have been shown to stimulate prolactin secretion via the H_1 receptor mechanism. Inhibition of prolactin secretion, however, occurs with the activation of the H_2 receptor (19). Other neurotransmitters, such as substance P and neurotensin, also affect prolactin secretion.

Although the principal hormonal regulatory pathway for prolactin involves neurotransmitters, the hormone appears to be able to regulate its own secretions through a short feedback. Bergland and Page demonstrated that the retrograde flow occurs within the portal system and, in fact, between lobes of the pituitary (20). The interventricular injection of prolactin in the rat increases the turnover of dopamine in the median eminence. Similarly, high rates of turnover have been demonstrated during both lactation and pregnancy, and these patterns are decreased after either hypophysectomy or treatment with bromocriptine. These observations support the existence of a short feedback loop at the level of the pituitary. The regulation of prolactin release is still more complicated because gonadotropin-releasing hormone (GnRH) has been shown to increase prolactin secretion in vitro (21). Lactotroph cell differentiation is shown to be stimulated by incubation of fetal tissue with the α chain of leutinizing hormone (LH). However, the incubation of the β chain of LH or follicle-stimulating hormone (FSH) in vitro using human pituitary cell cultures failed to stimulate prolactin secretion (22). The incubation of antiserum to the β chain of LH and FSH, however, inhibited the GnRH-mediated release of prolactin. GnRH-associated peptide (GAP), a peptide component of the precursor GnRH, has been reported to increase prolactin secretion in the rat. Such data suggest that prolactin secretion is controlled by multiple endocrine, paracrine, and autocrine mechanisms.

CONTROL OF LACTATION

Lactogenesis is divided into two stages: Stage 1 occurs prepartum and stage 2 occurs at about the time of parturition. Milk letdown occurs fairly abruptly during the second and fourth days postpartum in the human, although the transition from colostrum production to pure milk secretion occurs gradually. This process may take up to a month and coincides with a fall in plasma progesterone levels and the rise in serum prolactin. Twelve weeks before parturition, changes in milk composition occur (23). One finds increased production of lactose, proteins, and immunoglobulins and a decrease in sodium and chloride. There is an increase in blood flow, oxygen, and glucose uptake in the breast. There is also an increase in the amount of citrate present in the breast at about the time of parturition. Milk secretion occurs in the third trimester, and the composition of milk remains fairly stable until term. This is exemplified by the stable production of α-lactalbumin and milk-specific protein. At parturition there is a fall in placental lactogen production, and progesterone levels reach the nonpregnant range within several days. Estrogen falls to baseline levels in 5 days, whereas prolactin decreases over approximately 14 days. A fall in progesterone levels seems to be the most important event in the establishment of lactogenesis (24,25). This was confirmed by observations in the early nineteenth century that milk secretion would not occur until removal of the placenta. The administration of exogenous progesterone prevents lactose and lipid synthesis after oophorectomy in pregnant rats and in ewes (26). Further, progesterone administration inhibits casein and α-lactalbumin synthesis in vitro.

Table 1.2. *Regulators of lactation*

Prolactin	(major regulator)
Corticoids	
Thyroxine	
Growth hormone	
Insulin	
Estradiol	(priming)
Progesterone	(priming)

In the human, lactation is maintained by the interaction of numerous hormones (Table 1.2). After removal of either the pituitary or adrenal gland from a number of animal species, milk production is terminated (27). The species dictates the type of replacement therapy that is required to reinstitute milk production. For instance, in the rabbit and sheep, prolactin is effective alone. In the ruminant, milk secretion is restored by the addition of corticoids, thyroxin, growth hormone, and prolactin. Prolactin appears to be a key hormone in the maintenance of lactation, because the administration of bromocriptine, a dopamine agonist inhibitor of prolactin secretion, blocks lactogenesis (28). This effect varies with the species, inhibition of prolactin, in ruminants, shows very little effect on the establishment of lactation except in the ovine. The role of thyroid hormones in lactation is unclear. Thyroidectomy inhibits lactation, and replacement therapy with thyroxine increases milk yield. It has been suggested that growth hormone and thyroxine synergize to alter milk yield, and triiodothyronine has been shown to act directly on mouse mammary tissue in vitro to increase its sensitivity to prolactin (29).

During pregnancy, the integrated baseline of serum prolactin is elevated when compared to the nonpregnant state. Suckling or manipulation of the breast leads to an elevation in prolactin within about 40 minutes (30). This response can be duplicated by the application of electrical stimulation to rat mammary nerves (31). Both growth hormone and cortisol are also released by this stimulus. The response appears to be greatest in the immediate postpartum period and is attenuated over the next 6 months. The application of lidocaine (Xylocaine) to the nipple, blocking nerve conduction, obliterates the response of prolactin to stimuli. Further, if two infants suckle simultaneously, the rise in prolactin is amplified. Suckling increases the secretion of prolactin as well as the oxytocin. After the application of the stimulus, there is an 8- to 12-hour delay before milk secretion is fully stimulated. This response correlates with the frequency and duration of suckling. There is no correlation between the amount of prolactin released and milk yield.

Suckling of the breast results in an increase in intramammary pressure bilaterally. This occurs secondary to contraction of the myoepithelial cells in response to oxytocin and octapeptide. This occurs after application of a stimulus to the nipple, which activates sensory receptors transmitting impulses to the spinal cord and hypothalamus. Oxytocin is produced in neurons located in the supraoptic and paraventricular nuclei. It is estimated that about 2 ng of oxytocin is released per 2- to 4-second pulse intervals (32). Oxytocin is synthesized in the hypothalamus as part of a large prohormone that is cleaved and packaged into secretory granules. It is transported by exoplasmic flow and further cleaved into the native hormone and a neurophysin-like binding protein. The synthesis and release of oxytocin are rapid, and 1.5 hours after injection of a radioactive amino acid tracer into cerebrospinal fluid, labeled oxytocin is released by exocytosis. Electrical pulse activity has been measured in oxytocic neurons 5 to 15 seconds before milk ejection in the rat model system. The response is conditioned because the cry of an infant or various other perceptions associated with nursing can trigger activity in the central circuits.

BREAST SCREENING AND SELF-EXAMINATION

When and how the patient and physician attempt to detect early breast cancers is a matter of controversy. The imaging techniques, that is, mammography, sonography, and magnetic resonance imaging, are discussed in depth in later chapters. Several factors must be considered before instituting screening for a disease process. First, the disease must be important from a clinical perspective; that is, it should be common and be associated with significant morbidity or mortality. This prevalence may be influenced by sample size, race, sex, age, geography, and other parameters. Second, the screening test to be used must be available, acceptable to the patient population, and not too costly. It should be easy to perform, involve little or no patient discomfort, and be sensitive and specific, and it cannot yield false-positive or false-negative data. Third, the disease to be screened for should have a defined natural history and detectable presymptomatic stage. Fourth, the disease must have an available and efficacious treatment, and screening for untreatable diseases at this juncture in history is not cost effective.

Breast self-examination is one of the most important methods for diagnosis of breast diseases, either benign or malignant. A poll conducted for the American Cancer Society found that physicians play a pivotal role in encouraging patients to practice self-breast examination. When patients receive personal instruction from their physicians, 92% continue to practice self-breast examination regularly (33). Women should be taught breast self-examination by the age of 20 years. The patient needs to be aware of what is normal in terms of the look and feel of the breast, be aware of the changes that may occur, be encouraged to report changes without delay, and present for a physician's examination. It should be emphasized to patients that they need to look for any change in the size or contour of the breast, puckering or dimpling of the skin, any discrete lump, particularly one that is not movable, asymmetric nodularity of the breast that persists after menstruation, any pain or discomfort that deviates from normal, any discharge whether clear, serous or bloody, and any nipple contraction or distortion.

It is generally recommended that women examine their breasts at least once per month. Because the breasts are most tender before menstruation, often examination is done with the onset of menstruation or afterward. For women who are menopausal or who have undergone hysterectomy, examination at the first of each month is recommended. The technique of examination is standardized and consists of six steps. The first involves observation of the breasts for the aforementioned changes as well as visualization of the breasts during movement to accentuate contour. This could be carried out by placing the hands on the hips and flexing the shoulders forward and then raising the hands behind the head. Palpation of the breast should be carried out with the contralateral hand. It has been recommended by some physicians that the breast be moistened with soapy solution. Examination can be carried out systematically with the finger tips or in a circumferential fashion. Finally, the nipples should be inspected and the areola compressed to assess for the presence of discharge.

Despite the perceived benefit of self-breast examination, there are many reasons why women do not practice it (34). Many false-positive results occur, and many women are examined for benign lesions. Examination gives rise to anxiety and worry about finding lumps that may or may not represent a cancer, and some women feel guilty about not performing breast examinations or about not examining properly. The reward for carrying out thorough self-breast examinations is the detection of disease and is a negative reinforcement. The overall sensitivity of self-breast examination is poor, and the percentage of false-negative results is high (35,36) compared with the 80% to 90% sensitivity for mammography. The World Health Organization, Russian Federation, randomized self-breast examination study enrolled approximately 60,000 women in each group; 190 cancers were detected in the examination group and 192 in the control group. The detection rate was 3.15 per 1000 in the breast examination group and 3.19 per 1000 in the control group. The investigators concluded that there was no difference in cancer detection rate, no difference in tumor characteristics, a significantly higher rate of visits to specialists, a significantly higher rate of referral for further investigation by specialized institutions, and significantly more excisional biopsies in the breast self-examination group.

The positive predictive value of self-examination in younger women is poor (4% to 6%). The overwhelming majority of women who have positive results do not have breast cancer. This is in contrast to older women; studies in the United States show that 48% of the lumps detected in women older than 55 years were malignant compared with 3% in women younger than 44 years.

At present, there appears to be no compelling evidence that breast self-examination is effective in reducing the morbidity and mortality of breast cancer. However, because greater than 90% of breast cancers are found by women themselves, it seems that the teaching of effective breast cancer self-detection techniques continues to be investigated to maximize the results. There are those who believe that breast self-examination could be made more acceptable to women if the ritualistic exercise was de-emphasized and women were encouraged to take the opportunity to observe and feel their breasts while performing daily activities such as bathing or dressing.

Breast examination should be part of the annual examination rendered women by all primary care specialists. The patient should be asked about a family history of breast cancer, particularly in a mother or sister, the birth of their first child, and age of menarche. Attention should be paid to ethnic origin, a history of breast irradiation, alcohol consumption, a diet consisting of high fat intake, and menstrual regularity. The physical examination should be carried out in both the sitting and lying positions. The breasts should be inspected for symmetry at rest and symmetry during motion; thickening of the skin; any dimpling of the breast surface, areola, or nipple; nipple inversion; discharge from the nipple; and any discoloration of the skin. The breasts should be examined bilaterally using the finger tips, the axillae should be palpated, and an attempt made by both the physician and patient to express discharge from the nipples. Other variations include examining the breasts while wet and using a thin paper towel to slid over the breast surface to evaluate nodularity (Table 1.3).

All women older than 35 years should have an annual breast examination. It is recommended that a baseline mammographic examination be obtained by 40 years of age or earlier if the patient is at risk (Fig. 1.2) (37,38). Mammography should be performed every 1 to 2 years from age 40 to 50 years, and women older than 50 years

Table 1.3. Breast self-examination

Examination should begin by age 20 years.
Exams should be performed at least once per month.
The following factors should be assessed:
   Size and symmetry
   Symmetric movement
   Lumps that persist
   Skin puckering, dimpling, discoloration
   Nipple discharge
   Pain
   Nipple inversion

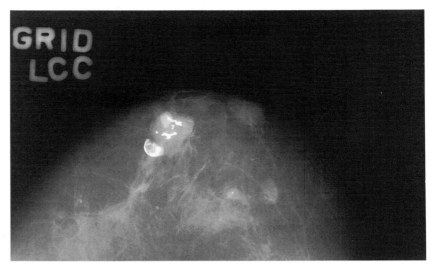

Figure 1.2. *Mammogram demonstrating calcification in a 40-year-old patient.*

should have an annual mammogram as well as an annual breast examination. Significant risk factors alter the frequency of examination and mammography. There is considerable controversy about the need for a baseline mammogram before 40 years of age in asymptomatic women and about the frequency with which mammography should be performed in women aged 40 to 50 years (39,40). The effect of mammography cannot be overemphasized as a means of reducing the mortality among breast cancer. The Health Insurance Plan Program of New York showed a 30% decrease in mortality in women older than 50 years who are screened (41). Studies from the Netherlands suggest a reduction in breast cancer rates by 50% in patients undergoing annual mammography (42).

Breast cancer is now considered to be an occult metastatic disease, with tumor dissemination often occurring before surgical therapy. Patients are generally diagnosed with breast cancers in the 1- to 2.5-cm range after the cancer has presumably been present for 10 years. Mammography can ordinarily detect lesions between 1 mm and 1 cm in size, and modern instruments can now detect clustered microcalcification smaller than 1 mm. However, care must be taken in applying mammography to younger women with dense breasts, because a negative examination may yield false-negative results.

DuPont argued that screening has saved the lives of women in the 50-year and older age group and, therefore, should detect a similar amount of disease in the 40-year and older age group. He pointed out that although studies have not been of sufficient power to show benefit of screening in women 40 to 49 years of age, studies likewise do not disprove benefit (37).

The breast screening study of Canada is the only trial that prospectively attempted to evaluate women in the fourth decade of life. It failed to show any advantage of screening women on the basis of a power calculation of 40%. In 7 years of follow-up of women aged 40 to 49 years, it was found that 25,214 received annual mammography and clinical examination and that they displaced a statistically insignificant excess of deaths resulting from breast cancer compared with 25,216 women who received a single clinical examination of the breasts and returned to normal community care. Unfortunately, normal community care might mean that patients received mammography as well as physician examination, and apparently some 26% of these women received mammograms, which could easily skew and obliterate any statistical difference.

Data analysis conducted by Elwood on all screening studies published before December 1992 indicated the total number of observed person-years at 7 years follow-up. In women 40 to 49 years of age, 601,380 person-years have been observed for screened women and 528,848 person-years for controlled subjects for a total of 1.13 million person-years in the age group. Despite these numbers, the efficacy of screening could not be demonstrated at least with the population-based technique.

As a result of these reports, the National Cancer Institute no longer recommends that women aged 40 to 49 years have routine mammographic screening. Proponents of the guidelines claim that screening mammography does not work for women in this age group because of their high breast density and the fact that lumps that are detected are usually benign and resolve without surgery. Although it has been demonstrated that five times as many cancers per 1000 first-screening mammographic examinations are diagnosed in women aged 50 years and older, compared with younger women, women aged 40 to 49 years with a positive family history of breast cancer had a higher positive predictive value compared with women without such a history: 0.13 versus 0.04, $p = 1.00$ (38). Therefore, it seems reasonable to recommend 1) frequent self-breast examinations to all women older than 20 years, 2) annual examinations beginning at least by the age of 35 years, 3) baseline mammography at approximately 40 years of age, 4) mammography every year after the age of 50 years, and 5) mammography used liberally in women aged 40 years and older with a positive family history of breast cancer.

References

1. McKiernan J, Coyne J, Canglone S. History of breast development in early life. Arch Dis Child 1988;63:136.

2. Cowie AT. Backward glances. In: Yokoyama A, Mizuno H, Nagasawa H, eds. Physiology of mammary glands. Baltimore: University Park Press, 1978:43.

3. Toneli G, Sorof S. Epidermal growth factor: requirement for development of cultured mammary glands. Nature 1980;285:250.

4. Ichinose R, Nandi S. Influence of hormones on lobulo-alveolar differentiation of mouse mammary glands in vitro. J Endocrinol 1966;35:331.

5. Cowie A, Tindal J, Yokoyama A. The induction of mammary growth in the hypophysectomized goat. J Endocrinol 1966;34:154.

6. Lyons WR. Hormonal synergism in mammary growth. Proc R Soc Biol 1958;149:303.

7. Going JJ, Anderson TJ, Battersby S, et al. Proliferative and secretory activity in human breast during natural and artificial menstrual cycles. Am J Pathol 1988;130:193.

8. Talwalker P, Meites T. Mammary lobulo-alveolar growth induced by anterior pituitary hormones in adreno-ovariectomized-hypophysectomized rats. Proc Soc Exp Biol Med 1961;107:880.

9. France J, Seddon R, Liggins G. A study of a pregnancy with low estrogen production due to placental sulfatase deficiency. J Clin Endocrinol Metab 1973;36:19.

10. Topper Y, Freeman C. Multiple hormone interactions in the developmental biology of the mammary gland. Physiol Rev 1980;60:1049.

11. Elias J. Effect of insulin and cortisol on organ cultures of adult mouse mammary gland. Proc Soc Exp Biol Med 1959;101:500.

12. Blackwell RE, Guillemin R. Hypothalamic control of adenohypophyseal secretions. Annu Rev Physiol 1973;35:357.

13. Gibbs OM, Neill JD. Dopamine levels in hypophyseal stalk blood in the rat are sufficient to inhibit prolactin secretion in vitro. Endocrinology 1978;103:1895.

14. Neill JD, Luque EH, Mulchahey JJ, Nagy G. Regulation of prolactin secretion. In: Blackwell RE, Chang RJ, eds. Prolactin-related disorders: proceedings of a symposium. Florham Park, NJ: MacMillan Healthcare, 1987.

15. MacLeod RM, Judd AM, Jarvis WD, et al. Receptor and post-receptor mechanisms for hypothalamic peptides at the pituitary level. In: Muller EE, MacLeon RM, eds. Neuroendocrine respectives, vol. 5. Amsterdam: Elsevier, 1986:45.

16. Matsushita N, Kato Y, Shimatsu A, et al. Effects of VIP, TRH, GABA and dopamine on prolactin release from superfused rat anterior pituitary cells. Life Sci 1983;32:1263.

17. Hagen TC, Arnaout MA, Scherzer WJ, et al. Antisera to vasoactive intestinal polypeptide inhibit basal prolactin release from disbursed anterior pituitary cells. Neuroendocrinology 1986;43:641.

18. Aguilear G, Hyde CL, Catt KJ. Angiotensin-II receptors and prolactin release to pituitary lactotrophs. Endocrinology 1987;111:1045.

19. Knigge U, Dejgaard A, Wollesen F, et al. Histamine regulation of prolactin secretion through H_1-H_2-receptors. J Clin Endocrinol Metab 1982;55:118.

20. Bergland R, Page R. Can the pituitary secrete directly to the brain? (affirmative anatomical evidence). Endocrinology 1978;102:1325.

21. Blackwell RE, Rogers-Neame NT, Bradley EL, et al. Regulation of human prolactin secretion by gonadotropin releasing hormone in vitro. Fertil Steril 1986;46:26.

22. Blackwell RE, Garrison PN. Inhibition of prolactin secretion by antiserum

to the alpha- and beta-subunits of gonadotropin. Am J Obstet Gynecol 1987;156:863.

23. Fleet J, Goode J, Hamon M, et al. Secretory activity of goat mammary glands during pregnancy and the onset of lactation. J Physiol (Lond) 1975;251:763.

24. Vonderhaar BK. Studies on the mechanism by which thyroid hormones enhance α-lactalbumin activity in explants from mouse mammary glands. Endocrinology 1977;100:1423.

25. Martin R, Glass M, Wilson G, Woods K. Human α-lactalbumin and hormonal factors in pregnancy and lactation. Clin Endocrinol 1973;13:223.

26. Hartmann P, Trevethan P, Shelton J. Progesterone and oestrogen and the initiation of lactation in ewes. J Endocrinol 1973;59:249.

27. Hearn J. Pituitary inhibition of pregnancy. Nature 1973;241:207.

28. Brun F, del Re R, del Pozo E, et al. Prolactin inhibition and suppression of puerperal lactation by a Br-ergocriptine (CB 154): a comparison with estrogen. Obstet Gynecol 1973;41:884.

29. Vance MI, Cragun JR, Reimnitz C, et al. Diagnosis and management of prolactinomas. Cancer Metastasis Rev 1989;5:125.

30. Gross B, Eastman C, Bowen C, McEldruff A. Integrated concentration of prolactin in breast-feeding mothers. Aust N Z J Obstet Gynaecol 1979; 19:150.

31. Tyson J. Nursing and prolactin secretion: principal determinants in the mediation of puerperal infertility. In: Crosignani P, Robyn C, eds. Prolactin and human reproduction. Orlando, FL: Academic Press, 1977:97.

32. Lincoln O, Wakerley J. Electrophysiological evidence for the activation of supraoptic neuronics during the release of oxytocin. J Physiol 1974; 242:533.

33. Dodd GD. 1988 American Cancer Society guidelines for breast cancer screening. Cancer 1992;69:1885.

34. Austoker J. Cancer prevention in primary care. BMJ 1994;309:168.

35. Kopans DB, Halpern E, Hulka CA. Statistical power in breast cancer screening trials and mortality reduction among breast cancer screening trials and mortality reduction among women 40–49 years of age with particular emphasis on the national breast screening study of Canada. Cancer 1994;74:1196.

36. Baines CJ. A different view on what is known about breast screening and the Canadian national breast screening study. Cancer 1974;74:1207.

37. Dupont WD. Evidence of efficacy of mammographic screening for women in their forties. Cancer 1994;74:1204.

38. Kerkikowske K, Grady D, Barclay J, et al. Positive predictive value of screening mammography by age and family history of breast cancer. JAMA 1993;270:2444.

39. Kopans DB, Halpern E, Hulka CA. Mammography screening for breast cancer. Cancer 1994;74:1212.

40. Noller K. ACOG Newsletter 1994;38:1.

41. Shapiro S, Venet W, Strax P, et al. Ten to fourteen year effect of screening on breast cancer mortality. J Natl Cancer Inst 1982;69:349.

42. Verbeck ALM, Holland R, Sturmans F, et al. Reduction of breast cancer mortality through mass screening with modern mammography. Lancet 1984;1:222.

Breast Dysfunction: Galactorrhea and Mastalgia

Gary W. DeVane

GALACTORRHEA AND NIPPLE DISCHARGE

Introduction and Classification

The frequency of discharges and secretions of the breast requires a thorough understanding of the cause and clinical significance of these findings in the management of breast disease. Nipple discharge, the spontaneous release of fluid, is a common presenting finding that may be caused by an underlying pathologic lesion, hormone imbalance, or merely a physiologic event.

The incidence of nipple discharge is difficult to ascertain because of differences in examination techniques. Nipple discharge was noted in 256 of 3287 (7.8%) women undergoing breast surgery (1). Papanicolaou et al (2) were able to obtain breast secretion from 170 of 917 (18.5%) normal women using either massage or a breast pump. However, when special care or suction devices are used, fluid can be obtained in approximately 50% to 70% of nonlactating normal women (3–5). The finding of nonspontaneous, usually physiologic discharge depends on many factors, including age, race, and menopausal status (Tables 2.1 and 2.2) (6).

Spontaneous nipple discharge must be regarded as abnormal, although in most cases the cause is usually benign. Chitty (7) proposed classifying nipple discharges on the basis of causative factors outside the breast that are predominately neuroendocrine or pharmacologic,

Table 2.1. Nipple aspirate fluid (NAF) availability among various racial groups

Group	Number with NAF	Number attempted (%)
Caucasian	158/225	(70.2)
Filipino	7/10	(70.0)
Black	23/37	(62.2)
Mexican-American	37/71	(52.1)
Asian	65/263	(24.7)

Reproduced by permission from King EB, Goodson W. Discharges and secretions of the nipple. Philadelphia: WB Saunders, 1991.

Table 2.2. Nipple aspirate fluid (NAF) availability and age

Age group (yr)	Number with NAF/number attempted (%)	
	All races	Caucasian
≤ 20	9/18 (50.0)	4/6 (66.6)
21–30	66/121 (54.5)	36/48 (75.0)
31–40	77/145 (53.1)	44/57 (77.2)
41–50	70/125 (56.0)	37/47 (78.7)
51–60	30/78 (38.5)	21/35 (60.0)
≥ 60	23/86 (26.7)	16/32 (50.0)
Total	275/573 (47.9)	158/225 (70.2)

Reprinted by permission from King EB, Goodson W. Discharges and secretions of the nipple. Philadelphia: WB Saunders, 1991.

those caused by disease of the nipple-areola complex, and those related to the ductal system.

Nipple Discharge

Physiologic breast secretion is nonspontaneous and frequently bilateral; arises from multiple ducts; and may be expressed by gentle manual massage using circumareolar pressure or a negative-pressure breast pump or other device. Physiologic discharge is usually serous in character and may be caused by frequent breast examination, sexual stimulation, hormone treatment, or medications. Galactorrhea is also a multiple-duct discharge that is differentiated from other physiologic discharges by the milk-like character of the secretion.

Pathologic discharge is usually unilateral and either spontaneous or intermittent. This type of discharge may be bloody, serosanguineous, serous, clear, or greenish-gray. Frequently, the pathologic discharge can be localized to a single duct. Discharge caused by carcinoma is usually bloody, although clear, serous fluid may be observed (7).

The first step in the evaluation of women with nipple discharge is to determine whether the discharge is pathologic or physiologic. Careful assessment of the breast discharge is mandatory, including testing for occult blood. If a discharge is physiologic, reassurance of its benign nature should be provided. When a pathologic nipple discharge is suspected, the main goal is to exclude the rare possibility of carcinoma. The evaluation of galactorrhea is primarily an assessment of endocrine and neuroendocrine factors requiring an evaluation of hormone abnormalities.

Galactorrhea

Galactorrhea is the inappropriate secretion of milk in nonpuerperal women and in men. The spontaneous leakage of milk from the breasts is viewed as more worrisome than milk-like secretion that must be manually expressed. The amount of milk secreted varies greatly as does its composition. When the secretion is white, opaque, or milky, further evaluation regarding pathologic breast disease is unnecessary. Rapid microscopic confirmation of milk secretion can be obtained by expressing the nipple discharge directly onto a glass slide, placing a coverglass, and viewing under low magnification. Multiple lipid droplets are diagnostic of milk (Fig. 2.1).

Galactorrhea may occur as an isolated finding or in association with amenorrhea, oligomenorrhea, and infertility. The association of inappropriate lactation and reproductive disorders has been well rec-

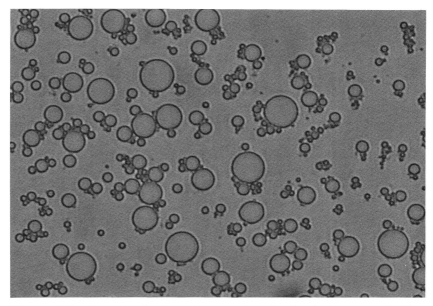

Figure 2.1. *Example of galactorrhea secretion visualized microscopically. Note characteristic lipid droplets. (Original magnification × 400.)*

ognized. Chiari et al (8) in 1855 and Frommel (9) in 1882 independently described a syndrome of postpartum amenorrhea with persistent lactation. Subsequently, Argonz and Del Castillo (10) described nonpuerperal lactation with associated hypoestrogenemia.

Ultimately, Forbes et al (11) observed patients with the syndrome of galactorrhea and amenorrhea associated with low urinary follicle-stimulating hormone. These were the first observations linking galactorrhea with pituitary dysfunction. Although at that time prolactin could not be measured, the subsequent development of sensitive radioimmunoassay (RIA) for prolactin demonstrated that pituitary micro- and macroadenomas are capable of secreting large amounts of prolactin, which causes the observed amenorrhea and galactorrhea previously described.

Physiologic Breast Changes During Pregnancy

Marked ductal, lobular, and alveolar growth takes place during pregnancy under the influence of luteal and placental sex steroids, placental lactogen, prolactin, and chorionic gonadotropin. Although prolactin is not critical in normal breast development, levels increase during the first half of pregnancy but then reach levels 10 to 15 times higher than normal in the third trimester. Terminal ductal sprouting with some branching and lobular formation occurs under estrogenic influence within the first 3 to 4 weeks of pregnancy (12). At 5 to 8 weeks, breast enlargement is observed with superficial vein dilatation and increasing pigmentation of the nipple-areola complex. During the second trimester, further ductal proliferation occurs under progesterone influence with increased invasion of the connective tissue surrounding the lobular-alveolar structures by lymphocytes and differentiation of epithelial stem cells. During the last trimester, fat droplets accumulate into the presecretory alveolar cells under prolactin influence with increased filling of the alveoli with colostrum as well as hypertrophy of myoepithelial cells, connective tissue, and fat (12). As pregnancy continues, colostrum is composed of desquamated epithelial cells with aggregates of lymphocytes, round cells, and desquamated phagocytic areolar cells (foam cells).

Hormonal Control of Breast Development During Pregnancy

Prolactin and human placental lactogen (HPL) increase markedly during pregnancy, reaching peak levels before delivery (Fig. 2.2). Human prolactin and HPL have approximately 13% amino acid homology with similar lactogenic activity (13). Although more than 80% of the amino acid sequence of HPL is similar to that of human growth hor-

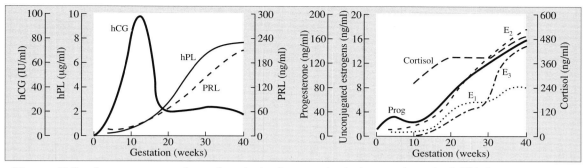

Figure 2.2. _Serum concentrations of prolactin, human chorionic gonadotropin (hCG), human placental lactogen (hPL), cortisol, progesterone, and unconjugated estrogens during pregnancy. The values have been obtained from several sources in the literature_ (E_1 = estrone; E_2 = estradiol; E_3 = estriol). _Reprinted by permission from Rebar RW. Gestational changes of the reproductive tract and breasts. Philadelphia: WB Saunders, 1991._

mone, HPL has very little somatotrophic activity (14). Growth hormone levels remain low during human pregnancy and do not have an important role in breast development and lactation in women (15).

Estrogen and progesterone levels increase dramatically during normal pregnancy (see Fig. 2.2) (16). It appears that estrogen promotes the formation of lactotrophic cells in the pituitary and increases the secretion of prolactin (17). Estrogen in the presence of prolactin promotes breast ductal development. Progesterone stimulates lobular-alveolar growth while suppressing secretory activity. High progesterone levels inhibit lactose synthetase and milk protein (casein) messenger ribonucleic acid synthesis in vitro (18). It is largely because of high levels of circulating estrogen and progesterone that women do not lactate during pregnancy (19). The abrupt withdrawal of estrogen and progesterone at delivery with the expulsion of the placenta triggers the onset of lactation.

Glucocorticoid levels increase during pregnancy (20,21) primarily as a result of a decreased clearance rate and an increase in corticosteroid-binding globulin. Although not essential for ductal or alveolar growth, glucocorticoids enhance growth of lobules during pregnancy (18). Insulin is required for prolactin and other hormones to exert their effects on breast tissue in vitro, and insulin or insulin-like growth factors are probably necessary in vivo as well (18). Thyroid hormones increase the responsiveness of breast cells to prolactin.

Lactation

In pregnant women, the breast is capable of milk secretion by the second trimester. The syntheses of lactose, casein, and α-lactalbumin increase as parturition approaches. The presence of α-lactalbumin, the regulatory subunit of the lactose synthetase enzyme complex (22), indicates that final differentiation has occurred. The final stage of lactogene-

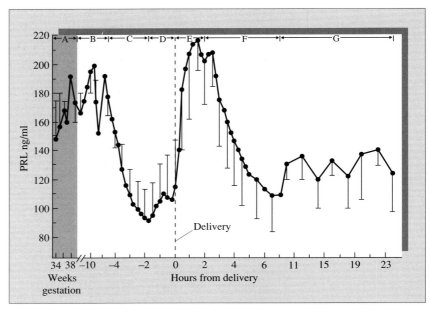

Figure 2.3. The multiphasic pattern of prolactin (PRL) levels (mean ± SE) during the periparturitional periods. During the last few weeks of pregnancy (phase A), PRL levels show frequent fluctuations. These levels are maintained during early hours of labor (phase B). However, during the ensuing hours of active labor, a remarkable decline in PRL levels occurs, reaching a nadir about 2 hours before delivery (phase C). There is some recovery during the last 2 hours before delivery (phase D), leading to a dramatic upward surge of PRL during the first 2 hours after delivery (phase E). PRL levels fall progressively during the subsequent 5 hours (phase F) and reach a relatively constant level with random fluctuation during the next 16 hours (phase G). Reprinted by permission from Endocrine regulation of the reproductive system in Reproductive Endocrinology: Physiology pathophysiology and clinical management, SSC Yen and RB Jaffe, eds. Philadelphia: WB Saunders, 1991, 373.

sis occurs after delivery when the presecretory alveolar epithelium is converted into active milk-synthesizing and milk-releasing cells.

As previously described, actual lactation is initiated after delivery and removal of the placenta, resulting in a dramatic decline in progesterone, estrogen, and placental lactogen levels. Rising hormone levels of prolactin and glucocorticoids are thought to play a part in this process. However, prolactin levels reach a peak just before delivery (23) and then rebound before initiation of lactation (Fig. 2.3). Furthermore, estrogen treatment after delivery inhibits postpartum lactation in the presence of elevated prolactin levels (24). Probably progesterone withdrawal is the most likely trigger mechanism for the initiation of lactation (25), but this action of falling progesterone concentration is only manifest in the presence of adequate prolactin levels. Exogenously administered progesterone is less effective than estrogen in stopping lactation once the process has become established.

With delivery, the hormonal environment consists of relatively high prolactin and low estrogen and progesterone levels. Colostrum is secreted in varying amounts during the first postpartum days. After colostrum secretion, transitional milk and then mature milk is produced under the influence of continued prolactin stimulation. Maintenance of lactation requires milk removal by periodic suckling, which provides an essential stimulus for the release of both oxytocin and prolactin (26). Without suckling, breast milk synthesis declines even with appropriate hormonal conditions.

Hormonal Mechanisms in Lactation

Prolactin is essential for the initiation of lactation in humans and most other species. Suckling in postpartum women is a potent stimulus for the release of prolactin, and in the first few weeks already high maternal serum prolactin levels undergo further elevation with each nursing episode. Later, between the third and seventh weeks after delivery, baseline prolactin levels decline, but nursing-induced increases are sustained. Suckling-induced prolactin secretion, although minimal, persists in most women for many months (Fig. 2.4) (27). This nursing-

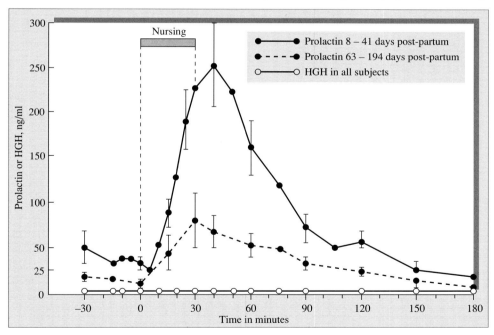

Figure 2.4. Plasma prolactin and growth hormone concentrations during nursing in postpartum women. Eight women were studied 8 to 41 days postpartum and six women were studied 63 to 194 days postpartum. Prenursing prolactin levels in the latter group are within the normal range. Plasma growth hormone showed no change in any of the subjects during nursing (HGH = human growth hormone). Reprinted by permission from the Endocrine Society and Noel GL, Suh HK, Frantz AG. Prolactin release during nursing and breast stimulation in postpartum and nonpostpartum subjects. J Clin Endocrinol Metab 1974;38:413–423. © The Endocrine Society.

induced rise is probably important in maintaining lactation (27) but does not occur in all women studied in the late postpartum period (28). High levels of prolactin appear to be required for the initiation of lactation, but once breast enzyme mechanisms are activated, lactation can continue with baseline prolactin concentrations that are normal or only minimally elevated. Nonetheless, prolactin is necessary for maintenance of lactation as indicated by the blockage of milk secretion in women by the administration of bromocriptine, a dopamine agonist, which causes an abrupt decline in prolactin concentration (24). The administration of bromocriptine to women at any time postpartum will reduce prolactin levels and completely inhibit lactation (24).

A necessary component of lactation is the expulsion of milk from the alveoli and ducts caused by contraction of myoepithelial cells under oxytocin influence. Oxytocin is synthesized within specialized magnocellular neurons of the paraventricular and supraoptic nuclei of the hypothalamus (29). The milk ejection reflex occurs when direct stimulation to areolar sensory neurons (suckling) triggers afferent nerve fibers via the spinal cord to the brain neurons (Fig. 2.5).

Oxytocin release can also be caused by psychic factors such as anticipation of nursing (30). Enhanced oxytocin secretion causes the sensation of milk letdown and the appearance of milk via ejection at the nipple. This is often associated with uterine cramping. Oxytocin release in response to nursing is maintained throughout the postpartum period in women (31). Although oxytocin and prolactin are both

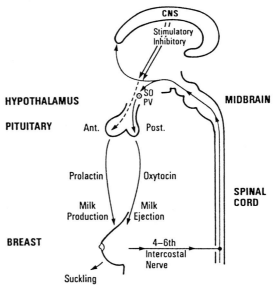

Figure 2.5.   Neuroendocrine reflexes initiated by suckling (CNS = central nervous system; PV = paraventricular nucleus; SO = supraoptic nucleus; ant. = anterior pituitary; post. = posterior pituitary). Reprinted by permission from Rebar RW. Gestational changes of the reproductive tract and breasts. In Creasy, RK and Resnik, R, eds. Maternal-Fetal Medicine: Principles and Practice. Philadelphia: WB Saunders, 1991.

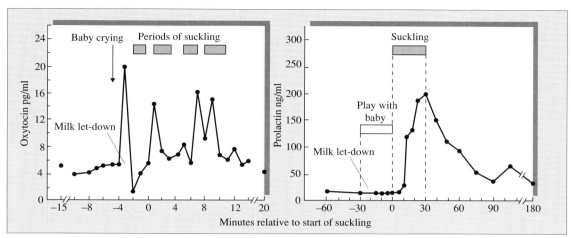

Figure 2.6. *Plasma oxytocin (left) and prolactin (right) concentrations in response to the anticipation of nursing and suckling in lactating women. Milk letdown occurred in association with acute release of oxytocin but no prolactin. Reprinted by permission from Yen SSC. Prolactin in human reproduction. Philadelphia: WB Saunders, 1991.*

released in response to suckling, the patterns of release are very different (32,33) (Fig. 2.6) (27,33). Oxytocin is normally released before or at the start of suckling as a conditioned response to tactile, auditory, or visual stimuli; prolactin release occurs only in response to direct stimulation of the nipple (27,33). Oxytocin release can be inhibited, with impairment of milk production, by stress and psychic factors that activate the sympathetic nervous system.

Nonphysiologic Lactation: Galactorrhea

Galactorrhea is the secretion by the nipple of a milky fluid under nonphysiologic circumstances in that it is not occurring in relation to a pregnancy or for the nourishment of a child. The amount of milk secreted is usually persistent and variable. The secretion may either be spontaneous or require manual expression. Spontaneous leakage of milk from the breasts is usally of more concern than milk that must be expressed. Although usually white or opaque, the color may be yellow, green, or brown. The darker colored discharges must be distinguished from blood or bloody discharges that might be caused by benign or neoplastic tumors of the breast. The actual quantity of milk-like secretion is not important because any galactorrhea demands evaluation in nulliparous women and in parous women if there is persistence of lactation after weaning or if 1 year has elapsed since delivery. Galactorrhea can involve one or both breasts and is associated with a variety of ovulatory disorders, including absence of menses.

Because the action of a lactogenic hormone is a necessary requirement for the initiation of milk production, galactorrhea should be considered a biologic marker of abnormal prolactin physiology. Lactation, as described previously, requires complex hormone interactions. Thus, hyperprolactinemia does not always lead to galactorrhea; therefore, hyperprolactinemia is more common than galactorrhea. Indeed, without necessary hormone priming, galactorrhea will not occur, even with very high circulating prolactin concentrations. Just as in normal lactation, once inappropriate prolactin secretion has initiated galactorrhea, this secretion may be maintained by minimal or intermittent prolactin elevation.

Prolactin Physiology

Prolactin-secreting cells constitute 10% to 25% of the normal pituitary and increase to 70% during pregnancy. The predominant biologic form of prolactin contains 198 amino acids (23,000 Mol wt) in a single polypeptide chain and is referred to as monomeric or "little" prolactin (34). Higher molecular weight forms of prolactin, referred to as "big" and "big-big" prolactin, circulate in varying amounts. The larger polymeric forms have substantially less biologic activity than the monomeric forms (35). Glycosylated prolactin also occurs in humans but has reduced immunologic activity compared with nonglycosylated forms as measured by RIA (36,37).

The awareness of the possibility that prolactin measured in an RIA may not be the native form is important. Generally, the higher molecular weight types are less biologically active but often have similar RIA activity compared with prolactin. Thus, the heterogeneous circulating forms may result in RIA measurement of serum prolactin that does not correlate well with clinical findings. Examples are women with galactorrhea who have normal serum prolactin levels as measured by RIA (38). Also, there are individuals with hyperprolactinemia as measured by RIA with no obvious clinical abnormalities (39,40).

Not only are there multiple circulating forms of prolactin with various biologic activities, but there are many physiologic conditions that lead to associated transient increases in prolactin release. These conditions include sleep, intake of high-protein meals, exercise, physical and emotional stress, and probably elevations associated with orgasm (Table 2.3).

Beyond these physiologic conditions associated with prolactin secretion, there are relative increases in circulating prolactin levels that fluctuate during the menstrual cycle. In certain assay systems, there is a late follicular increase in prolactin consistent with estrogen stimulation of prolactin release, and also luteal phase prolactin elevations are seen (41,42). These changes are usually not significant but should be appreciated if variable results are obtained with random sampling during the menstrual cycle.

Table 2.3. *Physiological conditions stimulating prolactin release*

Sleep	Ovulation
Feeding	Pregnancy
Exercise	Suckling
Stress	? Dehydration
Coitus	

Reprinted by permission from DeVane GW. Difficulty in the measurement and assessment of prolactin. Presented at the XIIIth World Congress on Fertility and Sterility, Marrakesh, 1989.

The evaluation of prolactin concentration is further complicated by the fact that certain drug therapies increase prolactin secretion. The effects of sedatives, tranquilizers, and other dopamine receptor–blocking agents lead to elevation of prolactin secretion (Table 2.4).

Under normal physiologic circumstances, prolactin secretion by the anterior pituitary is restrained by tonic hypothalamic inhibitory influence (43). Most of the inhibitory effects of the hypothalamus can be accounted for by hypothalamic dopamine. Dopamine acts directly on the pituitary via the hypophysial portal system (Fig. 2.7). Dopamine binds specifically to lactotroph cells, causing a cascade of membrane-associated and intracellular events, which results in inhibition of prolactin synthesis and release (44). Hypersecretion of prolactin occurs when the hypothalamic-pituitary portal vasculature is interrupted, as seen in pituitary stalk section (45) and mass lesions (see Fig. 2.7) (46).

There are stimulatory factors that cause prolactin synthesis and release. Thyrotropin-releasing hormone (TRH) is a hypothalamic tripeptide that causes rapid prolactin release in humans (47,48). Because TRH controls the release of thyroid-stimulating hormone (TSH) (49), and TSH levels do not rise during physiologic hyperprolactinemia (i.e., lactation), the role of TRH as a physiologic releasing factor is unclear. There are many other stimulatory releasing factors (Table 2.5), but none of these appear to have a physiologic function.

The presence of galactorrhea is always directly or indirectly related to inappropriate prolactin release or action. There should be no real concern regarding breast disease; rather, a search for one of the multiple factors involved in the control of prolactin secretion must be undertaken. The evaluation of galactorrhea must exclude the rare possibility of a pituitary tumor. The following section provides an overview regarding various causes of galactorrhea.

Differential Diagnosis

The finding of galactorrhea is associated with prolactin excess; when galactorrhea occurs with amenorrhea, hyperprolactinemia is present

Table 2.4. Conditions associated with inappropriate prolactin secretion

Pharmacologic causes	Pathologic causes
Estrogen therapy	Hypothalamic lesions
Anesthesia	Craniopharyngioma
DA receptor blocking agents	Glioma
Phenoghiazones	Granulomas
Haloperidol	Histocytosis disease
Metoclopramide	Sarcoid
Domperidone	Tuberculosis
Pimozide	Stalk transection
Sulpiride	Postsurgical or head injury
DA re-uptake blocker	Irradiation damage of the hypo-
Nomifensine	thalamus
CNS-DA depleting agents	Pseudocyesis (functional)
Reserpine	Pituitary tumors
α-methyldopa	Cushing's disease
Monoamine oxidase inhibitor	Acromegaly
Inhibition of DA turnover	Prolactinoma
Opiates	Mixed GH or ACTH- and PRL-
Stimulation of serotoninergic system	secreting adenomas
Amphetamines	"Nonfunctional" adenomas
Hallucinogens	Reflex causes
Histamine H_2-receptor antagonists	Chest wall injury and herpes
Cimetidine	zoster neuritis
	Upper abdominal surgery
	Hypothyroidism
	Renal failure
	Ectopic production
	Bronchogenic carcinoma
	Hypernephroma

DA = dopamine; CNS = central nervous system; GH = growth hormone; ACTH = corticotropin; PRL = prolactin.
Reprinted with permission from Yen SSC. Prolactin in human reproduction. Philadelphia: WB Saunders, 1986.

in more than 80% of patients (38). Prolactin elevation has several mechanisms, including the following: 1) autonomous production by pituitary tumors or hyperplastic tissue; 2) decreased dopamine or dopamine action as caused by hypothalamic disease or drugs that block dopamine syntheses, release, or action; 3) direct stimulatory effects on the lactotroph (estrogen or TRH secretion in hypothyroidism); and 4) decreased clearance of prolactin as seen in renal failure.

Pharmacologic Causes of Hyperprolactinemia

A careful medication history should be obtained from hyperprolactinemic patients. Oral contraceptives and postmenopausal hormone replacement therapy may increase circulating prolactin concentration (50,51) and result in proliferation of breast glandular elements.

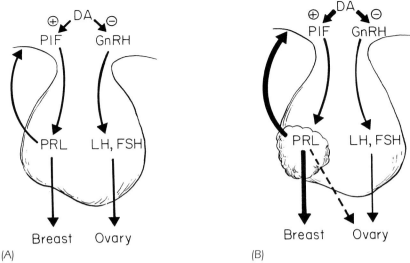

Figure 2.7. (A) Conceptualized model of the role of dopamine (DA) in regulation of prolactin (PRL) secretion and gonadotropin-releasing hormone (GnRH)–mediated gonadotropin release in normal women. (B) In the presence of hyperprolactinemia (prolactinoma), a short-loop feedback effect increases dopamine production in the hypothalamus, which inhibits GnRH activity and leads to gonadotropin suppression. (PIF = prolactin-inhibiting factor; LH = leutinizing hormone; FSH = follicle-stimulating hormone.) Reprinted by permission from Chang RJ. Anovulation of CNS origin: anatomic causes. Norwalk, CT: Appleton & Lange, 1993.

Galactorrhea with oral contraceptives usually occurs during menses, when withdrawal of estrogen and progestin simulates hormone withdrawal at the time of parturition (52). Dopamine-blocking drugs (e.g., phenothiazines, butyrophenones, metoclopramide) and dopamine-

Table 2.5. Peptides with prolactin-releasing activity

TRH
Vasoactive intestinal peptide (VIP)
Serotonin
Endogenous opiates
Epidermal growth factor
Fibroblast growth factor
Gonadotropin-releasing hormone (GnRH)
Cholecystokinin
Vasopressin
Angiotensin II
Vitamin D
Substance P
Neurotensin
Bombesin

TRH = thyroid-releasing hormone.
Reprinted by permission from Melmed S. Control of prolactin synthesis and secretion. New York: Thieme Medical Publishers, 1993.

depleting drugs (e.g., methyldopa and reserpine) are important causes of hyperprolactinemia via their ability to reduce dopamine availability at the lactotroph, thus decreasing the normal inhibition of prolactin. Other drugs known to increase prolactin secretion include opiates, amphetamine, verapamil (53), cimetidine (54), and cocaine (55). The mechanism of action of several of these drugs is demonstrated in Table 2.4.

Pathologic Causes of Hyperprolactinemia

Hypothalamus

Infiltrative or degenerative lesions of the hypothalamus may result in hyperprolactinemia and galactorrhea by a reduction in hypothalamic dopamine production (56). Tumors such as craniopharyngioma or germinoma may cause amenorrhea and other ovulatory disturbances via increased prolactin release or abnormalities of gonadotropin-releasing hormone (GnRH) secretion. Hypothalamic stalk lesions and stalk compression, which causes a reduction of hypothalamic dopamine delivery to the pituitary, result in hyperprolactinemia and often galactorrhea (see Table 2.4).

Pituitary

Pituitary tumors occur with relative frequency ranging from 10% to 23% in large autopsy series (57,58). Pituitary tumors that secrete prolactin are referred to as prolactin-secreting adenomas and account for at least 70% of all pituitary adenomas (59). A microadenoma refers to tumors 10 mm or smaller; macroadenomas are larger than 10 mm in diameter. Upward expansion can lead to visual field defects caused by optic nerve compression. The use of computed tomographic (CT) scans or magnetic resonance imaging (MRI), together with assessment of circulating prolactin concentration, allows for the diagnosis of "prolactinoma" with high accuracy. Patients with these prolactin-secreting adenomas usually present with galactorrhea and menstrual irregularities, including amenorrhea. Subtle changes in ovulatory function such as luteal phase defects may occur with only modest prolactin excess (60,61). The likelihood of finding an adenoma is correlated to the level of prolactin measured. Any value greater than 75 to 100 ng/mL should be regarded with suspicion and probably merits radiologic evaluation. Values greater than 200 to 300 ng/mL invariably are associated with prolactin-secreting tumor (38,62). Rarely, tumors are found in patients with normal prolactin levels (52).

Because galactorrhea and amenorrhea are such obvious clinical features of prolactin excess, evaluation of these patients must be undertaken to determine whether a prolactin tumor is present. The diagnosis of a prolactinoma is based on serum prolactin concentration and the radiologic appearance of the pituitary gland. The diagnosis of pituitary tumor in males is more difficult because galactorrhea rarely occurs even with extremely high prolactin levels (63).

Hypothyroidism

Severe primary hypothyroidism may cause hyperprolactinemia either because of elevated TRH levels or by decreased dopaminergic influence. This may lead to a condition in which prolactin levels are slightly above normal or even within the upper normal range (64). Untreated hypothyroidism of longer duration is associated with higher prolactin levels and often galactorrhea (65). Enlargement of the sella turcica may occur in association with hypothyroidism; if hyperprolactinemia is present, the condition may mimic a prolactinoma (66). Administration of thyroid hormone to restore euthyroidism usually lowers the prolactin level and stops the galactorrhea, leading to resolution of the pituitary enlargement (67). Elevated TSH is the earliest laboratory abnormality associated with hypothyroidism and should be obtained to screen for primary hypothyroidism (68). Thyroid replacement does not cause a reduction in prolactin levels or cessation of galactorrhea in euthyroid patients.

Other Endocrine and Metabolic Disorders

Adrenal Disorders

Galactorrhea and amenorrhea may occur in patients with Addison's disease (adrenal insufficiency), and symptoms resolve with glucocorticoid treatment (69). Galactorrhea and hyperprolactinemia may occur in patients with Cushing's syndrome, which may represent a direct effect of glucocorticoids on the breast (70), although dopaminergic mechanisms are probably involved.

Acromegaly

Galactorrhea is present in approximately 20% of patients with acromegaly, and about 33% of patients also have hyperprolactinemia in addition to growth hormone excess (71). Elevated prolactin may be caused by pituitary stalk compression resulting from expansion of the growth hormone tumor with resultant reduction in available dopamine suppression at the lactotroph.

Renal Failure

Hyperprolactinemia occurs in 20% to 37% of renal disease patients and in almost 80% of patients undergoing hemodialysis (72,73) and is often associated with galactorrhea. Reduced clearance of prolactin accounts for the hyperprolactinemia.

Chest Wall Lesions

Galactorrhea can be associated with disease affecting the chest walls, such as herpes zoster, or can occur after thoracotomy (74). The hyperprolactinemic response is probably caused by stimulation of afferent neural pathways. Excessive stimulation of the nipple or areola may also result in hyperprolactinemia and galactorrhea (27) presumably via the same mechanism.

Ectopic Prolactin Production

Galactorrhea may be seen with underlying carcinoma. Bronchogenic carcinoma and hypernephroma have been demonstrated to secrete prolactin (75).

Idiopathic Galactorrhea

The actual clinical significance of the presence of galactorrhea is complex because the true prevalence is unknown. Most women with minimal galactorrhea and normal menstrual cycles do not seek a physician's care unless there is concern regarding breast cancer. Furthermore, galactorrhea may be missed on physical examination unless it is specifically sought.

After careful evaluation, the cause of galactorrhea will usually be identified in most patients. Nonetheless, in many large series of patients presenting with galactorrhea, a high percentage of women will have no obvious cause for this finding (38,76–79). In the majority of patients, the galactorrhea is associated with normal menses and in parous women may represent a residue of postpartum lactation that has never disappeared. Some of these women have normal prolactin levels, and the galactorrhea is the result of increased sensitivity of the breast tissue to normal levels of circulating prolactin (80). In one large series, when galactorrhea occurred spontaneously, the incidence of hyperprolactinemia was 55%, but when galactorrhea was found on manual expression, only 20% of these women had elevated prolactin levels (79). Serum prolactin levels as measured by RIA correlate poorly with milk secretion because the hormonal milieu of the patient must be appropriate for galactorrhea to occur. Furthermore, as described previously, there is heterogeneity of the prolactin molecule, including dimers and glycosylated forms, which have altered immunologic and biologic activity (81).

Clinically, the presence of galactorrhea with associated regular menses and normal serum prolactin should be classified as idiopathic, and no further evaluation such as MRI or CT scans in these patients is required (80), although serum prolactin level should be obtained on one or more occasions. In those women with galactorrhea, hyperprolactinemia, and associated amenorrhea without a radiographic present pituitary tumor, more careful surveillance is required. Long-term studies of patients with idiopathic hyperprolactinemia indicate either no change or a reduction in prolactin levels in most cases with a low incidence of tumor development (82).

Other Causes

Galactorrhea has been observed in patients with hepatic cirrhosis, upon refeeding after starvation (83), and even in adolescent boys with gynecomastia (84).

Diagnosis of Galactorrhea

The evaluation of patients with galactorrhea is directed toward excluding physiologic and pharmocologic causes of hyperprolactinemia. Elevation of prolactin is necessary in pregnancy and occurs during sleep, exercise, and nipple stimulation and after food ingestion (see Table 2.3). Prolactin concentration is best measured in the fasting state and at least 2 hours after awakening to avoid sleep-related prolactin release (85). A careful drug history will elicit use of pharmacologic agents that increase prolactin secretion (see Table 2.4). Drug-induced elevated prolactin concentration is usually less than 75 to 100 ng/mL and returns to normal when the specific medication is discontinued.

Once physiologic and pharmacologic causes of galactorrhea and hyperprolactinemia have been excluded, pathologic causes must be considered (see Table 2.4). Symptoms suggestive of pituitary or hypothalamic diseases include headaches, visual disturbances, and changes in temperature, thirst, and appetite regulation (80). On physical examination, visual fields should be checked by confrontation, and signs of hypothyroidism, acromegaly, and Cushing's syndrome should be noted. Laboratory and radiologic studies are required if specific indications are present to identify the cause. A serum TSH is necessary to detect primary hypothyroidism. Depending on clinical suspicion, corticotropin, growth hormone response, or gonadotropin levels should be measured (80). Ovulatory function should be evaluated in any patient with menstrual irregularity or infertility when galactorrhea is present.

The diagnosis of pituitary tumor is dependent on the level of serum prolactin and on radiographic findings, particularly on MRI and CT scans, which have generally replaced polytomography of the sella turcica (58). Cone-down views and hypocycloidal tomography of the sella have been recommended to assess the status of the pituitary in patients with mild to modest hyperprolactinemia (86). However, small tumors may be missed, and variations in sellar configuration result in a high incidence of false-positive results, requiring corroboration with CT scanning (87).

MRI or CT scans should be performed if the serum prolactin is elevated or even slightly elevated if there are any other signs suggestive of a pituitary tumor. As previously noted, such scans are not mandatory in cases of minimal galactorrhea if the serum prolactin value is within the normal range and menses are regular (80). Although serum prolactin levels are related to tumor size, there is variability among patients, and normal or minimally elevated prolactin levels are also seen in patients with prolactinoma (87).

Treatment of Galactorrhea

If there is no evidence of pituitary tumor or menstrual dysfunction, treatment for elevated prolactin is not necessary because there are no data to indicate that prolonged hyperprolactinemia in the absence of amenorrhea (and hypoestrogenemia) is harmful (83). With amenorrhea and hyperprolactinemia, patients are at increased risk for the development of osteoporosis (88–90).

Patients with idiopathic hyperprolactinemia should undergo treatment only if galactorrhea is bothersome or if fertility is impaired (83). The treatment of choice is the reduction of circulating prolactin level with bromocriptine or other dopamine agonists (91). Bromocriptine has also been used in patients with otherwise unexplained infertility and expressible galactorrhea who are normoprolactinemic. These patients may have subtle increases in prolactin secretion or increased sensitivity to normal circulating prolactin as manifested by the biologic marker of galactorrhea. In these women, very-low-dose bromocriptine therapy (1.25–2.5 mg at bedtime) may correct subtle ovulatory dysfunction and result in improved fertility (92).

Pituitary Tumors

Therapy for prolactin-secreting tumors is based on whether the adenoma is stable or expanding (symptomatic) and the patient's desire to have fertility restored or unpleasant galactorrhea eliminated. Choices of treatment include surgery, drug therapy, radiotherapy, and close periodic observation to detect a growing tumor.

Before the availability of dopamine agonists, transsphenoidal surgery was the most widely used treatment for removal of a prolactinoma; when performed by experienced neurosurgeons, it remains an excellent procedure with low morbidity (93). Unfortunately, even in the best of hands, hyperprolactinemia recurs in 50% of patients with micro-adenoma within approximately 4 years after surgery and in 80% of patients with macroadenoma withing 2.5 years (94).

Conventional radiation therapy (45 Gy) over 25 days causes a slow decline in prolactin levels over 2 to 5 years. Radiotherapy is used mainly for inoperative macroadenoma and in patients who are intolerant of medical therapy. Radiotherapy is rarely curative and may lead to long-term complications such as hypopituitarism (95).

Bromocriptine and other dopamine agonists, including pergolide, have been used successfully for the treatment of hyperprolactinemia (96). Bromocriptine treatment is effective in lowering prolactin concentration in patients with microadenoma and macroadenoma as well as persistent postoperative hyperprolactinemia (97). On the basis of the excellent results with bromocriptine therapy in most patients, this treatment should be the primary therapy for all symptomatic pituitary adenomas.

For those patients with stable microadenoma, close observation, including yearly prolactin levels and CT scan every 2 to 5 years, is appropriate. Long-term studies of patients with untreated microadenoma have shown that only 10% have significant growth and spontaneous regression; resumption of menses and cessation of galactorrhea may occur (98,99). For macroadenomas, some form of therapy is usually advisable to prevent further growth and to shrink the tumor if it is symptomatic.

Prolactinomas and Pregnancy

Under normal circumstances, the pituitary gland enlarges as much as twofold during pregnancy probably as a result of rising levels of placental estrogen, which induces lactotroph hyperplasia and hypertrophy (100). Treatment of patients with idiopathic or tumor-related hyperprolactinemia is often aimed at restoration of fertility. The outcome of pregnancy in hyperprolactinemic women is generally good, but controversy regarding management exists (83).

Patients with intrasellar microadenomas are at minimal risk for complications, with only 1% having significant tumor enlargement (101). If bromocriptine was used to restore ovulation with a resultant pregnancy, this treatment should be discontinued once pregnancy has been confirmed. If a rare complication occurs, bromocriptine should be reinstituted because there has been no reported increase in spontaneous abortions, congenital malformations, or prematurity even when it is administered throughout pregnancy (102,103).

The risk of symptomatic enlargement in pregnancy with macroadenoma ranges from 15% to 35% (104). Tumor expansion is associated with headache, nausea, and vomiting with the onset of visual field compromise or loss of acuity. Reinstitution of bromocriptine reverses the clinical symptoms (103). Some patients with macroadenoma and hyperprolactinemia may not respond to medical therapy (105,106). Thus, before women with macroadenoma contemplate pregnancy, bromocriptine responsiveness should be demonstrated.

Breast-feeding does not appear to increase the risk of tumor expansion. In non-nursing mothers, inhibition of lactation can be achieved by reinstituting bromocriptine in doses of 5 to 10 mg daily for 2 weeks followed by gradual tapering (83). Resumption of ovarian function after delivery is often observed in patients with idiopathic hyperprolactinemia and in those patients who received chronic bromocriptine therapy before pregnancy (107).

Nipple Discharge and Breast Disease

Physiologic Secretion

As previously discussed, breast secretion is present in the ducts of 50% to 70% of asymptomatic women when careful examination or nipple aspiration by pump expression is performed (see Figs. 2.1 and 2.2). This physiologic fluid has many of the characteristics of colostrum and milk in that it contains exfoliated epithelial cells and nonepithelial cells of hematogenous and immune system origin. The fluid varies in color and appearance depending on its composition.

Physiologic breast secretion contains lactose, α-lactalbumin, immunoglobulin, cholesterol, fatty acids, and steroids (108). Substances from exogenous sources are also found in physiologic fluid, including caffeine, pesticides, and nicotine (6). These findings demonstrate that breast fluid is a true secretory product.

Papanicolaou and colleagues analyzed the "normal" cytology of nonspontaneous breast secretion and noted that the two benign cell types most often encountered were foam cells and duct epithelial cells (2). Benign epithelial cells consist of a few ductal cells, with only rare apocrine metaplastic cells present. There is a preponderance of foam cells showing predominantly histiocytic characteristics and a moderate number of cells of hematogenous origin.

Histologic Changes

Histologic changes in breast tissue occur during the menstrual cycle. Breast secretion obtained for cytology is most easily obtained during the premenstrual and menstrual intervals in normal women (2). Some increase in total cellularity and in the percentage of lymphocytes occurs in the periovulatory phase of the cycle. Changes in total cellularity and cell morphology during the menstrual cycle have revealed no significant differences that would interfere with cytologic evaluation of normal versus abnormal breast secretion (108).

Secretions Associated with Breast Disease

Abnormal nipple discharge is usually unilateral, spontaneous, and frequently localized to a single duct. Pathologic discharge may be bloody, serosanguineous, serous, or greenish-gray. The significance of bloody discharge is its association with intraductal papilloma, other papillary lesions, duct ectasia, and carcinoma.

The cytologic presence of erythrocytes and papillary clusters of 30 ductal cells or more suggests a malignant process (109). Haagensen (110) described a colorless, thin, watery discharge as specific for cancer, but this is extremely uncommon and rarely mentioned by other authors.

Although spontaneous pathologic nipple discharge is abnormal, less than 5% of new patients referred to a breast clinic in Edinburgh complained primarily of breast secretion (7). Much of the confusion regarding abnormal breast discharge is historic in that early series reported a high association of breast discharge with carcinoma (111). In most of these cases, a coexistent breast mass was found. If a palpable breast mass is present, a biopsy of the mass should be performed for diagnosis. The clinical significance of nipple discharge becomes most important when there is no palpable mass. Classification of nipple discharge then provides information regarding usually a benign cause for the abnormal discharge.

Discharge Caused by Areolar Disease

Discharge and crusting of the areolar tissue are relatively uncommon but are important to differentiate from more serious causes (Table 2.6).

Nipple Adenoma

A nipple adenoma presents with a bloody discharge, associated erythema, and often ulceration of the nipple skin. Examination reveals an indiscrete, superficial mass. This lesion is similar in appearance to Paget's disease requiring an excisional biopsy for diagnosis.

Table 2.6. Nipple discharges resulting from causes within the breast

Nipple & areola	Breast duct
1. Nipple adenoma	1. Duct papilloma(s)
2. Eczema	2. Duct ectasia
3. Paget's disease	3. Cancer *in situ,* or early invasive cancer
4. Ulcerating carcinoma	4. Cystic disease
5. Inversion of nipple and maceration	5. Idiopathic

Reprinted by permission from Chitty V. Nipple discharge. Baltimore: Urban & Schwarzberg, 1990.

This is not a precancerous lesion. Extensive local excision with conservation of the nipple is possible (110).

Nipple Eczema and Paget's Disease

Eczema or dermatitis of the nipple is usually caused by irritation and may become secondarily infected. This causes a weeping, crusty discharge similar in appearance to Paget's disease, which is a more serious entity. These conditions can be easily differentiated by the fact that eczema occurs rapidly and spreads to most of the areola within a few weeks. Eczema never destroys the nipple as Paget's disease can. Eczema involves the nipple-areola complex. Diagnosis must be made by wide excision under local anesthesia. Eczema is treated by avoidance of the irritant and a short course of topical steroids (7).

Nipple Eversion with Maceration

This rare condition is usually seen in elderly women. The inverted nipple forms a cavity, which becomes macerated and produces a discharge. This condition is resolved by eversion and cleaning of the nipple.

Nipple Discharge and Ductal Diseases

Most pathologic nipple discharges are caused by ductal disease (see Table 2.6). Nipple discharge has been reported in 10% to 15% of women with benign breast disease and in 2.5% to 3% of those with carcinoma (112,113). By far, the most common benign lesions are duct ectasia and duct papilloma, but in situ ductal or early invasive cancer is the most important. Cytology may be indicated when the discharge is bloody or serous and there is no clinically evident mass or significant mammographic findings.

Duct Ectasia

Duct ectasia is a benign disease complex consisting of dilatation with loss of elastin in duct walls and the presence of chronic inflammatory cells, especially plasma cells, around the walls, described as periductal mastitis (114). The cause is uncertain, and theories range from collection followed by transudation of secretions in ducts dilated from previous pregnancy to primary periductal inflammation. The fact that inflammatory causes of the disease predominate in younger women indicates that periductal inflammation may be the primary abnormality, with duct dilatation resulting (115,116).

Anaerobic bacteria may have a role in the pathogenesis of "periductal mastitis," but more likely bacterial infection develops secondary to stasis in large ducts, resulting in secondary complications such as fistula, nonlactation abscess, and inflammatory masses (117).

Nipple discharge is the most common symptom of duct ectasia. It is usually bilateral and arises from multiple ducts. The color may be pale yellow, green, or brown with a paste-like consistency. The discharge is not blood stained but may be weakly guaiac positive. Patients are usually postmenopausal and present because the discharge is a nuisance and because of their concern that this might indicate cancer. Other than expressed discharge, there are no other findings. A mammogram should be performed to exclude coexistent carcinoma.

Further treatment depends on personal preference. If the discharge is bothersome, a retroareolar major duct excision is recommended (7).

Duct Papilloma

Papilloma is a benign lesion of epithelium, usually with supportive stroma, growing within ducts independently of the walls. Most common is solitary intraductal papilloma located in the major ducts near the nipple. It is almost always benign and only rarely associated with carcinoma. The peripheral variety of papilloma is uncommon, usually originating within lobular units and extending along small ducts. This type is usually multifocal and related to epithelial hyperplasia (118). Multiple peripheral papillomas are associated with an increased risk for breast cancer (119), but this is probably because of the epithelial hyperplasia and atypia associated with this condition (120).

Both central and more peripheral papillomas present with discharge from a *single duct* of the nipple, which may be serous or bloody. Pressure over the area of breast harboring the papilloma results in discharge from the nipple (110). Occasionally, the papilloma is close to the duct orifice and may prolapse out of the ostium. Cytology of single or unilateral nipple discharge is worthwhile if expert cytology is available. A definite diagnosis of carcinoma is almost always reliable, but negative results should be regarded with caution. Cytology alone cannot be the basis for diagnosis of duct papilloma.

The treatment of choice for either central or more peripheral papilloma is microdochectomy. After cannulating the single duct involved, the duct and segment that drain are completely excised.

Early Ductal Carcinoma

In most modern series, in situ ductal carcinoma is responsible for between 5% and 10% of unilateral nipple discharge (7). This may be either serous or bloody, but the color presentation is not of prognostic significance. In one report, nipple discharge alone or in association with a mass or Paget's disease was observed in about one third of unscreened patients with in situ ductal cancer (121). An associated mass should always be sought because this finding is a strong indicator of possible cancer. Leis et al (122) found palpable masses in 59 (88%) of 67 patients with nipple discharge and cancer.

The optimum treatment of occult or in situ disease after biopsy confirmation is unknown, but mastectomy is indicated for most cases, especially when disease is extensive and multifocal (7).

Management of Breast Discharge

As previously described, the vast majority of nipple discharges is caused by benign conditions. Among women with nipple discharge, malignancy is found in only a small percentage. Chaudary et al (123) reported that only 16 (0.6%) of 2476 patients with breast cancer presented with discharge and no other finding. Furthermore, nipple discharge is common in the general female population; yet spontaneous nipple discharge is the chief complaint in only 3% to 6% of women coming to breast specialty services. Despite these facts, breast secretion or discharge is always listed on health educational brochures as an important sign of breast cancer; therefore, the finding of nipple discharge by self-examination may cause much unwarranted anxiety.

The management of nipple discharge is straightforward and depends on a clear description of the macroscopic appearance of the secretion. Only spontaneous, persistent, and nonlactational discharges are of significance (124).

The most important feature of a discharge is the presence of blood. Blood-related discharges can be serous, serosanguineous, or bloody and are associated in a minority of women with underlying carcinoma. All other discharges, such as multicolored, opalescent, or milky types, are not associated with cancer (125). The only exception is the rare crystal-clear water type (7,110). Therefore, the majority of women can be reassured, by the appearance of their breast secretion on initial breast examination that there is no concern regarding malignancy.

Blood-related discharges are due to duct ectasia or hyperplastic epithelial lesions. Rough estimates of the incidence indicate that 50% are caused by intraductal papilloma, 35% by duct ectasia, and 5% to 15% by cancer (124). The likelihood of a nipple discharge being caused by malignancy increases appreciably with age. Seltzer et al (126) noted a 32% incidence of carcinoma in women older than 60 years presenting with discharge and no palpable mass compared with a 7% incidence in women younger than 60 years. Although the single most important point in the patient history is whether the discharge is spontaneous or expressed, the number of ducts producing discharge is also important because discharges from multiple ducts are rarely malignant, whereas single-duct discharge can represent a true risk factor indicating cancer. Also, if there is a palpable mass, the appropriate evaluation of the mass takes precedence over the secretion. Devitt (127) found that a breast mass was usually present when nipple discharge was associated with cancer. Careful breast examination is obviously important in the assessment of breast discharge and will sometimes reveal a "trigger point" at which pressure will maximize the nipple discharge. Mammography is used to identify abnormalities such as an impalpable carcinoma or linear calcifications indicative of ductal carcinoma in situ.

Summary: Treatment of Breast Secretion

For patients with physiologic discharge, reassurance is sufficient. For galactorrhea, an evaluation for endocrinologic abnormality or pharmacologic causes should be undertaken. For women with pathologic discharge, an attempt should be made to localize the source of the discharge to one quadrant by examination and mammography. Surgical treatment should be performed when appropriate.

The management of blood-related discharge is surgical. Intraductal papilloma is usually seen when there is a relatively profuse discharge from a single duct. If a palpable breast mass is present, biopsy of the mass should be performed for diagnosis. Terminal duct excision is the procedure of choice for the surgical treatment of noncancerous single-duct nipple discharge (see Fig. 2.8). If the bloody discharge is from multiple ducts or in a patient older than 40 years, total duct excision as described by Hadfield is the operation of choice (128).

MASTALGIA

Introduction and Classification of Breast Pain

Many women present with a history of breast pain, tenderness, and nodularity. This symptom complex is usually termed mastalgia, which literally means "breast pain." Mastalgia is reported to be the most common breast-related symptom causing women to consult physicians and surgeons (110,129–131). It is estimated that at least 50% of all women have palpably irregular breasts (127). Furthermore, cyclic discomfort and nodularity of the breast are so common as to be considered a normal physiologic occurrence. Haagensen advised that cyclic bilateral breast pain and nodularity represent physiologic problems that should not be confused with pathologic entities (110). This leads to confusion regarding when breast pain constitutes a disease. Yet there are extremes of the normal cyclic changes such that severe mastalgia and nodularity can become debilitating.

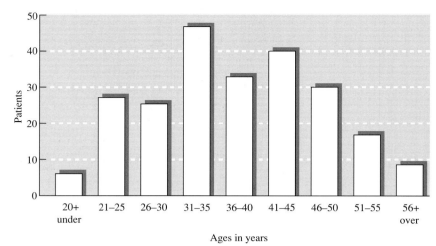

Figure 2.8. *Distribution, by age, of patients presenting with mastalgia. Reprinted by permission from Preece R, Mansel R, Bolton P, et al. Clinical syndromes of mastalgia. © by The Lancet Ltd. Lancet 1976;2:670.*

The incidence of mastalgia remains uncertain because of the difficulty in distinguishing it from the cyclic breast pain many women experience premenstrually. Preece et al (132) distinguished cyclic mastalgia by its intensity or persistence, which is often difficult to quantitate. In their large series, patients with mastalgia ranged in age from 13 to 66 years at the time of referral (Fig. 2.8). Cyclic mastalgia occurred most commonly during the third decade of life. Noncyclic mastalgia tended to present a decade later, with shorter duration symptoms and a high spontaneous reduction rate.

Normal Breast Changes

Because mastalgia appears to be an aberration of normal physiology, a consideration of the normal processes occurring within the breast may provide an understanding of this benign breast disorder.

Breast Development

The premenstrual breast consists of only a few ducts. At menarche, duct development within lobular structures begins, with mature lobules developing between 15 and 25 years of age. This explains the increased frequency of fibroadenoma during this interval because it is a condition analogous to gross hypertrophy of a lobule. Until about 35 years of age, the progesterone dominance in the luteal phase is associated with increased acinar sprouting from the ductules.

Cyclic Changes

Vorrher (133) described changes occurring during the menstrual cycle. Both epithelial and stromal tissues of the lobule are under balanced estrogen and progesterone control. Cyclic changes are associated with clinical symptoms of heaviness and premenstrual fullness almost never associated with detectable histologic changes. Any imbalance in this hormonal relationship is usually responsible for exaggerated symptoms. Superimposed on normal cyclic changes are the much more striking effects of pregnancy and lactation (see Physiologic Breast Changes During Pregnancy). With the cyclic breast changes responsive to ovarian steroids and dramatic alterations occurring during pregnancy, there is abundant opportunity for minor aberrations to occur. Indeed, on histologic examination of an asymptomatic woman in her 30s, fibroses and adenomas can usually be identified (134).

Breast Involution

Involutional changes are seen by 35 years of age or even earlier. For the remaining 15 to 20 years of ovarian function, cyclic hormonal change and involution are occurring simultaneously, increasing the chance of abnormalities of breast structure (134). This coincides with the peak incidence by age of women presenting with mastalgia. The involutional process involves an orderly regression of lobules and surrounding fibrous tissue. Intralobular connective tissue is replaced by interlobular-type fibrous tissue. By menopause, only a few ducts remain with no evidence of lobular structures. If specialized stroma disappear prematurely, the epithelial acini remain and may form microcysts. With mechanical obstruction, macrocysts can occur.

Aberrations of Normal Development and Involution

Hughes and colleagues (134) proposed the term "aberrations of normal development and involution" (ANDI) to classify most common benign breast disorders within a physiologic setting (Table 2.7). This approach recognizes that most breast symptoms and disorders are based on the normal processes of development, cyclic change, and involution. Within this conceptual framework, conditions that affect a large portion of the population should be regarded as normal or, at worst, a disorder but certainly not a disease. An example is the presence of perimenstrual mastalgia and nodularity, which is a "normal" event. The breast pain of women with gross exaggeration of these physiologic symptoms with no pathologic findings is termed, using the ANDI classification, "cyclic pronounced mastalgia" or "severe

Table 2.7.   *A broad classification of benign breast disorders*

1.   ANDI
      Development
         Adolescent hypertrophy
         Fibroadenoma
      Cyclic change
         Mastalgia
         Clinical nodularity
      Involution
         Cyst formation
         Sclerosing adenosis
2.   Duct ectasia and periductal mastitis
3.   Epithelial hyperplasias
4.   Conditions with well-defined etiology (e.g., lactational abscess, trau-
      matic fat necrosis)

ANDI = aberration of normal development and involution.
Adapted by permission from Hughes LE, Mansel RE, Webster DJT. Aberrations
of normal development and involution (ANDI): a concept of benign breast disorders based on pathogenesis. London: Baillière Tindall, 1989.

painful nodularity." This is the clinical presentation often termed
"fibrocystic disease," a term that is no longer considered appropriate
(135). The ANDI approach stresses the importance of a broad view of
benign breast disorder, especially when dealing with problems such
as mastalgia when there are no histologic changes. A more traditional
classification will be followed regarding evaluation and management
of mastalgia, but, in fact, most benign breast disorders could be considered as aberrations of normal development and involution.

Classification of Mastalgia

A complete and detailed description of breast pain is important to
guide diagnostic evaluation and to assess the results of therapy. One
method to classify breast pain was established in the Cardiff Mastalgia
Clinic using a protocol describing several features of presenting symptoms (Table 2.8) (136). Preece et al (132) determined the incidence of
various causes of mastalgia in 232 patients referred to their center
after initial breast examination and mammogram to exclude a dominant mass of carcinoma (Table 2.9). In their patient sample, three
patterns of breast pain were identified: cyclic, noncyclic, or nonbreast
mastalgia.

Cyclic Mastalgia

Cyclic pain is the most common type of breast pain among women
seeking specialty consultation for painful breasts with or without nodu-

Table 2.8. Contents of the Cardiff mastalgia protocol

Feature	Examples
Descriptive terms	Tenderness/heaviness/burning
Periodicity	Continuous, intermittent
Duration	
Distribution in breast	
Radiation	
Aggravating factors	Physical contact
Relieving factors	Analgesics/drugs/well-fitted brassière
Diurnal pattern	
Disturbance of lifestyle	Sleep loss/marital problem/can't hug children
Dominant hand	

Reprinted by permission from Hughes LE, Mansel RE, Webster DJT. Breast pain and nodularity. London: Baillière Tindall, 1989.

larity. Cyclic pain is usually maximal premenstrually and is relieved with the onset of menses. Cyclic mastalgia may be unilateral or bilateral and is not well localized. The upper outer quadrants of the breast are most usually involved, and the pain is described as heaviness, aching, and soreness. The most severely affected have been referred to as "cyclically pronounced" patients (136). This terminology is used to denote the increased intensity of the symptom defined either by duration (>1 week per cycle) or by severity, as determined by the use of a breast pain calendar, which provides a semiquantitative means of assessing pain (Fig. 2.9). Cyclic mastalgia frequently radiates to the ipsilateral axilla and arm (131,132). The mean age of women with cyclic mastalgia ranges from 33 to 35 years (Fig. 2.10) (137). Cyclic mastalgia is a disease affecting premenopausal women, although it has been reported in postmenopausal women on replacement hormone therapy (138). Mammography is not helpful in cyclic mastalgia because no specific radiologic appearance correlates with the area of discomfort.

The natural history of cyclic mastalgia is variable. Wisbey et al stud-

Table 2.9. Frequency of patterns in 232 prospectively documented mastalgia patients

Pattern/diagnosis	Number (%)
Cyclic, pronounced	93 (40.0)
Noncyclic	62 (27.0)
Tietze's syndrome	25 (11.0)
Trauma (postbiopsy)	19 (8.0)
Sclerosing adenosis	11 (4.7)
Cancer	1 (0.5)
Miscellaneous and nonbreast	21 (9.0)

Adapted with permission from Preece R, Mansel R, Bolton P, et al. Clinical syndromes of mastalgia. Lancet 1976;2:670. © The Lancet Ltd.

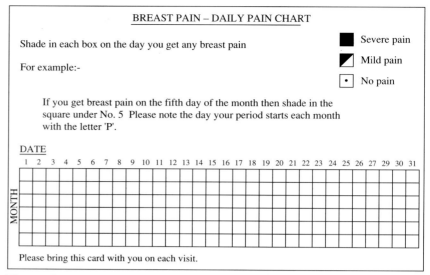

Figure 2.9. Daily breast pain chart (215). *Reprinted by permission from Preece PE. Mastalgia. Baltimore: Urban & Schwarzberg, 1990.*

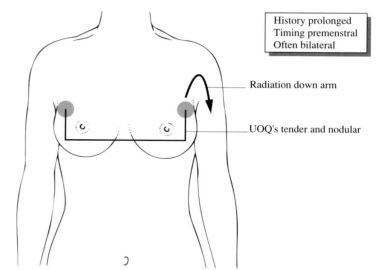

Figure 2.10. *Diagram showing the clinical features of cyclic mastalgia. It is premenopausal; mean age of onset is 34 years. Descriptive terms are "heaviness" and "tenderness to touch"; it is relieved by menstruation and menopause (UOQ = upper outer quadrant). Reprinted by permission from Hughes LE, Mansel RE, Webster DJT. Breast pain and nodularity. London: Baillière Tindall, 1989.*

ied 174 women with this disorder for a mean duration of 6.8 years (137). Sixty percent of these women had spontaneous resolution of breast pain without therapy. In 44% of patients, this resolution occurred at menopause. Pregnancy and oral contraceptive use resulted in pain relief in 17% and 13%, respectively. Geschickter (139) reported that half of patients with bilateral mastalgia continued to experience pain 3 to 4 years after presentation, and one third of these women had symptoms at 8 years.

Noncyclic Mastalgia

Noncyclic mastalgia is breast pain that is not associated with cyclic ovarian function. In the Cardiff study, 27% of women presented with this noncyclic pattern (see Table 2.9). This type of mastalgia is associated with a wide range of conditions occurring in the breast or chest wall. This is in contrast to cyclic mastalgia, which is always linked to pituitary-ovarian function. Most cases of noncyclic mastalgia are idiopathic and occur in both pre- and postmenopausal women. The noncyclic pain tends to be well localized in the breast and is present more frequently in the subareolar or inner quadrant. This type of pain may be intermittent or constant. Unilateral pain is more frequent than in cyclic mastalgia, and the description of the pain is different, described as having a burning, stabbing, or throbbing characteristic (Fig. 2.11). Other terms describe a transient, sharp quality lasting for minutes or days at a time (136). Mammography may be of some assistance in the noncyclic group because coarse calcification and ductal dilatation are radiographic changes seen in duct ectasia. In the Cardiff study, 42 of 62 patients who underwent mammography showed radiologic evi-

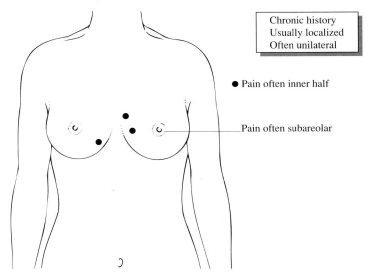

Chronic history
Usually localized
Often unilateral

● Pain often inner half

——— Pain often subareolar

Figure 2.11. *Diagram showing the clinical features of noncyclic mastalgia. It is premenopausal or postmenopausal; mean age of onset is 43 years. Descriptive terms are "drawing" and "burning"; it is not relieved by reproductive events. Reprinted by permission from Hughes LE, Mansel RE, Webster DJT. Breast pain and nodularity. London: Baillière Tindall, 1989.*

Table 2.10. Frequency of breast pain as a presenting symptom of operable breast cancer

Study	Percentage of cancers presenting with pain
Preece	7
River	24
Haagensen	5
Smallwood	18
Yorkshire Group	5

Reprinted by permission from Hughes LE, Mansel RE, Webster DJT. Breast pain and nodularity. London: Baillière Tindall, 1989.

dence of duct ectasia within their painful breast; of these, 20 showed calcification of secretory disease at the site of complaint (136).

Noncyclic mastalgia includes a wider range of clinical problems. Although uncommon, Preece and associates found that 17 (7%) of 240 patients with breast cancer had pain as their only initial complaint (140). The pain tended to be well localized in the breast and continuous. Pain as the initial symptom of breast cancer is rare but was observed in both premenopausal and postmenopausal women (Table 2.10) (136).

Noncyclic mastalgia is most common in the fourth decade of life; yet in 8 (12%) of 67 cases reported by Wisbey et al pain developed after the menopause (137). Thirty-two (48%) of the 67 women had relief of breast pain during the follow-up period; relief was spontaneous in one half.

Other Noncyclic Causes of Breast Pain

Noncyclic mastalgia may also be caused by benign lesions of the breast, including macrocysts, fibroadenoma, and duct ectasia. Duct ectasia should be suspected when pain is persistently localized to the subareolar area in the presence of pasty nipple discharge and dilated ducts that are palpable or visualized by mammography as prominent ducts or clusters of coarse calcifications (141). Breast pain caused by these lesions responds well to cyst aspiration or excision of the fibroadenoma or ectatic ducts.

Pain described as noncyclic mastalgia may also arise from the musculoskeletal structure of the chest wall or may be referred from other sites. Tietze's syndrome (142), or painful costochondritis, is not true breast pain but rather pain felt in the region of the breast that overlies the costal cartilage (Fig. 2.12). This pain is always localized to the medial aspect of the breast, and one or several costal cartilages are tender and feel enlarged. In large series, this is the third most frequent cause of breast pain (see Table 2.9). It is chronic

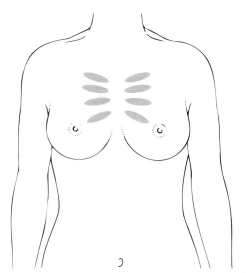

Tender over costal cartilage

Figure 2.12. Diagram showing the clinical features of Tietze's syndrome. It is often unilateral and occurs at any age; there is no time pattern and no palpable abnormality; it has a chronic course. Reprinted by permission from Hughes LE, Mansel RE, Webster DJT. Breast pain and nodularity. London: Baillière Tindall, 1989.

and may occur at any age. No abnormalities of the rib are seen on chest x-ray film.

Breast pain can also arise from physical exertion with subsequent soreness of the pectoral muscle, which mimics true mastalgia. A presenting complaint of breast pain may also be reported in women with cervical radiculopathy (143). Breast pain caused by radiculopathy is unilateral and is usually associated with symptoms of cervical, occipital, hand, or arm discomfort. The diagnosis is confirmed by cervical spine x-ray films demonstrating narrowing of C6–7 interspaces.

Trauma to the breast is a cause of persistent noncyclic pain that can be localized to resolving hematoma or to prior benign biopsy sites (see Table 2.9). Often the biopsy site might have been complicated by infection or hematoma formation. Fat necrosis may occur in the breast. The pain from trauma or at biopsy sites probably is caused by scarring. Care in performing biopsy incisions that do not cross Langer's lines usually avoids subsequent biopsy site pain.

Sclerosing adenosis is also a minor cause of breast pain (see Table 2.9). Sclerosing adenosis consists of proliferative glandular epithelium in which fibrosis distorts the normal pattern of the lobule (144,145). The proliferating epithelial cells have been described as invading both nerves and blood vessels (146,147). Preece et al (148) speculated that either the epithelial proliferation or the pronounced fibrosis causes the pain. The finding of sclerosing adenitis is seen in patients with well-localized noncyclic mastalgia whose mammogram shows small areas of calcification at the site of breast pain.

Occasionally, noncyclic breast pain is associated with breast cancer.

When cancer is actually painful, early detection of this disease is possible. Preece et al (140) suggested that lobular carcinoma has a special propensity to cause pain.

Clinical Evaluation of Patients with Mastalgia

Clinicians, particularly surgeons, have long considered the symptom of mastalgia as an expression of neurosis. Atkins stated that women with mastalgia were irritable and suggestive (149). More recently, mastalgia has been said to occur more frequently in "frustrated unhappy nulliparae" (150), and Haagensen described women with severe breast pain as unstable and hypochondriacal but not frankly psychotic (110). Preece and associates (151) used a questionnaire to measure psychoneurotic traits in patients with mastalgia; women undergoing outpatient treatment for varicose veins and actual psychiatric outpatients served as controls. The frequency of psychiatric traits in women with mastalgia did not differ significantly from that of women with varicose veins, and both groups scored well below the psychiatric group (Table 2.11). There is little support for the view that most breast pain is psychosomatic.

A careful history detailing the character, location, intensity, and duration of the breast pain is an essential beginning in the evaluation of mastalgia. An attempt to determine whether a relationship to the menstrual cycle exists should be undertaken because this will indicate cyclic mastalgia. A physical examination must be performed to rule out a dominant mass. A mammogram is a routine part of the evaluation of women with breast pain who are older than 35 years.

If the physical examination and mammogram fail to reveal breast cancer, the woman should be reassured that her pain is not caused by cancer. In more than 85% of women, reassurance that mastalgia is not a symptom of cancer and an explanation that it is an exaggerated form of

Table 2.11.   Neuroticism scores of mastalgia patients compared with patients with varicose veins or psychiatric disease

Factor	Mastalgia (n = 300)	Varicose veins (n = 156)	Psychiatric outpatients (n = 173)
Anxiety	7.6 ± 0.23	7.8 ± 0.30	11.0 ± 0.26*
Depression	4.2 ± 0.16	5.1 ± 0.21	7.6 ± 0.29*
Phobia	5.0 ± 0.16	5.7 ± 0.22	6.8 ± 0.29*

Values represent mean ± SD.
*Significantly greater than mastalgia or varicose vein groups. High scores imply abnormality (Mastalgia health questionnaire).
Adapted by permission from Hughes LE, Mansel RE, Webster DJT. Breast pain and nodularity. London: Baillière Tindall, 1989.

a normal physiologic process (132) is all that is necessary. In the remaining patients, medical treatment has to be considered (152). The single most important test in the evaluation and treatment of mastalgia is a breast pain chart (see Fig. 2.9). Careful documentation of symptoms permits an accurate estimation of the severity of pain as well as a precise relationship to the patient's menstrual cycle.

Etiology of Mastalgia

Although fibrocystic changes can be demonstrated in the breasts of many women with mastalgia, there is no convincing evidence that these types of changes are causally related to breast pain. Watt-Boolsen and associates examined histologic specimens from women with cyclic and noncyclic mastalgia as well as pain-free controls and found no difference in intraductal proliferation, adenosis, or proliferation of periductal connective tissue between groups (153). Because there appears to be no histologic changes characteristic of breast pain, other causes, including diet and hormonal abnormalities, have been proposed.

Minton and colleagues were the first to popularize the relationship between caffeine ingestion and breast pain and nodularity (154). In initial studies, 45 women with fibrocystic, painful breasts stopped all methylxanthine consumption (caffeine, theophylline, and theobromine, or chocolate), and 37 had complete resolution of fibrocystic changes; 7 improved. Minton and colleagues' studies did not have control groups, the amount of methylxanthine intake was variable, and no systematic method to record severity of pain was used. In a well-controlled study by Heyden and Muhlbaier, the presence of breast pain could not be correlated with methylxanthine intake (155). Marshall and associates failed to demonstrate a difference in caffeine intake in 323 women with fibrocystic disease and 1458 controls (156). No benefit from caffeine restriction was noted by Allen and Froberg in a study of 56 women randomized to a caffeine-restricted diet or having no dietary restrictions (157). Both pain and nodularity were assessed over a 4-month period, and no improvement was noted. Thus, the available data do not support a role for caffeine as a cause of mastalgia or a therapeutic benefit from caffeine restriction.

A possible relationship between mastalgia and endogenous hormones has been postulated for many years. The cyclic nature of most breast pain and the usual resolution at the menopause further indicate that ovarian hormones may play a role in mastalgia causation.

However, most studies failed to show any consistent abnormality in basal levels of reproductive hormones. Nonetheless, at least three theories of causes of hormonal imbalance have been proposed: increased estrogen production of the ovary, diminished progesterone secretion, and hyperprolactinemia. Geschickter, in 1945, suggested that breast pain might be caused by a hyperestrogenic condition (139). More recent studies have failed to confirm that mastalgia and nodularity have abnormal estrogen levels (158–161). Mauvais-Jarvis and colleagues (162) reported that luteal phase progesterone levels were significantly lower in women with mastalgia compared with asymptomatic controls. Additional studies have failed to reveal a defect in luteal phase progesterone values between mastalgia patients and controls (161,163). Sitruk-Ware and associates proposed that it is the estrogen-progesterone ratio in the luteal phase that may cause breast pain, not the absolute value measured (158,162).

Prolactin is the other hormone that has been postulated to play a role in the cause of mastalgia. Peters and associates measured baseline prolactin levels in 193 women with breast pain and nodularity and found a significant increase in prolactin levels compared with controls (164). This study was biased by the fact that 101 of the women in the study group also had galactorrhea. Women with diffusely nodular, painful breasts were observed to have elevated prolactin levels, but an even greater elevation was observed in women with macrocysts and no pain (165). Others have been unable to confirm an abnormality in basal prolactin levels in women with mastalgia (158,166). Nonetheless, a disturbance in hypothalamic feedback control of prolactin secretion may play a subtle or indirect role in the cause of cyclic mastalgia.

Water retention in the breasts premenstrually has been suggested as a cause of cyclic mastalgia and is the rationale for the use of diuretics in the treatment of breast pain. Preece and associates (167) examined changes in body water during the menstrual cycle and compared this to breast pain perception. There was no correlation between total body water and the occurrence of breast pain.

The finding that women with mastalgia have low plasma levels of the essential fatty acid γ-linolenic acid and its metabolites, which are important components of the cell membrane, has led to the hypothesis that essential fatty acid deficiency may alter the functioning of cell membrane receptors, producing a hypersensitive condition (168,169). This has led to a consideration of essential fatty acid supplementation to improve clinical symptoms of mastalgia.

Medical Management of Mastalgia

Because breast pain may spontaneously resolve (137) and patients respond dramatically to placebo treatment (152), double-blind, placebo-controlled therapeutic trials are required to prove drug efficacy. Before medical therapy is contemplated, simple reassurance that the patient's breast pain is not caused by cancer or other serious breast conditions usually is sufficient treatment for 85% of patients (132).

Diet Control

As previously noted, Minton and colleagues' report of an association between caffeine ingestion and painful breasts and fibrocystic changes (154) has been challenged because the study groups were poorly defined and indistinct parameters were used. Several case-control studies have examined the association of methylxanthine consumption and benign breast disease (155–157,170) and have failed to demonstrate any real correlation. Nonetheless, most physicians recommend a modified "Minton diet" for patients who have fibrocystic changes or mastalgia.

Supplementation with Evening Primrose Oil

The serendipitous finding that evening primrose oil caused a reduction in breast pain in schizophrenic patients has led to studies investigating the role of fats in mastalgia (171). The oil of the evening primrose is unique in that it contains 7% linolenic acid and 72% linoleic acid. The oil of the flower represents the richest source of essential fatty acids known. Women with cyclic and noncyclic mastalgia have normal blood levels of linoleic acid but reduced levels of the metabolite γ-linolenic acid, dihomo-γ-linolenic acid, and arachidonic acid, suggesting a relative block at the rate-limiting desaturation step between linoleic acid and γ-linolenic acid (168).

Horrobin (172) postulated that, as a result of the high consumption of saturated fats, there may be a disruption of the normal ratio of saturated fats in cell membranes. As a result, steroid hormone receptors in the breast have a higher affinity for estrogen, resulting in increased target tissue effect with no change in circulating estrogen levels. This situation may cause breast pain that could be relieved by providing γ-linolenic acid, which shifts the balance of membrane fatty acid toward normal. This would reduce steroid receptor affinity and excessive sensitivity with resultant reduction in breast pain.

One clinical, placebo-controlled trial showed that treatment with evening primrose oil at a dose of 3 g per day (three 500-mg capsules twice a day) over a 4-month interval significantly reduced breast pain, tenderness, and nodularity compared with placebo (173). This treatment was associated with an elevation of essential fatty acids toward normal. Overall, in British clinical experience, evening primrose oil causes a favorable response in 44% of patients with cyclic mastalgia and an improvement in 27% of patients with noncyclic pain (152).

There is no known side effect, except for rare bloating, and patient compliance is generally good because evening primrose oil is viewed as a natural, holistic approach to treatment rather than a drug. This polyunsaturated fatty acid compound is not approved for use in the United States but is available in health food stores. In the United Kingdom, evening primrose oil (EFAMAST) is licensed for prescription by the Committee of Safety of Medicine and is, therefore, available for use when prescribed (171). In that country this treatment is preferred for young women who may require long-term treatment, women taking birth control pills, and those who wish to avoid the potential risks and side effects of other medications to be discussed.

Vitamin Supplementation

Vitamin E

Abrams reported that vitamin E produced relief of moderate to severe breast pain in 16 of 25 women studied (174). In two other placebo-controlled studies involving a total of 201 women, there were no significant differences between vitamin E and placebo in the resolution of symptoms of benign breast disease when evaluated radiographically and clinically (175,176).

Vitamin B

Smallwood et al studied the effect of vitamin B_6 on 42 women with severe cyclic mastalgia (177). There was no difference between patients with breast pain undergoing vitamin treatment and placebo-treated controls.

Vitamin A or Retinoids

The use of vitamin A or retinoids has been advocated as a means of cancer chemoprevention. Band et al reported that 50,000 U/day decreased breast proliferative changes as seen by mammography in 5 of 12 women (178). Daily β-carotene supplementation with intermittent retinol (all-*trans*-retinol 300,000 IU per day) 7 days before each menses was administered in 25 women with moderate to severe cyclic mastalgia (179). After 6 months of treatment, there was marked reduction in breast pain with no adverse side effects. Unfortunately, there was no control group. Noncyclic mastalgia was not improved with this treatment. This therapeutic approach will need substantiation in an appropriate study but does suggest a possible synergism between β-carotene and retinol.

Properly controlled studies fail to demonstrate a role for vitamins in the treatment of mastalgia. Thus, there is no solid evidence to support vitamin therapy in patients with benign breast symptoms. Nonetheless, many physicians prescribe these supplements as a safe, nontoxic therapy because of their placebo effect (180).

Hormone Suppression

Oral Contraceptives

Because fibrocystic changes may be affected by normal changes in estrogen and progesterone during the ovarian cycle, oral contraceptive usage has been proposed as a treatment on the basis of associated cyclic hormone suppression. In their study of women who had used oral contraceptives for 4 years, LiVolsi et al (181) reported a 50% reduction in fibrocystic changes with minimal ductal atypia compared with women who had never taken birth control pills. Ory noted a reduction in breast biopsy rate in women who take oral contraceptives (182). In at least one study, high-dose estrogen birth control pills decreased breast pain and fibrocystic changes (183). Present-day oral contraceptives contain much lower amounts of hormone and may not be as effective in reducing benign proliferative changes. However, considering their safety, a therapeutic trial may be warranted in symptomatic cyclic breast pain.

Danazol

Danazol is a synthetic derivative of testosterone and is the only drug approved by the Food and Drug Administration for the treatment of mastalgia. Danazol may have significant side effects because of its mild androgenic properties and its direct effect on hypothalamic-pituitary function. Side effects include menstrual irregularities or amenorrhea, water retention, and rare androgenic changes, including growth of facial hair and voice changes. Mansel and associates (184) reported the first controlled study of danazol therapy in which 28 premenopausal women with cyclic breast pain were randomized to treatment with 200 mg or 400 mg daily or placebo for 3 months. Regardless of the treatment schedule used, danazol significantly decreased pain scores compared with placebo.

In a large Scandinavian study, the effect of danazol therapy on 109 women with moderate to severe breast pain was evaluated (185). In this comprehensive 30-month project, patients received either 200 mg or 400 mg of danazol per day. Most patients noted rapid relief of breast pain regardless of the dosage. Breast pain was totally eliminated in 90% of patients. A significant reduction in the amounts of mammographic density was observed beginning 3 months after therapy started. Of note, 67% of women treated with the 200-mg dose experienced a relapse, with a mean interval of 9.2 months; the higher dose group time to relapse was 12.2 months, but only 52% had recurrence of pain within a 27-month observation period. There was also a dramatic reduction in new breast cyst development. Pye and associates treated 120 women with cyclic mastalgia with danazol and noted a 71% total or significant pain reduction (152). In 48 women with noncyclic mastalgia, only 17 (35%) experienced major improvement.

Sutton and O'Malley decreased the dose to 100 mg every other day and noted complete pain relief in 37 (83%) of 44 women, with fewer side effects than previously reported (186). A low-dose danazol regimen for long-term or recurrent treatment has been used (187). An initial response is induced at a dose of 200 mg/day for 2 months, and then the dose is reduced to 100 mg/day. If the beneficial response is maintained for 4 months, the dose is further reduced to 100 mg on alternate days during the entire cycle or daily during the luteal phase only. Various low-dose modification therapy for patients with recurrence of pain has been tried, but because of the spontaneous resolution of cyclic mastalgia, low-dose danazol should be stopped every 12 months to assess whether further treatment is necessary. Because of possible teratogenic effects of danazol (Danocrine), women on a low-dose regimen should use some form of contraception.

Currently, danazol appears to be an excellent drug for the treatment of breast pain and nodularity, with an overall improvement rate of approximately 70%. If no improvement in symptoms is seen after 2 months, a different drug should be tried. For women who experience relapse after therapy, repeated courses of danazol seem to be effective. The main side effects of danazol are dose-related weight gain and menstrual irregularity.

Bromocriptine

The prolactin inhibitor bromocriptine has been used in the treatment of breast pain because of studies suggesting that elevation of basal prolactin levels (161,164,165) or an exaggerated prolactin response (188–190) may be the hormonal abnormality responsible for mastalgia. Dogliotti and colleagues found an 89% decrease in pain and 92% reduction in nodularity in 150 patients treated with bromocriptine (191). Nine percent of patients experienced recurrence of symptoms after 3 months and 30% experienced recurrence at 1 year. In placebo-controlled studies, similar improvement was noted (192,193); however, 30% of the patients had significant side effects, including nausea, headaches, dizziness, and hypotension. They concluded that, although there are patients with severe mastalgia who benefit from bromocriptine, in patients with less severe pain the side effects are greater than the benefit (193).

Mansel and coworkers studied 29 women with cyclic pain and 11 with noncyclic pain over six menstrual cycles (194). A significant improvement was observed in patients with cyclic symptoms, but no improvement was noted in patients with noncyclic mastalgia. The lack of efficacy of bromocriptine in noncyclic mastalgia was confirmed in a larger series in which only 20% of women with noncyclic pain responded, which was similar to the rate associated with placebo (152). In this study, there was a 33% incidence of side effects, most commonly nausea, headache, dizziness, and constipation. Therapy with bromocriptine should be started at a dosage of 1.25 mg (one-half tablet) at night for 1 week and then increased to 2.5 mg at night for 2 months. If a response is seen, bromocriptine should be continued for an additional 3 months. A study comparing danazol and bromocriptine in 34 women with cyclic mastalgia showed that danazol produced a greater reduction in breast pain than bromocriptine and placebo, but both active agents had significant side effects (195).

Tamoxifen

Tamoxifen acts as both an estrogen antagonist and an agonist and has been used in 60 women with mastalgia in a randomized, placebo-controlled study (196). Mastalgia resolved in 71% of women receiving tamoxifen, 20 mg daily, and in 38% of those taking placebo. The most common side effects with tamoxifen were hot flashes, nausea, and vaginal discharge. In a similar study, 16 (89%) of 18 women treated with tamoxifen, 10 mg daily for 6 months, had complete resolution of breast pain. Twelve months after completion of therapy, 53% did not have recurrence of symptoms (197).

Generally, this drug is not considered a first-line medication because of unresolved questions regarding long-term effects when used in young women with benign disease. Administration for short intervals does not measurably change spinal or femoral bone density and thus can probably be given safely for short-term treatment of mastalgia (198). Nonetheless, tamoxifen should be used for cancer treatment and only used for recalcitrant benign disease unresponsive to safer medications.

GnRH Agonist

This class of drugs is derived by amino acid replacement of the native GnRH molecule, causing a stronger, longer lasting effect on gonadotropin receptors. This leads to a downregulation of the receptor with resultant suppression of ovarian function. This causes a hypoestrogenic condition. In an open study, one of these agonists (goserelin) was administered as a monthly depot injection. Eighty-one percent of patients with both cyclic and noncyclic mastalgia showed improvement after 6 months of treatment (199). In another nonrandomized study, this agonist was used to treat 21 premenopausal women with severe recurrent or refractory breast pain; beneficial results were achieved in this very difficult group of patients (200). This study was expanded, and 54 women with moderate to severe mastalgia were treated for six cycles. The overall response rate was 85%; almost all of the women with cyclic pain responded to the agonist treatment, but only 70% of those women with noncyclic mastalgia ultimately responded. The major problem was the high incidence of side effects reported by most patients (hot flushes, 87%;

headache, 57%; decreased libido, 37%; nausea and vomiting, 28%; and depression or irritability, 24%). The relapse rate after stopping goserelin was 80%, with a mean follow-up of 6 months. The investigators indicate that this agent will not be useful for the majority of mastalgia patients because of the high incidence of side effects and the very high recurrence rate.

Gestrinone

Gestrinone is a synthetic C-19 progestin with androgenic, antiestrogenic, and antiprogestigenic properties that has been used as a midcycle and weekly oral contraceptive for women (201). In a multicenter study, gestrinone (2.5 mg twice per week) and placebo were administered in a double-blind fashion to women with cyclic mastalgia (202). The average percentage of reduction in mean analogue pain reduction scores was 80% with gestrinone and 37% with placebo. Forty-one percent of gestrinone-treated and 14% of placebo-treated patients experienced at least one side effect. Androgen-mediated side effects were the most common, including oily complexion, hirsutism, and intermenstrual bleeding. Only one patient withdrew from the study because of side effects. Gestrinone is similar in its action to danazol; however, the dose of gestrinone required is much less than that of danazol, and no other contraceptive is necessary in women who wish to avoid pregnancy. This drug is not available in the United States.

Hormone Treatment for Mastalgia

Progesterone

The possibility that mastalgia may be due to relative progesterone insufficiency or may increase estrogen influence has led to the use of progesterone treatment for this condition. Geschickter first reported the successful treatment of 13 of 15 women with mastalgia using progesterone extract therapy in 1943 (139). Studies on the use of percutaneous progestin alone (203) or in combination with oral progesterone (204) to treat mastalgia have proven successful. Two randomized, placebo-controlled studies have shown a beneficial effect of oral progesterone on mastalgia (205,206). Pye and coworkers found progesterone to be no more effective than placebo in relieving mastalgia in 39 women (152). Another study using progesterone cream application for cyclic mastalgia found that the active steroid was no better than placebo cream in relieving breast discomfort (207). Yet Nappi and associates showed that vaginal micronized progesterone treatment achieved 65% improvement in breast pain scores compared with 22% of patients receiving placebo (208). These same patients showed no improvement in breast nodularity. Also, medroxyprogesterone acetate (20 mg/day) administered during the luteal phase in 26 women with mastalgia was no more effective than placebo in the relief of breast pain or nodularity as assessed by linear analogue scale (209). The weight of evidence from placebo-controlled studies indicates that progesterone is not an effective therapy for mastalgia.

Testosterone

Anecdotal reports indicate that injection of testosterone propionate or other androgens can rapidly resolve acute breast pain (86,210). Testosterone undecanate (Organon), an oral preparation of testosterone (40 mg/day), was compared with placebo in 30 women with mastalgia over a 3-month interval. There was a significant reduction of pain scores for both treatments, but the greatest reduction was with testosterone administration (210). Only nausea in two patients and an increased libido and facial hair in another patient were caused by the androgen treatment. This form of treatment probably should not be used because of the proven efficacy of other proven therapies.

Thyroid Hormone

Several studies have demonstrated an improvement of breast pain and nodularity in patients with clinical hypothyroidism treated with thyroxine (211,212). In an uncontrolled study, Estes treated 19 women with mastalgia with levothyroxine, 0.1 mg daily for 2 months, and reported significant or complete relief in 73% (213). More recently, Peters and coworkers studied the effect of thyroxine in patients with mastalgia who demonstrated exaggerated prolactin responsiveness to TRH stimulation (214). During 8 weeks of thyroxine supplementation, mastalgia was significantly improved in the treatment group. Of note, 13 of the 18 mastalgia patients had diffuse goiter, suggesting that the TRH-induced exaggerated prolactin response might be an indicator of subclinical hypothyroidism. Further evaluation of the effect of thyroid hormone on mastalgia is required before this can be recommended as a standard therapy, except for those few women with mastalgia and subclinical hypothyroidism.

Other Treatments: Diuretics

Diuretics and salt restriction have been clinically used to relieve premenstrual bloating in patients with benign breast disease. The only study to evaluate this premise clearly showed that there were no changes in total body water premenstrually in patients with mastalgia (167). Thus, there is little scientific basis for treating cyclic mastalgia with diuretics. Diuretic therapy may actually be detrimental by causing rebound edema or rare depression (215).

Treatment for Noncyclic Breast Pain

In severe noncyclic mastalgia, routine measures to rule out cancer must be undertaken. Any dominant mass that does not yield fluid on aspiration should be evaluated by biopsy. Nonetheless, surgery should be avoided as an approach to the treatment of breast pain in the absence of dominant masses or duct ectasia. Although pain may be localized to one area of the breast, excision of this area most commonly leads to migratory pain elsewhere in the breast. If pain is localized to one area of the breast or chest wall, costochondritis and cervical radiculopathy should be considered and appropriately treated with anti-inflammatory agents, physiotherapy, or a cervical collar. Persistent, idiopathic, noncyclic pain may require symptomatic analgesia.

In 1989, Galea and Blamey reported their experience in treating patients with noncyclic breast pain at the Nottingham Mastalgia Clinic (216). They categorized noncyclic breast pain as "true" or pain of musculoskeletal origin. In their experience, 90% of women with unilateral noncyclic breast pain had musculoskeletal pain. This was usually characterized by normal breast examination despite severe breast pain symptoms. Women with localized pain or chest wall or breast "trigger spot" discomfort were treated with injection of local anesthetic and 40 mg of methylprednisolone acetate into the site of maximal tenderness. Patients with diffuse lateral chest wall pain were treated with nonsteroidal anti-inflammatory drugs (NSAIDs), usually naproxen, 250 mg three times per day. Those patients with cervical spondylosis were treated with physiotherapy and NSAIDs. Patients with duct ectasia were managed with reassurance and analgesia. This selective approach to the treatment of noncyclic breast pain led to a beneficial response in approximately 70% of women. This compares favorable to response rates seen in women with cyclic mastalgia treated with hormone manipulation.

Breast Clinic Approach to Management of Mastalgia

In 1971, a specialty research clinic was established within the Cardiff Mastalgia Clinic to develop a classification based on clinical symptoms defining the different patterns of breast pain (132) and its natural history (137). Three discrete patterns of breast pain were defined: cyclic mastalgia, noncyclic mastalgia, and Tietze's syndrome (costochondritis). This clinical approach to an essentially neglected symptom (breast pain) has led to improvement in clinical classification and treatment.

The most effective treatment for breast pain has proven to be exclusion of serious disease, reassurance, and an explanation of the condition. This is successful in 85% of patients initially presenting with breast pain (152,171). In the remaining 15%, the pain is of such severity that a disruption of the patient's lifestyle results and drug therapy is required.

Initially, assessment of pain was documented using a pain chart (see Fig. 2.9). Precise documentation of the frequency and severity of pain before treatment provides a baseline documentation of the severity of pain and a basis for comparison of symptoms after treatment is instituted. Some form of visual analogue system for recording pain and menstrual bleeding is useful in classifying the degree of pain and its relationship to ovarian function. Patients who have demonstrated mastalgia after 2 to 3 months of charting (allowing enough time for spontaneous remission) should be classified and treated by one of three main agents.

The Cardiff study's (217) first choice for cyclic pain is evening primrose oil because it has an acceptable efficacy and is almost free of side effects. The next drug is danazol, which has the best overall response (80%) but has definite side effects. The next agent is bromocriptine, which has efficacy between danazol and evening primrose oil but also has side effects in almost 20% of patients (Table 2.12) (217).

The overall response to the three main drug therapies is much lower in noncyclic mastalgia patients: approximately 45%. Danazol is the preferred treatment because both bromocriptine and evening primrose oil are equivalent to placebo in noncyclic patients (217). Those patients with localized symptoms are well served by local anesthetic and steroid injection. The only side effect is mild local discomfort, which is quickly relieved by the local anesthetic.

At Cardiff Clinic, the current policy is to treat for 3 months initially and then discontinue the medication to determine whether symptoms recur. At least 50% of symptoms recur but usually will not require

Table 2.12. Side effects of the principal therapies

Therapy	Common side effects	Incidence (%)
Danazol, 100–400 mg	Weight gain	
	Acne	
	Amenorrhea	25
	Hirsutism	
	Reduction in breast size	
	Voice change	
Bromocriptine, 2.5 mg twice daily	Nausea	
	Dizziness	20
	Headache	
Evening primrose oil, 6 500-mg-capsules daily	Mild nausea	<2

Adapted by permission from Hughes LE, Mansel RE, Webster DJT. Breast pain and nodularity. London: Baillière Tindall, 1989.

further treatment because the pain is milder. Patients with severe recurrences can be placed on the original therapy if a prior good response was noted or on alternative treatment if the response had been poor (152).

Special Issues Regarding Breast Pain

An interesting study was performed in 1990; a questionnaire was sent to a random sample of consultant general surgeons (more than 25% of the United Kingdom's total) regarding management of cyclic mastalgia (218). This study, which had an 89% response rate, revealed that danazol was the most commonly used agent. Initial treatments by nonspecialist surgeons included danazol (31%), analgesia (19%), and diuretics (17%), and those by breast surgeons included evening primrose oil (30%), tamoxifen (13%), and vitamin B_6 (13%). For persistent pain, nonspecialist surgeons prescribed danazol (46%) and surgery in 18% of cases, whereas breast surgeons prescribed danazol (65%) and bromocriptine in 30% of cases. Breast specialists tended to use treatment initially associated with fewer side effects and almost never used surgical excision of local trigger points. The specialist surgeons used danazol and bromocriptine only for severely resistant patients, because these drugs have clearly been shown to be effective in multiple placebo-controlled studies. In most studies of mastalgia, the placebo response is about 19% (152).

Although most patients with mastalgia are not neurotic or psychotic (151), in a selected group of patients with severe mastalgia unresponsive to drugs, a subset of patients have symptoms that reflect an underlying depressive disorder (219). These patients should be evaluated by a psychiatrist, and a trial of antidepressants should be prescribed before proceeding to surgical treatment.

Surgery should be avoided as an approach to the therapy of breast pain in the absence of a dominant mass or duct ectasia. In those rare drug-resistant patients with severe cyclic mastalgia, subcutaneous mastectomy followed by breast reconstruction is considered with caution (138). As for noncyclic mastalgia, breast resection either by excisional biopsy or excision of collecting ducts may be performed (127,220). Even subcutaneous mastectomy does not guarantee pain relief (130). Thus, surgery, if used at all, should be an option only after thorough patient counseling, including psychiatric consultation.

There have also been reports of phantom breast pain syndrome after mastectomy (221,222). In a more recent study, the incidence rates of phantom pain and nonpainful phantom sensations were 17.4% and 11.8%, respectively, 6 years after surgery. Pain in the scar that persisted for 6 years was reported in 31% of patients. This is a remarkably high incidence of pain in women undergoing mastectomy for cancer and underscores the recommendation not to perform surgery for be-nign breast disease.

Menopausal Changes

In a 10-year review of severe cyclic and noncyclic mastalgia, chronic pain may change with time because mastalgia in more than half of the patients initially classified as cyclic became noncyclic in nature over time (223). Cyclic mastalgia almost always resolves at menopause, but in those patients whose pain has changed, the menopause may have no effect on severity. Although resolution of cyclic mastalgia is nor-mally associated with hormonal events such as the menopause, spon-taneous resolution otherwise is rare.

Women who have never experienced breast pain and nodularity may develop aching pain with commencement of hormone replacement therapy. Because these are older women at greater risk for breast can-cer, these symptoms tend to cause more concern than in the younger patient. Postmenopausal women who experience pain with replace-ment therapy should use a low-dose regimen for a limited duration of time only (171).

Despite the fact that only 7% of patients with operable cancer have mastalgia as the presenting symptom (140), it is important to care-fully exclude cancer in patients with mastalgia so that adequate reas-surance can be given to these anxious patients. Cancer must be seriously considered as a diagnosis in patients presenting with well-localized breast pain of recent onset (140). A large percentage of patients with pain and cancer had lobular cancers that were not recognized by mammogram. This suggests that lobular carcinoma may elicit pain at a preclinical stage, allowing for early diagnosis and treatment.

Generalized nodularity alone, usually in the upper outer quadrant of the breast, does not require therapy unless the nodule persists as a dominant mass that requires excisional biopsy to exclude malignancy. Usually, the pain and lumpiness are part of the spectrum of normal breast physiology. A reduction in nodularity is observed with the same suppressive agents used for mastalgia (danazol and bromo-criptine). When areas of painful nodularity (trigger spots) are excised, the relief of pain is only transitory, and excision often leads to scarring and breast deformity (217). Thus, a dominant mass must undergo biopsy, but a painful nodule should be excised ony as a last resort for the management of breast pain with nodularity. This often proves a conundrum for the clinician, who must always be aware that cancer can be present when there is pain in the breast and that a new, persistent, noncyclic pain usually is benign, but cautious observation in women older than 30 years is required.

References

1. Leis H, Pilnik S, Dursi J, Santoro E. Nipple discharge. Int Surg 1973;58:162.
2. Papanicolaou G, Holquist D, Bader G, et al. Exfoliative cytology of the human mammary gland and its value for the diagnosis of cancer and other diseases of the breast. Cancer 1958;11:377.
3. Petrakis NL, Mason L, Lee R. Association of race, age, menopausal status, and cerumen type with breast fluid secretion in nonlactating women, as determined by nipple aspiration. J Natl Cancer Inst 1975;54:829–834.
4. Sartorius O, Smith H, Morris P, et al. Cytologic evaluation of breast fluid in the detection of breast disease. J Natl Cancer Inst 1977;59:1073.
5. Love S, Schnitt S, Connolly J, Shirley R. Benign breast disorders. In: Harris JR, Hellmans, Henderson IC, Kinne DW, eds. Breast diseases. Philadelphia: JB Lippincott, 1987:22.
6. King EB, Goodson WH. Discharges and secretions of the nipple. In: Bland KI, Copeland EM, eds. The breast. Philadelphia: WB Saunders, 1991:47–48.
7. Chitty V. Nipple discharge. In: Smallwood JA, Taylor I, eds. Benign breast disease. Baltimore: Urban & Schwarzenburg, 1990:85–87.
8. Chiari J, Braun C, Spaeth J. Report of two cases of puerperal atrophy of the uterus with amenorrhea and persistent lactation. In: Klinik der Geburtshilfe und Gynackologie. Erlangen: Enke, 1855:371.
9. Frommel R. Ueber puerperale atrophie des uterus. Gynakologe 1982; 7:305.
10. Argonz J, Del Castillo E. A syndrome characterized by estrogenic insufficiency, galactorrhea and decreased urinary gonadotropins. J Clin Endocrinol Metab 1953;13:79.
11. Forbes A, Henneman P, Griswold G, Albright F. Syndrome characterized by galactorrhea, amenorrhea and low urinary FSH: comparison with acromegaly and normal lactation. J Clin Endocrinol Metab 1954;14:265.
12. Vorherr H. Human lactation and breast feeding. In: Larson BL, ed. Lactation: a comprehensive treatise. New York: Academic Press, 1978:181–280.
13. Cowie AT, Forsyth IA, Hart IC. Hormonal control of lactation. In: Monographs on Endocrinology, vol. 15. New York: Springer-Verlag, 1980.
14. Niall HD, Hogan ML, Sauer R, et al. Sequences of pituitary and placental lactogenic and growth hormones: evolution from a primordial peptide by gene reduplication. Proc Natl Acad Sci USA 1971;68:866–869.
15. Kletzky OA, Rossman F, Bertolli SI, et al. Dynamics of human chorionic gonadotropin, prolactin, and growth hormone in serum and amniotic fluid throughout normal human pregnancy. Am J Obstet Gynecol 1985; 151:878–884.
16. Tulchinsky D, Hobel CJ, Yeager E, Marshall JR. Plasma estrone, estradiol, estriol, progesterone, and 17-hydroxyprogesterone in human pregnancy: 1. Normal pregnancy. Am J Obstet Gynecol 1972;112:1095–1100.
17. Frantz AG, Kleinberg DL, Noel GL. Studies on prolactin in man. Recent Prog Horm Res 1972;28:527–590.
18. Topper YJ, Freeman CS. Multiple hormone interactions in the developmental biology of the mammary gland. Physiol Rev 1980;60:1049–1106.
19. Kleinberg DL, Todd J, Babitsky G, et al. Estradiol inhibits prolactin induced α-lactalbumin production in normal primate mammary tissue in vitro. Endocrinology 1982;110:279–281.

20. Carr BR, Parker CR, Madden JD, et al. Maternal plasma adrenocortico-tropin and cortisol relationships throughout human pregnancy. Am J Obstet Gynecol 1981;139:416–422.

21. Vleugels MP, Eling WM, Rolland R, deGraaf R. Cortisol levels in human pregnancy in relation to parity and age. Am J Obstet Gynecol 1986;155:118–121.

22. Brodbeck U, Denton WL, Tanahashi N, Ebner KE. The isolation and identification of the B protein of lactose synthetase as α-lactalbumin. J Biol Chem 1967;242:1391–1397.

23. Rigg LA, Yen SSC. Multiphasic prolactin secretion during parturition in human subjects. Am J Obstet Gynecol 1977;128:215–218.

24. Brun del Re R, del Pozo E, deGrandi P, et al. Prolactin inhibition and suppression of puerperal lactation by a bromocryptine (CB 154). Obstet Gynecol 1973;41:884–890.

25. Kuhn NJ. Lactogenesis: the search for trigger mechanisms in different species. Symp Zool Soc London 1977;41:165–192.

26. Vorherr H. Suppression of lactation. In: The breast. New York: Academic Press, 1974:198–217.

27. Noel GL, Suh HK, Frantz AG. Prolactin release during nursing and breast stimulation in postpartum and nonpostpartum subjects. J Clin Endocrinol Metab 1974;38:413–423.

28. Tyson JE, Friesen HG, Anderson MS. Human lactational and ovarian response to endogenous prolactin release. Science 1972;177:897–900.

29. Brownstein MJ, Russell JT, Gainer H. Synthesis transport and release of posterior pituitary hormones. Science 1980;207:373–378.

30. Dawood MY, Khan-Dawood FS, Wahi RS, et al. Oxytocin release and plasma anterior pituitary and gonadal hormones in women during lactation. J Clin Endocrinol Metab 1981;52:678–683.

31. Leake RD, Waters CB, Rubin RT, et al. Oxytocin and prolactin responses in long-term breast-feeding. Obstet Gynecol 1983;62:565–568.

32. Johnston JM, Amico JA. A prospective longitudinal study of the release of oxytocin and prolactin in response to infant suckling in long-term lactation. J Clin Endocrinol Metab 1986;62:653–657.

33. McNeilly AS, Robinson ICAF, Houston MJ, Howie PW. Release of oxytocin and prolactin in response to suckling. BMJ 1983;286:257–259.

34. Shorne B, Parlow A. Human pituitary prolactin: the entire amino acid sequence. J Clin Endocrinol Metab 1977;45:1115.

35. Farkouh NH, Packer MG, Frantz AG. Large molecular size prolactin with reduced receptor activity in human serum: high proportion in basal state and reduction after thyrotropin-releasing hormone. J Clin Endocrinol Metab 1979;48:1026.

36. Sinha YN, Gilligan TA, Lee DW. Detection of a high molecular weight variant of prolactin in human plasma by a combination of electrophoretic and immunological techniques. J Clin Endocrinol Metab 1984;58:752.

37. Lewis UJ, Singh RNP, Sinha YN, VanderLaan WP. Glycosylated human prolactin. Endocrinology 1985;116:359.

38. Kleinberg DL, Noel GL, Frantz AG. Galactorrhea: a study of 235 cases including 48 with pituitary tumor. N Engl J Med 1977;296:579.

39. Whittaker PG, Wilcox T, Lind T. Maintained fertility in a patient with hyperprolactinemia due to "big-big" prolactin. J Clin Endocrinol Metab 1981;53:863.

40. Larrea F, Excorza A, Valero A, et al. Heterogeneity of serum prolactin throughout the menstrual cycle and pregnancy in hyperprolactinemic

women with normal ovarian function. J Clin Endocrinol Metab 1989; 68:982.

41. Ben-David M, Schenker JG. Transient hyperprolactinemia: A correctable cause of ideopathic female infertility. J Clin Endocrinol Metab 1983;57: 442–444.

42. Vekeman M, Delvoye P, L'Hermite M, Robyn C. Serum prolactin levels during the menstrual cycle. J Clin Endocrinol Metab 1977;44:989.

43. MacLeod RM. Regulation of prolactin secretion. In: Martini L, Ganong WF, eds. Frontiers in neuroendocrinology. New York: Raven Press, 1976:169–194.

44. Goldsmith PC, Cronin MJ, Weiner RI. Dopamine receptor sites in the anterior pituitary. J Histochem Cytochem 1979;27:1205–1207.

45. Turkington RW, Underwood LE, Van Wyk JJ. Elevated serum prolactin levels after pituitary stalk section in man. N Engl J Med 1971;285:707–710.

46. Frohman LA. Diseases of the anterior pituitary. In: Felig P, Baxter JD, Broadus AE, Frohman LA, eds. Endocrinology and metabolism. New York: McGraw-Hill, 1981:151–232.

47. Bowers CY, Friesen HG, Hwang P, et al. Prolactin and thyrotropin release in men by synthetic pyroglutamyl-hystadyl-prolinamide. Biochem Biophys Res Commun 1971;45:1033–1041.

48. Jacobs LS, Snyder PJ, Wilbur JF, et al. Increased serum prolactin after administration of synthetic thyrotropin releasing hormone (TRH) in man. J Clin Endocrinol Metab 1971;33:996–998.

49. Gautvik LM, Tashjian AH Jr, Kourides IA, et al. Thyrotropin-releasing hormone is not the sole physiologic mediator of prolactin release during suckling. N Engl J Med 1974;290:1162–1166.

50. Yen SSC, Ehara Y, Siler TM. Augmentation of prolactin secretion by estrogen in hypogonadal women. J Clin Invest 1974;53:652–655.

51. Abu-Fadil S, DeVane GW, Siler TM, Yen SSC. Effects of oral contraceptive steroids on pituitary prolactin secretion. Contraception 1976;13:79.

52. Frantz AG. Prolactin secretion in physiologic and pathologic human conditions measured by bioassay and radioimmunoassay. In: Josimovich JB, Reynolds M, Cobo E, eds. Lactogenic hormones, fetal nutrition, and lactation. New York: Wiley, 1974:379–412.

53. Gluskin LE, Strasberg B, Shah JH. Verapamil-induced hyperprolactinemia and galactorrhea. Ann Intern Med 1981;95:66–67.

54. Ehrinpreis MN, Dhar R, Narula A. Cimetidine-induced galactorrhea. Am J Gastroenterol 1989;84:563–565.

55. Mendelson JH, Mello NK, Teoh SK, et al. Cocaine effects on pulsatile secretion of anterior pituitary, gonadal, and adrenal hormones. J Clin Endocrinol Metab 1989;69:1256–1260.

56. Archer DF. Current concepts of prolactin physiology in normal and abnormal conditions. Fertil Steril 1977;28:125–134.

57. Costello RT. Subclinical adenoma of the pituitary gland. Am J Pathol 1936;12:205.

58. Burrow GN, Wortzman G, Rewcastle NB, et al. Microadenomas of the pituitary and abnormal sellar tomograms in an unselected autopsy series. N Engl J Med 1981;304:156–158.

59. Franks S, Jacobs HS, Nabarro JDN. Studies of prolactin in pituitary disease. J Endocrinol 1975;67:55.

60. Schlechte J, Sherman B, Halmi N, et al. Prolactin-secreting pituitary

tumors in amenorrheic women: a comprehensive study. Endocr Rev 1980;1:295–308.

61. Keye WR, Chang RJ, Wilson CB, Jaffe RB. Prolactin-secreting pituitary adenomas: III. Frequency and diagnosis in amenorrhea-galactorrhea. JAMA 1980;244:1329–1332.

62. Cooper PE, Martin JB. Neuroendocrinology. In: Rosenberg RN, ed. Comprehensive neurology. New York: Raven Press, 1991:605–621.

63. Brenner SH, Lessing JB, Quagliarello J, Weiss G. Hyperprolactinemia and associated pituitary prolactinomas. Obstet Gynecol 1985;65:661–664.

64. Honbo KS, Van Herle AJ, Kellett KA. Serum prolactin levels in untreated primary hypothyroidism. Am J Med 1978;64:782–787.

65. Contreras P, Generini G, Michelsen H, et al. Hyperprolactinemia and galactorrhea: spontaneous versus iatrogenic hypothyroidism. J Clin Endocrinol Metab 1981;53:1036–1039.

66. Groff TR, Shilkin BL, Utiger RD, Talbert LM. Amenorrhea-galactorrhea, hyperprolactinemia, and suprasellar pituitary enlargement as presenting features of primary hypothyroidism. Obstet Gynecol 1984;63:86S–89S.

67. Tolis G, Hoyte K, McKenzie JM, et al. Clinical, biochemical, and radiologic reversibility of hyperprolactinemic galactorrhea-amenorrhea and abnormal sella by thyroxine in a patient with primary hypothyroidism. Am J Obstet Gynecol 1978;131:850–852.

68. Katz E, Adashi EY. Hyperprolactinemic disorders. Clin Obstet Gynecol 1990;33:622–639.

69. Kelver ME, Nagamani M. Hyperprolactinemia in primary adrenocortical insufficiency. Fertil Steril 1985;44:423–425.

70. Mahesh VB, Dalla Pria S, Greenblatt RB. Abnormal lactation with Cushing's syndrome, a case report. J Clin Endocrinol Metab 1969;29:978–981.

71. Nabarro JDN. Acromegaly. Clin Endocrinol 1987;26:481–511.

72. Sievertsen GD, Lim VS, Nakawatase C, Frohman LA. Metabolic clearance and secretion rates of human prolactin in normal subjects and in patients with chronic renal failure. J Clin Endocrinol Metab 1980;50:846–852.

73. Lim VS, Kathpalia SC, Frohman LA. Hyperprolactinemia and impaired pituitary response to suppression and stimulation in chronic renal failure: reversal after transplantation. J Clin Endocrinol Metab 1979;48:101–107.

74. Richardson GS. Reflex lactation (thoracotomy) and reflex ovulation (intercostal block): case report, review of the literature, and discussion of mechanisms. Obstet Gynecol Surv 1970;25:1021–1036.

75. Turkington RW. Ectopic production of prolactin. N Engl J Med 1971;285:1455–1458.

76. Tolis G, Somma M, Van Campenhout J, et al. Prolactin secretion in 65 patients with galactorrhea. Am J Obstet Gynecol 1974;118:91–101.

77. Boyd AE III, Reichlin S, Tuskoy RN. Galactorrhea-amenorrhea syndrome: diagnosis and therapy. Ann Intern Med 1977;87:165–175.

78. Gomez F, Reyes FI, Fairman C. Nonpuerperal galactorrhea and hyperprolactinemia: clinical findings, endocrine features, and therapeutic responses in 56 cases. Am J Med 1977;62:648–660.

79. Yen SSC. Prolactin in human reproduction. In: Yen SSC, Jaffe RB, eds. Reproductive Endocrinology. Philadelphia: WB Saunders, 1986:237–263.

80. Frantz AG, Wilson JD. Endocrine disorders of the breast. In: Wilson JD, Foster DW, eds. Textbook of endocrinology. 8th ed. Philadelphia: WB Saunders, 1990:958.

81. Pellegrini I, Gunz G, Ronin C, et al. Polymorphism of prolactin secreted

by human prolactinoma cells: immunological, receptor binding, and biological properties of the glycosylated and nonglycosylated forms. Endocrinology 1988;122:2667.

82. Martin TL, Kim M, Malarkey WB. The natural history of idiopathic hyperprolactinemia. J Clin Endocrinol Metab 1985;60:855–858.

83. Kaplan CR, Schenken RS. Endocrinology of the breast. In: The female breast. Baltimore: Williams & Wilkins, 1990:22–44.

84. Rohn RD. Benign galactorrhea/breast discharge in adolescent males probably due to breast self-manipulation. J Adolescent Health Care 1984;5:210–212.

85. Frantz AG. Prolactin. N Engl J Med 1978;298:201–207.

86. Speroff L, Glass RH, Kase NG. Clinical gynecologic endocrinology and infertility. 4th ed. Baltimore: Williams & Wilkins, 1983:291–296.

87. Blackwell RE. Diagnosis and management of prolactinomas. Fertil Steril 1985;43:5–16.

88. Klibanski A, Neer RM, Beitins IZ, et al. Decreased bone density in hyperprolactinemic women. N Engl J Med 1980;303:1511–1514.

89. Schlechte JA, Sherman B, Martin R. Bone density in amenorrheic women with and without hyperprolactinemia. J Clin Endocrinol Metab 1983;56:1120–1123.

90. Koppelman MCS, Kurtz DW, Morrish KA, et al. Vertebral body bone mineral content in hyperprolactinemic women. J Clin Endocrinol Metab 1984;59:1050–1053.

91. Chang RJ. Hyperprolactinemia and menstrual dysfunction. Clin Obstet Gynecol 1983;26:736.

92. DeVane GW, Guzick DS. Bromocriptine therapy in normoprolactinemic women with unexplained infertility and galactorrhea. Fertil Steril 1986; 46:1026–1031.

93. Post K, Biller B, Adelman L, et al. Selective transsphenoidal adenomectomy in women with galactorrhea-amenorrhea. JAMA 1979;242:158.

94. Serri O, Rasio E, Beauregard H, et al. Recurrence of hyperprolactinemia after selective transsphenoidal adenomectomy in women with prolactinoma. N Engl J Med 1983;309:280–283.

95. Tan SL, Jacobs HS. Management of prolactinomas—1986. Br J Obstet Gynecol 1986;93:1025–1029.

96. Vance ML, Evans WS, Thorner MO. Diagnosis and treatment: drugs five years later. Bromocriptine. Ann Intern Med 1984;100:78–91.

97. Molitch ME, Elton RL, Blackwell RE, et al. Bromocriptine as primary therapy for prolactin secreting macroadenomas: results of a prospective multicenter study. J Clin Endocrinol Metab 1985;60:698–705.

98. Weiss MH, Teal J, Gott P, et al. Natural history of microprolactinomas: six year follow-up. Neurosurgery 1983;12:180–183.

99. Koppelman MCS, Jaffe MJ, Rieth KG, et al. Hyperprolactinemia, amenorrhea, and galactorrhea: a retrospective assessment of 25 cases. Ann Intern Med 1984;100:115–121.

100. Goluboff LG, Ezrin C. Effect of pregnancy on the somatotroph and the prolactin cell of the human adenohypophysis. J Clin Endocrinol Metab 1969;29:1533.

101. Melmed S, Braunstein GD, Chang RJ, et al. Pituitary tumors secreting growth hormone and prolactin. Ann Intern Med 1986;105:238.

102. Turkalj I, Braun P, Krupp P. Surveillance of bromocriptine in pregnancy. JAMA 1982;247:1589.

103. Konopka P, Raymond JP, Meceron RE, et al. Continuous administration

of bromocriptine in the prevention of neurologic complications in pregnant women with prolactinomas. Am J Obstet Gynecol 1983;146:935.

104. Molitch ME. Pregnancy and the hyperprolactinemic woman. N Engl J Med 1985;312:1364–1370.

105. Boulanger CM, Mashchak CA, Chang RJ. Lack of tumor reduction in hyperprolactinemic women with extrasellar macroadenomas treated with bromocriptine. Fertil Steril 1985;44:532.

106. Pellegrini I, Rasolonjannahary R, Gunz G, et al. Resistance to bromocriptine in prolactinomas. J Clin Endocrinol Metab 1989;69:500.

107. Ruiz-Velasco F, Tolis G. Pregnancy in hyperprolactinemic women. Fertil Steril 1984;41:793–805.

108. Petrakis NL. Physiologic, biochemical, and cytologic aspects of nipple aspirate fluid. Breast Cancer Res Treat 1986;8:7–19.

109. Takeda T, Suzuki M, Sato Y, et al. Cytologic studies of nipple discharges. Acta Cytol 1982;26:35.

110. Haagensen CD. Diseases of the breast. Philadelphia: WB Saunders, 1971:102–103.

111. Adair FE. Sanguineous discharge from the nipple and its significance in relation to cancer of the breast. Ann Surg 1930;91:197.

112. Leis HP Jr, Dursi MD, Mersheimer WL. Nipple discharge: significance and treatment. N Y State J Med 1967;67:3105–3110.

113. Urban JA, Egeli RA. Non-lactational nipple discharge. CA Cancer J Clin 1978;28:130–140.

114. Azzopardi JG. Problems in breast pathology. Philadelphia: WB Saunders, 1979.

115. Dixon JM, Anderson TJ, Lumbsden AB, et al. Mammary duct ectasia. Br J Surg 1983;70:601–603.

116. Rees BI, Gravelle IH, Hughes LE. Nipple retraction in duct ectasia. Br J Surg 1977;64:577–580.

117. Browning J, Bigrigg A, Taylor I. J R Soc Med 1986;79:715–716.

118. Ohuchi N, Abe R, Takahashi T, Tezuka F. Origins and extension of interductal papillomas of the breast—a three-dimensional reconstruction study. Breast Cancer Res Treat 1984;4:117–218.

119. Murad TM, Contesso G, Mouriesse H. Nipple discharge from the breast. Ann Surg 1982;195:259–264.

120. Page DL, Anderson TJ. In: Diagnostic histopathology of the breast. Edinburgh: Churchill Livingstone, 1987: – .

121. Fentiman IS, Fagg N, Millis RR, Hayward JL. In situ carcinoma of the breast: implications of disease pattern and treatment. Eur J Surg Oncol 1986;261–266.

122. Leis HP, Cammarata A, LaRaja RD, Higgins H. Breast biopsy and guidance for occult lesions. Int Surg 1985;70:115–118.

123. Chaudary MA, Millis RR, Davies GC, Hayward JL. Nipple discharge: the diagnostic value of testing for occult blood. Ann Surg 1982;196:651–655.

124. Hughes LE, Mansel RE, Webster DJT. In: Benign disorders of the breast. London: Baillière Tindall, 1989:133–142.

125. Horgan K. Management of nipple discharge.

126. Seltzer M, Perloff L, Kelley R, Fitts W. The significance of age in patients with nipple discharge. Surg Gynecol Obstet 1970;131:519.

127. Devitt JE. Clinical benign disorders of the breast and carcinoma of the breast. Surg Gynecol Obstet 1981;152:437.

128. Hadfield J. Excision of the major duct system for benign diseases of the breast. Br J Surg 1960;48:472–477.

129. Boston Women's Health Collective. Our bodies, ourselves. New York: Simon & Schuster, 1976:125.

130. Nichols S, Water W, Wheeler M. Management of female breast disease by Southampton general practitioners. BMJ 1980;281:140.

131. Dowle CS. Breast pain: classification, aetiology and management. Aust N Z J Surg 1987;57:423.

132. Preece R, Mansel R, Bolton P, et al. Clinical syndromes of mastalgia. Lancet 1976;2:670.

133. Vorherr H. The breast: morphology, physiology and lactation. New York: Academic Press, 1974.

134. Hughes LE, Mansel RE, Webster DJT. Aberrations of normal development and involution (ANDI): a concept of benign breast disorders based on pathogenesis. In: Benign disorders and diseases of the breast: concepts and clinical management. London: Baillière Tindall, 1989:15–26.

135. Love SM, Gelman RS, Silen W. Fibrocystic "disease" of the breast—a non disease. N Engl J Med 1982;307:1010–1014.

136. Hughes LE, Mansel RE, Webster DJT. Breast pain and nodularity. In: Benign disorders and diseases of the breast: concepts and clinical management. London: Baillière Tindall, 1989:75–92.

137. Wisbey J, Mansel R, Pye J. Natural history of breast pain. Lancet 1983;2:672.

138. Blichert-Toft M, Watt-Boolsen S. Clinical approach to women with severe mastalgia and the therapeutic possibilities. Acta Obstet Gynecol Scand Suppl 1984;123:185.

139. Geschickter CF. Mastodynia (painful breasts). In: Diseases of the breasts. 2nd ed. Philadelphia: JB Lippincott, 1945:183–199.

140. Preece P, Baum M, Mansel R, et al. Importance of mastalgia in operable breast cancer. BMJ 1982;284:1299.

141. Ingelby H, Gershon-Cohen J. Comparative anatomy, pathology and roentgenology of the breast. Philadelphia: University of Pennsylvania Press, 1960:247.

142. Tietze A. A peculiar accumulation of cases with dystrophy of the cartilages of the ribs. Berliner Klinische Wochenschrift 1921;30:829–831.

143. LeBan M, Meersehaert J, Taylor R. Breast pain: a symptom of cervical radiculopathy. Arch Phys Med Rehabil 1979;60:315.

144. Davies JD. Neural invasion in benign mammary dysplasia. J Pathol 1973;109:225–231.

145. Foote FW, Stewart FW. Comparative studies of cancerous versus non-cancerous breasts. Ann Surg 1945;121:6–53.

146. Taylor HB, Norris HJ. Epithelial invasion of nerves in benign disease of the breast. Cancer 1967;20:2245–2249.

147. Eusebi U, Azzopardi JC. Vascular infiltration in benign breast disease. J Pathol 1976;118:9–16.

148. Preece PE, Fortt RW, Gravelle IH, et al. Some clinical aspects of sclerosing adenosis. Clin Oncol 1979;2:192.

149. Atkins H. Treatment of chronic mastitis. Lancet 1938;1:707.

150. Jeffcoate N. Principles of gynaecology. 4th ed. London: Butterworths, 1975:550.

151. Preece R, Mansel R, Hughes L. Mastalgia: psychoneurosis or organic disease? BMJ 1978;1:29.

152. Pye JK, Mansel RE, Hughes LE. Clinical experience of drug treatments for mastalgia. Lancet 1985;ii:373–377.

153. Watt-Boolsen S, Emus H, Junge J. Fibrocystic disease and mastalgia. Dan Med Bull 1982;29:252.
154. Minton JP, Abou-Issa H, Reiches N, Roseman J. Clinical and biochemical studies on methylxanthine-related fibrocystic breast disease. Surgery 1981;90:299.
155. Heyden S, Muhlbaier L. Prospective study of fibrocystic breast disease and caffeine consumption. Surgery 1984;96:479.
156. Marshall J, Graham S, Swanson M. Caffeine consumption and benign breast disease: a case control comparison. Am J Public Health 1982; 72:610.
157. Allen S, Froberg D. The effect of decreased caffeine consumption on benign proliferative breast disease: a randomized clinical trial. Surgery 1987;101:720.
158. Sitruk-Ware R, Terkers N, Mauvais-Jarvis P. Benign breast disease: I. Hormonal investigation. Obstet Gynecol 1979;53:457.
159. Walsh P, McDickens I, Bulbrook R, et al. Serum oestradiol-17β and prolactin concentrations during the luteal phase in women with benign breast disease. Eur J Cancer Clin Oncol 1984;20:1345.
160. England P, Skinner L, Cottrell K, Sellwood R. Sex hormones in breast disease. Br J Surg 1975;62:806.
161. Watt-Boolsen S, Andersen A, Blichert-Toft M. Serum prolactin and oestradiol levels in women with cyclical mastalgia. Horm Metab Res 1981;13:700.
162. Sitruk-Ware L, Sterkers N, Mowiszowicz I, Mauvais-Jarvis P. Inadequate corpus-luteal function in women with benign breast diseases. Clin Endocrinol Metab 1977;44:771.
163. Walsh P, Bulbrook R, Stell P, et al. Serum progesterone concentration during the luteal phase in women with benign breast disease. Eur J Cancer Clin Oncol 1984;20:1339.
164. Peters F, Schuth W, Scheurich B, Breckwoldt M. Serum prolactin levels in patients with fibrocystic breast disease. Obstet Gynecol 1984;4:381.
165. Cole E, Sellwood R, England P, Griffiths K. Serum prolactin concentrations in benign breast disease throughout the menstrual cycle. Eur J Cancer 1977;13:597.
166. Golinger R, Krebs J, Fisher E, Danowski T. Hormones and the pathophysiology of fibrocystic mastopathy: elevated luteinizing hormone levels. Surgery 1978;84:212.
167. Preece R, Richards A, Owen G, Hughes L. Mastalgia and total body water. BMJ 1975;4:498.
168. Horrobin DF. Cellular basis of prolactin action: involvement of cyclical nucleotides, polyamines, prostaglandins, steroids, thyroid hormones, NA K ATPases and calcium: relevance to breast cancer and the menstrual cycle. Med Hypoth 1979;5:599–614.
169. Horrobin DF, Manku MS. Clinical biochemistry of essential fatty acids. In: Horrobin DF, ed. Omega-6 essential fatty acids; pathophysiology and roles in clinical medicine. New York: Wiley-Liss, 1990:21–53.
170. Lubin F, Ron E, Wax Y, et al. A case-control study of caffeine and methylxanthine in benign breast disease. JAMA 1985;253:2388.
171. Gateley CA, Mansel RE. Management of the painful and nodular breast. Br Med Bull 1991;47:284–294.
172. Horrobin DF. The effects of gamma-linolenic acid on breast pain. Prostaglandins Leukot Essent Fatty Acids 1993;48:101–104.

173. Mansel RE, Pye JK, Hughes LE. Effects of essential fatty acids on cyclical mastalgia and noncyclical breast disorders. In: Horrobin DF, ed. Omega-6 essential fatty acids; pathophysiology and roles in clinical medicine. New York: Wiley-Liss, 1990:557–566.

174. Abrams A. Use cf vitamin-E in chronic cystic mastitis. N Engl J Med 1965;272:1080.

175. London R, Sundaram S, Murphy L, et al. The effect of vitamin-E on mammary dysplasia: a double blind study. Obstet Gynecol 1985;65:104.

176. Ernster V, Goodson W, Hunt T, et al. Vitamin E and benign breast disease: a double-blind, randomized clinical trial. Surgery 1985;97:490.

177. Smallwood J, Ah-Key D, Taylor I. Vitamin B_6 in the treatment of premenstrual mastalgia. Br J Clin Pract 1986;40:532.

178. Band PR, Deschamps M, Falardeau M, et al. Treatment of benign breast disease with vitamin A. Prev Med 1984;13:549.

179. Santamaria L, Dell'Orti M, Bianchi-Santamaria A. Betacarotene supplementation associated with intermittent retinal administration in women with premenopausal mastodynia. Boll Chim Farm 1989;128:284–287.

180. Murtagh J. Mastalgia. Aust Fam Physician 1991;20:818–819, 823.

181. LiVolsi VA, Stadel BV, Kelsey JL, et al. Fibrocystic breast disease in oral contraceptive users: a histopathological evaluation of epithelial atypia. N Engl J Med 1978;299:381.

182. Ory H. Oral contraceptives and reduced risk of benign breast disease. N Engl J Med 1976;294:419.

183. Ariel IM. Enovid therapy (norethynodrel with mestranol) for fibrocystic disease. Am J Obstet Gynecol 1973;117:453.

184. Mansel R, Wisbey J, Hughes L. Controlled trial of the antigonadotropin danazol in painful nodular benign breast disease. Lancet 1982;1:928.

185. Tobiassen T, Rasmussen T, Doberl A, Rannevik O. Danazol treatment of severely symptomatic fibrocystic breast disease and long-term follow-up—the Hjorring project. Acta Obstet Gynecol Scand Suppl 1984; 123:159.

186. Sutton G, O'Malley V. Treatment of cyclical mastalgia with low-dose short term danazol. Br J Clin Pract 1986;40:68.

187. Gateley CA, Mansel RE. Management of cyclical breast pain. Br J Hosp Med 1990;43:330–332.

188. Kumar S, Mansel R, Scanlon M, et al. Altered response of prolactin, luteinizing hormone and follicle stimulating hormone secretion to thyrotrophin releasing hormone/gonadotrophin releasing hormone stimulation in cyclical mastalgia. Br J Surg 1984;71:870.

189. Kumar S, Mansel R, Hughes L, et al. Prolactin response to thyrotropin-releasing hormone stimulation and dopaminergic inhibition in benign breast disease. Cancer 1984;53:1311.

190. Watt-Boolsen S, Eskildsen P, Blaehr H. Release of prolactin, thyrotropin and growth hormone in women with cyclical mastalgia and fibrocystic disease of the breast. Cancer 1985;56:500.

191. Dogliotti I, Mussa A, Sandrucci S. Prolactin and benign breast disease with special emphasis on bromocriptine therapy. In: Angeli A, et al, eds. Endocrinology of cystic breast disease. New York: Raven Press, 1983: – .

192. Blichert-Toft M, Andersen A, Henriksen O, Mygind T. Treatment of mastalgia with bromocriptine: a double-blind crossover study. BMJ 1979;1:237.

193. Durning P, Sellwood R. Bromocriptine in severe cyclical breast pain. Br J Surg 1982;69:248.

194. Mansel R, Preece P, Hughes L. A double blind trial of the prolactin inhibitor bromocriptine in painful benign breast disease. Br J Surg 1978;65:724.

195. Hinton C, Bishop F, Holliday H. A double-blind controlled trial of danazol and bromocriptine in the management of severe cyclical breast pain. Br J Clin Pract 1986;40:326.

196. Fentiman I, Caleffi M, Brame K, et al. Double-blind controlled trial of tamoxifen therapy for mastalgia. Lancet 1986;i:287.

197. Messinis I, Lolis D. Treatment of premenstrual mastalgia with tamoxifen. Acta Obstet Gynecol Scand 1988;67:307.

198. Fentiman IS, Caleffi M, Rodin A, et al. Bone mineral content of women receiving tamoxifen for mastalgia. Br J Cancer 1989;60:262–264.

199. Hamed H, Chaudary MA, Caleffi M, Fentiman IS. LHRH analogue for treatment of recurrent and refractory mastalgia. Ann R Coll Surg Engl 1990;72:221–224.

200. Fentiman IS, Hamed H, Caleffi M. Experiences with tamoxifen and goserelin in women with mastalgia. In: Mansel R, ed. Goserelin—the British multicentre trial. Br J Clin Pract 1989;68:33, 49–53.

201. Tamaya T, Fujimoto J, Watanabe Y, et al. Gestrinone (E2323) binding to steroid receptors in human uterine endometrial cytosol. Acta Obstet Gynecol Scand 1986;65:439–441.

202. Peters F. Multicentre study of gestrinone in cyclical breast pain. Lancet 1992;339:205–208.

203. Lafaye C, Aubert B. Action de la progesterone locale dans les mastopathies benignes. J Gynecol Obstet Biol Reprod 1978;7:1123.

204. Mauvais-Jarvis P, Sterkers N, Kuttenn F, et al. Traîtement des mastopathies benignes par la progesterone, et les progestatifs. J Gynecol Obstet Biol Reprod 1978;7:477.

205. Colin C, Gasparou, Lambotte R. Relationship of mastodynia with its endocrine environment and treatment in a double blind trial with lynestrenol. Arch Gynakol 1978;225:7.

206. Dennerstein L, Spencer-Gardiner C, Gotts G, et al. Progesterone and the premenstrual syndrome: a double blind crossover trial. BMJ 1985;290:1617.

207. McFadyen IJ, Raab GM, Macintyre CCA, Forrest APM. Progesterone cream for cyclic breast pain. BMJ 1989;298:931.

208. Nappi C, Affinito P, DiCarlo C. Double-blind controlled trial of progesterone vagicream treatment for cyclical mastodynia in women with benign breast disease. J Endocrinol Invest 1992;15:801–806.

209. Maddox PR, Harrison BJ, Horobin JM, et al. A randomized controlled trial of medroxyprogesterone acetate in mastalgia. Ann R Coll Surg Eng 1990;72:71–76.

210. Laidlaw IJ, Gateley C, Gray P, et al. The Manchester Restandiol trial. Br J Clin Pract 1989;68:35–41.

211. Daro A, Gollin H, Samos F. The effect of thyroid on cystic mastitis. J Int Coll Surg 1964;41:58.

212. Love SM, Schmitt SJ, Connolly JL, Shirley RL. Benign breast disorders. Philadelphia: JB Lippincott, 1987:15–53.

213. Estes N. Mastodynia due to fibrocystic disease of the breast controlled with thyroid hormone. Am J Surg 1981;142:764.

214. Peters F, Pickardt R, Breckwoldt M. Thyroid hormones in benign breast disease. Cancer 1985;56:1082.

215. Preece PE. Mastalgia. In: Smallwood JA, Taylor I, eds. Benign breast disease. Baltimore: Urban & Schwarenberg, 1990:50.

216. Galea MH, Blamey RW. Non-cyclical breast pain: 1 year audit of an improved classification. Br J Clin Pract 1989;68:75–80.
217. Maddox PR, Mansel RE. Management of breast pain and nodularity. World J Surg 1989;13:699–705.
218. Pain JA, Cahill CJ. Management of cyclical mastalgia. Br J Clin Pract 1990;44:454–456.
219. Jenkins PL, Jamil N, Gateley C, Mansel RE. Psychiatric illness in patients with severe treatment-resistant mastalgia. Gen Hosp Psychiatry 1993;15:55–57.
220. Urban JA. Excision of the major duct system of the breast. Cancer 1963;16:516.
221. Kroner K, Krebs B, Skov J, Jorgensen HS. Immediate and long-term phantom breast syndrome after mastectomy: incidence, clinical characteristics and relationship to pre-mastectomy breast pain. Pain 1989;36(3):327–334.
222. Kroner K, Knudsen UB, Lundby L, Hvid H. Long-term phantom breast syndrome after mastectomy. Clin J Pain 1992;8:346–350.
223. Gateley CA, Miers M, Skone JF, Mansel RE. The Cardiff mastalgia clinic experience of the natural history of mastalgia. In: Benign breast disease. NJ: Parthenon Publishing, 1991:17–21.

3

Breast Dysfunction: Congenital Anomalies of the Breast

Eli Reshef, Joseph S. Sanfilippo, and Norman S. Levine

Breast development and maturation are initiated in utero and continue until full maturity is attained at the end of the second decade of life. Because of this uniquely prolonged time course, some congenital and developmental abnormalities will not become apparent until after the onset of puberty. The cause of most breast abnormalities of shape and size such as asymmetry, hypoplasia, and hypertrophy is unknown. External factors such as trauma or neoplasms are uncommon, and the role of environmental factors is unclear. Hence, most breast anomalies are presumed to be the result of factors present before birth. Such factors may be primary disorders of embryonic breast and chest wall development or endocrinopathies or chromosomal abnormalities that secondarily affect the breast. It is quite possible, however, that certain events in childhood may adversely affect breast development despite normal embryonic and prenatal assignment. In most cases, such postnatal events cannot be identified, and the disorder is, therefore, categorized as "congenital." Table 3.1 outlines the classification of congenital breast abnormalities.

Minor breast anomalies, in particular those of asymmetry and polythelia, are quite common. It is fortunate that severe, disfiguring congenital breast anomalies are rare. The psychological impact of a disfiguring breast abnormality on the affected individual may be devastating, especially when superimposed on the physical and psychosocial turmoil already present at puberty. An individual affected by congenital breast anomalies, therefore, requires special attention and empathy. A clear understanding of the natural time course of breast development, sensitivity to the psychological issues involved, and

Table 3.1. *Classification of primary congenital breast anomalies*

Congenital anomalies of the nipple and areola	Congenital anomalies of breast tissue
1. Disorders of absence and excess: athelia, polythelia 2. Disorders of shape and size: inversion, herniation, hypertrophy, hypoplasia	1. Disorders of absence and excess: amastia, polymastia 2. Disorders of shape and size: hypertrophy, hypoplasia, combined hypertrophy and hypoplasia, asymmetry (with and without associated musculoskeletal anomalies), abnormal shape (tuberous, cone shaped, goat udder) 3. Congenital breast hemangioma

utilization of modern surgical techniques with meticulous attention to aesthetics are all prerequisites for providing the best results to the affected individual.

EMBRYOLOGY

The origin of the breast is from both ectodermal and mesodermal embryonic layers. The stromal component is derived from mesoderm and the parenchymal segment from ectoderm. Growth and development of the mammary glands start during fetal life and extend to the end of the second decade of life, when final breast maturation is attained. At 5 to 6 weeks after conception, initial development begins in the form of solid down-growths of the epidermis in the area of the embryonic mammary line ("milk line"), with subsequent extension into the underlying mesenchyme. The mammary line is composed of two thickened strips of ectoderm that extend from the axilla to the inguinal region on each side (Fig. 3.1). Under normal circumstances, these epithelial lines or ridges eventually disappear, except for a small segment that persists in the thoracic region bilaterally.

The breast stroma is derived from the mesoderm and consists of dense mesenchyme and fat pad precursor tissue. The breast parenchyma, which consists of lumina formed by layers of epithelial cells with surrounding myoepithelial elements, is derived from the ectoderm. The luminal epithelium will eventually develop into ducts and alveoli, in which milk will be synthesized, stored, and transported. Invagination of the ectodermal mammary anlage downward into the mesenchyme starts at the seventh week of gestation (1). Proliferation of the parenchymal component of the mammary anlage continues in all directions. Branching and canalization of the ectodermal elements between the thirteenth and twentieth week lead to formation of milk

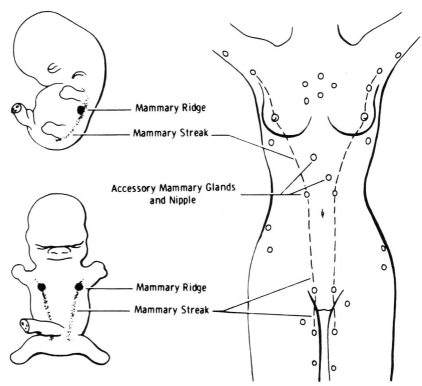

Figure 3.1. *The embryonic mammary ridge and the milk line in the adult female. The embryonic ridge, which extends from the axilla to the groin, develops at 5 to 6 weeks gestation and later involutes in all but the thoracic area. Remnants of this anlage, in the form of accessory nipples or breasts or both, may be found along this line. (Reproduced by permission from Vorherr H. The breast: morphology, physiology, and lactation. New York: Academic Press, 1974.)*

ducts between the twentieth and thirty-second weeks (1). Differentiation of these elements into lobular-alveolar structures occurs between the thirty-second and fortieth weeks of pregnancy (1). Phylogenetically, the breast parenchyma is a modified sweat gland with additional special apocrine and holocrine glands, the glands of Montgomery, which are situated around the mammary anlage. Only the main ducts are formed at birth, and the mammary glands remain underdeveloped until puberty.

BREAST DEVELOPMENT AFTER BIRTH

As a target organ for estrogen and other placental sex steroids, the mammary gland of the fetus and newborn responds by growth and elevation of the gland in both males and females. Histologically, there is evidence that the alveoli have secretory activity early in the neonatal period. Stimulation of this activity can lead to the appearance of milky discharge ("witch's milk") in 80% to 90% of newborns (1). This phenomenon is a manifestation of hormone withdrawal coupled with stimulation by prolactin, resulting in secretion of milk for up to 3 to 4 weeks postpartum. Subsequently, maternal prolactin secretion diminishes, and the neonatal breasts involute in a manner similar to postpartum maternal breast involution.

Suppression of the hypothalamic-pituitary-gonadal axis during early childhood leads to a minimal amount of ductal branching. In the typical sequence of pubertal development, thelarche (onset of visible breast growth) is the earliest symptom, with a median age of onset of 9.8 years in the United States (2). The endocrinologic events associated with breast development are a reflection of estrogen production from ovary. The actual onset of pubertal development is a complex entity that requires complicated interactions within the hypothalamic-pituitary-ovarian axis and its peripheral target tissues. Reduction in the sensitivity of the hypothalamus and pituitary to negative feedback of estrogen leads to increased hypothalamic-pituitary activity, ultimately resulting in elevated estrogen levels. This process in initiated, on the average, 1 year before onset of thelarche (2). Estrogens stimulate the mammary ducts to elongate and duplicate their epithelial lining and induce proliferation of the terminal ducts. This results in the formation of breast lobules. The volume and elasticity of the periductal tissues appear to be estrogen responsive, as are mammary vascularization and fat deposition.

At puberty, the breast develops in a horizontal "disk-like" fashion as well as in a vertical direction, with sprouting of primary and secondary milk ducts. Mammary ducts branch and differentiate into lobular-alveolar structures. Development occurs in five distinct phases (1):

Phase I: preadolescent elevation of the papilla (nipple)
Phase II: breast tissue growth with further development of subareolar tissue and formation of the breast bud
Phase III: further growth and development of the papilla
Phase IV: accelerated development of subareolar tissue with elevation of the nipple and areola, with the breast taking on a "globular" shape
Phase V: mature breasts under estrogen-progesterone effect

Once a normal balance of hypothalamic-pituitary-ovarian interaction occurs, which frequently requires 18 months after the onset of menarche (average age, 12.8 years in the United States) (2), the breasts will undergo cyclic changes in response to ovarian hormones. Final breast maturity and form are usually attained toward the end of the second decade of life, a time course that has to be considered when one contemplates surgical correction of congenital anomalies of the breast.

CONGENITAL BREAST ANOMALIES

Absence or Deficiency of Breast Tissue

Amastia and Athelia

Absence of one or both breasts (amastia) and absence of one or both nipples (athelia) are the rarest congenital breast anomalies (Figs. 3.2 and 3.3). The condition is usually unilateral and is often associated with other anomalies of the ipsilateral chest, shoulder girdle, and arm (Poland's syndrome). Amastia and athelia may also be associated with multiple congenital deformities of the head and neck, including ear, mouth, and nose malformations (3,4) (see Fig. 3.2), as well as with

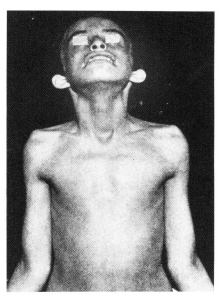

Figure 3.2. Congenital absence of breasts and nipples (combined amastia and athelia). This 12-year-old girl also had low-set ears, micrognathia, large mouth, increased carrying angle of the elbows, and chronic glomerulonephritis. (Reproduced by permission from Tawil HM, Najjar S. Congenital absence of breasts. J Pediatr 1968;73:752.)

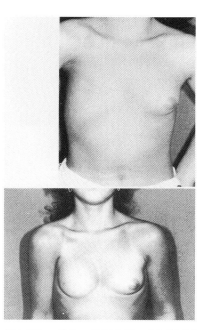

Figure 3.3. Poland's syndrome and athelia. The right breast in this 13-year-old girl was reconstructed using a tissue expander that was inflated gradually as her normal breast developed. A permanent prosthesis was inserted after final breast size and contour were achieved. (Reproduced by permission from Argenta LC, VanderKolk C, Friedman RJ, Marks M. Refinements in reconstruction of congenital breast deformities. Plast Reconstr Surg 1985;76:73–80.)

congenital ectodermal dysplasia (5). A few familial cases have been described (5), but it is primarily an isolated, noninheritable phenomenon. Amastia, but not athelia, may result from insufficient estrogen breast stimulation, as in the case of hypergonadotropic hypogonadism (e.g., Turner's syndrome), hypogonadotropic hypogonadism (e.g., Kallmann's syndrome), or constitutional delay of puberty. The precise embryonic event leading to amastia or athelia is not known. The embryonic mammary ridge, which develops between the bases of the upper and lower limb buds at approximately 5 to 6 weeks, regresses later in gestation (6 to 10 weeks) (7), with the exception of the thoracic region. Uncontrolled recession or regression of this embryonic structure, perhaps from segmental vascular compromise, may lead to absence of breast or nipple tissue.

One must consider the final maturation phases of breast development when surgical correction of amastia, especially of the unilateral variety, is contemplated. If augmentation of the deficient side is undertaken too early, seemingly satisfactory early results may become unsatisfactory as the contralateral breast changes size and contour. The main dilemma for the patient and her physician is to time augmentation of the deficient side appropriately, weighing the negative psychological impact of asymmetric lack of breast tissue on a teenage girl versus premature timing of surgical correction. The introduction of tissue expanders helps alleviate this dilemma by allowing early correction of asymmetry with gradual inflation to keep up with the growth of the contralateral breast followed by replacement with a permanent implant once full breast maturity is attained on the opposite side.

The use of synthetic implants for augmentation mammaplasty has been the subject of increased attention and controversy. Until the issues surrounding silicone breast implants are studied further, it might be prudent to consider alternatives such as saline implants. Augmentation may be performed with or without interposing latissimus dorsi muscle flaps between the implant and the nipple-areola complex. The implants may be placed in a subglandular or submuscular location. The reader may refer to Riefskohl (8), Georgiade (9), and others for a detailed discussion of augmentation techniques, including choice of incisions and the pros and cons of subglandular and submuscular implant placement at mammaplasty. In the case of athelia, nipple reconstruction can be performed using a graft from the earlobe or ear cartilage or from the contralateral nipple, by local flap techniques such as the "skate flap" or the "Maltese cross," or from pigmented skin in the upper inner thigh crease. The reconstructed areola may be made from inner thigh skin graft or may be tattooed later for a proper color match. To initiate and support breast growth in the case of lack of breast development resulting from hormonal deficiency (as in gonadal dysgenesis, congenital hypothalamic-pituitary aberrations, or constitutional delay of puberty), hormonal replacement with estrogens and progestins is used.

Hypoplasia

Decreased quantity of breast tissue is a subjective perception by the affected individuals. Whereas amastia may be an obvious end of the spectrum of breast size, and breast size may be defined as "too small" by its beholder. Therefore, the incidence of true breast hypoplasia cannot be accurately determined. Breast hypoplasia is more obvious when breast asymmetry occurs. Once the hypoplastic breasts reach final maturity (Fig. 3.4), augmentation mammaplasty may be performed. Tissue expanders are rarely needed. Generally, a single-stage procedure with a permanent prosthesis is used (8–10).

Excess Breast Tissue

Polythelia and Polymastia

Retention of accessory breast tissue (polymastia; Fig. 3.5A, B) or accessory nipple tissue (polythelia; Fig. 3.6) may be the result of abnormal regression of the mammary ridge. This phenomenon was considered by Darwin in his book *Descent of Man* as an example of *atavism* (inheritance of a characteristic from a remote rather than an immediate ancestor; evolutionary reversion). Polythelia (from the Greek *poly* meaning "many" and *theles* meaning "nipple") is the most common congenital breast anomaly, occurring in 1% to 6% of infants (6,11–13). It is more common in females as well as in people of Oriental and African heritage (6). No clear hereditary pattern has been described for these disorders even though familial occurrence has been reported, in one

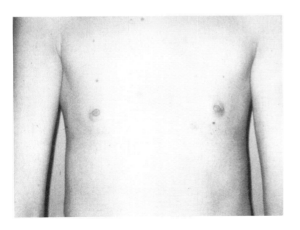
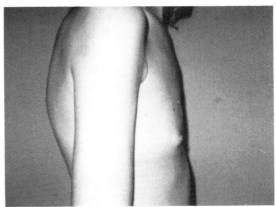

Figure 3.4.   Bilateral breast hypoplasia in an 18-year-old woman with normal serum estradiol and cyclic menses.

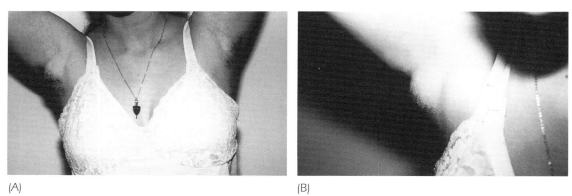

(A)   (B)

Figure 3.5. (A) Bilateral accessory breast tissue (polymastia). Both are in an axillary location. (B) Axillary polymastia (close-up view of right axillary area of patient in Figure 3.5A).

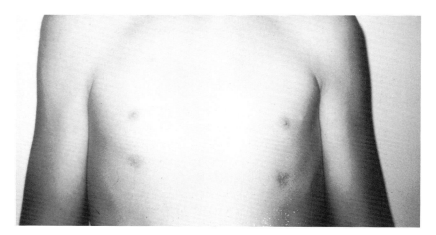

Figure 3.6. Accessory nipples (polythelia).

case in four successive generations (6). Polythelia and polymastia can occur in any combination. Most commonly, a small, pigmented nipple, with or without areola, can be found along the embryonic milk line (see Fig. 3.1), most commonly in the axilla and just below the breast. Two thirds of accessory nipples occur on the anterior thorax and abdomen. Uncommon locations along the embryonic milk line are the vulva, groin, and thigh. Accessory nipples have also been found in locations outside the mammary line, such as on the face, back, and neck. In one third to one half of cases, accessory nipples are bilateral.

Polymastia (from the Greek *poly* meaning "many" and *mastos* meaning "breast") is less common than polythelia. The accessory breast tissue is most commonly located in the axilla (see Fig. 3.5A, B), may or may not have a nipple, and is often bilateral. Accessory breast tissue may enlarge premenstrually or during pregnancy. It is more commonly a cosmetic problem rather than a source of bothersome symptoms. Excision of accessory breast tissue can be performed if indicated, especially in pregnancy or during lactation when the accessory tissue is well outlined. An association of polymastia and polythelia with other congenital anomalies has been reported (14–16). Renal anomalies (agenesis, renal cell carcinoma, supernumerary kidneys, and others), cardiac anomalies (septal defects, conduction defects), limb abnormalities (arthrogryposis multiplex congenita), and vertebral anomalies have all been associated with increased incidence of polymastia or polythelia. Whether the presence of accessory breast tissue implies an increase in other congenital anomalies is still under debate. A study of 1691 neonates (12) found the incidence of supernumerary nipples to be 2.5% but failed to detect any increase in congenital anomalies in the affected individuals. A study of 4113 school-age children found the incidence of polythelia to be 6% but failed to detect an increased rate of associated renal anomalies (13). Routine intensive diagnostic procedures beyond a thorough physical examination, therefore, are not warranted in an individual with accessory breast tissue unless other anomalies are also apparent.

Hypertrophy

Excess breast growth may be unilateral or bilateral (Figs. 3.7 and 3.8A). Unilateral hypertrophy with contralateral hypoplasia or amastia can also occur. The exact cause of breast hypertrophy is unknown. The most frequent type of true hypertrophy occurs during adolescence and is not associated with obvious pubertal or endocrine aberrations. Excessive breast growth poses both psychological and physical difficulties for the developing adolescent. The enlarged breasts are often

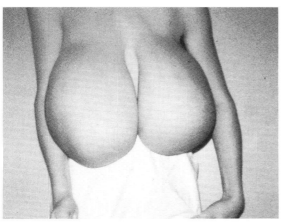 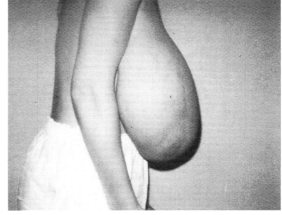

Figure 3.7. *Massive adolescent breast hypertrophy in a 17-year-old girl.*

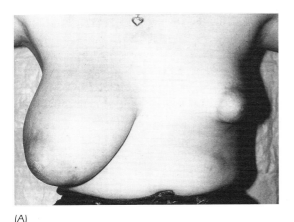 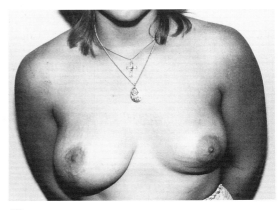

(A)   (B)

Figure 3.8. (A) Breast asymmetry with right breast hypertrophy and sharply tapered hypoplastic left breast. (B) Same patient as in Figure 3.8A after surgical correction. Right breast reduction mammaplasty and left breast augmentation mammaplasty were performed.

subject to ridicule and may cause significant neck and back discomfort as well as mastalgia. Adolescent breast hypertrophy does not regress, and reduction mammaplasty may be the only option available for severe physical symptoms and cosmetic concerns. Massive breast hypertrophy may occur in pregnancy as an abnormal response to the altered hormonal milieu. The precise cause for this disorder in pregnancy is unclear.

Careful planning, with close attention to the patient's physical and emotional concerns, is required before initiation of surgical treatment for breast hypertrophy. The preoperative examination must include examination of the breasts in the standing position. Unilateral hypertrophy and contralateral hypoplasia may be corrected in one or two steps (Fig. 3.8B). It may be advantageous to perform unilateral breast augmentation and a subsequent contralateral reduction mammaplasty once the final contour and size of the corrected hypoplastic breast are established (17). Several techniques of reduction mammaplasty are currently practiced, using superiorly or inferiorly placed dermal pedicle, vertical bipedicle dermal flap, or a free nipple graft. For a detailed discussion of surgical options and techniques, one may refer to Georgiade and coworkers' study (18).

Disorders of Breast Symmetry

Disorders of breast symmetry often become apparent only after the onset of puberty. In most cases, the cause is undetermined and, therefore, presumed to be congenital. Chest surgery, trauma (including burns), and irradiation involving the breast bud in childhood are obvious, albeit uncommon, causes for breast asymmetry. Poland's syndrome (see later discussion) may be classified as either a qualitative or a quantitative abnormality of one breast, depending on whether the affected side of the thorax has a breast at all or whether that breast is hypoplastic or deformed. Abnormalities of breast size are often subjective and are strongly hinged on cultural, social, and psychological factors. Any breast deformity, although arbitrary to some, may be of paramount importance to others.

Asymmetry

Although discrepancy in breast size is common, breast asymmetry sufficient to warrant surgical correction is rare. Noticeable asymmetry has been detected in 56 (4%) of 1400 patients presenting for mammoplasty evaluation (19). Discrepancy greater than 33% between the breasts is difficult to conceal (20). Variants of Poland's syndrome (see later discussion) represent more extreme versions of breast asymmetry. The continuum of breast asymmetry is composed of various combinations, including unilateral hypoplasia, unilateral hypertrophy, or a combination thereof (see Fig. 3.8A); asymmetric hypertrophy or hypoplasia; and unilateral hypoplasia with associated chest wall abnormalities (Figs. 3.3, 3.9A, B). Sternal anomalies, including pectus excavatum (Fig. 3.10) and pectus carinatum (Fig. 3.11A, B), may be associated with breast asymmetry. Surgical repair may be unilateral or bilateral depending on the type and severity of the abnormality.

Final breast maturation and the negative psychological impact of asymmetry on the patient must be considered. Satisfaction from surgi-

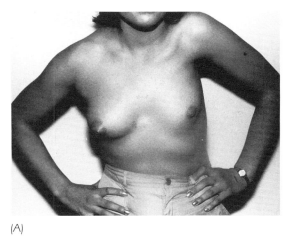
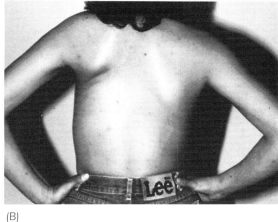

(A)   (B)

Figure 3.9.   (A) Poland's syndrome with hypoplastic left breast and absence of the left pectoralis major muscle. (B) Posterior view of the same patient in Figure 3.9A. Note the absence of the left latissimus dorsi muscle.

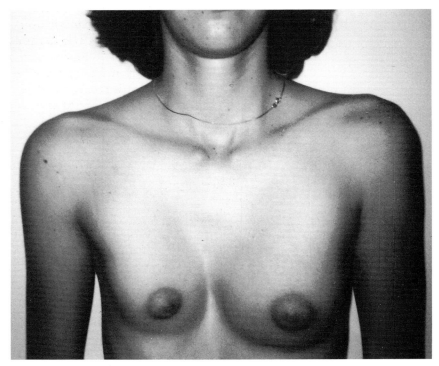

Figure 3.10.   Breast asymmetry associated with pectus excavatum abnormality.

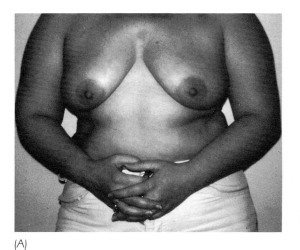

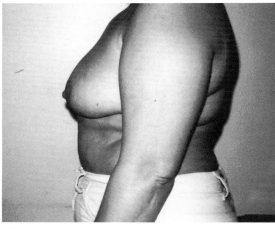

(A)   (B)

Figure 3.11.   Pectus carinatum abnormality without associated breast abnormality. (A) Frontal view. (B) Lateral view.

cal correction depends more on the patient's perception of attained symmetry than on the actual achievement of equal breast volume. Identical nipple placement is very important, as is the creation of symmetric breast mounds (17). For breast hypoplasia, various techniques of augmentation mammoplasty may be used (see prior discussion). If a tissue expander on the deficient side is used, it is placed beneath the nipple-areola complex and filled at bimonthly intervals until the volume exceeds the other side by approximately 200 mL (10). After an adequate amount of ptosis on the expanded side is achieved, the device is replaced with a permanent prosthesis (10). Reduction mammoplasty may be indicated for hypertrophic asymmetry (see Fig. 3.8B).

Poland's Syndrome

Originally described by Froriep in 1839 (21) and later by Poland in 1841 (22) as absence of the pectoral muscle associated with limb abnormalities, Poland's syndrome includes abnormalities of the torso and upper limb. Absence of the sternal head of the pectoralis major muscle is considered the minimal expression of Poland's syndrome. The condition is rarely bilateral and in most cases consists of unilateral amastia, breast hypoplasia, or even athelia (Figs. 3.3, 3.9A and B). The incidence of this syndrome is 1 in 30,000 births. It is more common in males and occasionally has a familial association. Chest wall anomalies include deformity or absence of ribs and cartilage on the involved side as well as deficiencies or absence of the pectoralis muscles, serratus, latissimus dorsi, and the external oblique muscle. Limb anomalies occur ipsilaterally and include syndactyly, absent phalanges, shortened forearm, and carpal bone deformities. Poland's syndrome is thought to be due to either disruption of the lateral embryonic plate mesoderm or vascular disruption of the subclavian artery before 6 weeks gestation.

The main concern for surgical correction is aesthetics because the absence of pectoral muscles does not usually cause significant functional problems. After correction of the chest wall deformity by selective osteotomies or chondrotomies (23), the soft tissue deformity can be corrected in various ways depending on the severity of the defect. Unilateral breast hypoplasia can be corrected by an implant that is custom-made to recreate the anterior axillary fold. The use of latissimus dorsi muscle has been advocated to augment or cover the implant as well as to replace the missing sternal head of the pectoralis muscle (24). The use of tissue expanders to develop a plane for a permanent implant has also been described (10).

Disorders of Breast Shape

Numerous variations of breast and nipple shape exist. The nipple-areola complex may enlarge and make up much of the substance of the breast ("nipple breast"; Fig 3.12) (25). The areola complex may herniate and produce a sessile protrusion from the breast mound (Fig.

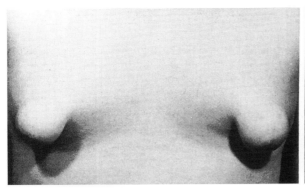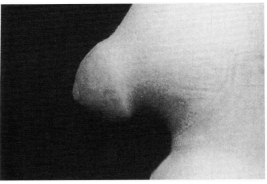

Figure 3.12. "Nipple breast" anomaly in hypoplastic, tuberous breasts with herniated breast tissue into the areola. (Reproduced by permission from Georgiade NG. Aesthetic breast surgery. Baltimore: Williams & Wilkins, 1983:24–87.)

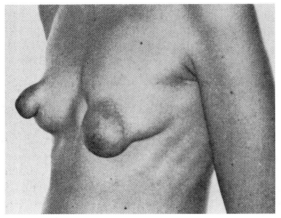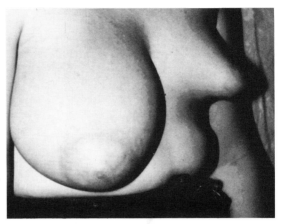

Figure 3.13. Abnormal nipples with herniation of breast tissue. (Reproduced by permission from Haagensen CD. Diseases of the breast. 2nd ed. Philadelphia: WB Saunders, 1971.)

Figure 3.14. Breast asymmetry with abnormal sharply tapered, hypoplastic left breast and right breast hypertrophy (same patient as in Figure 3.8A and 3.8B).

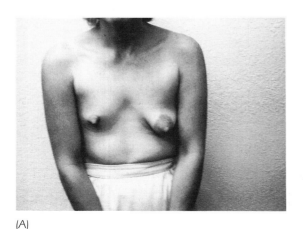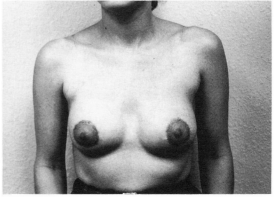

(A)   (B)

Figure 3.15. Breast asymmetry with bilateral "snoopy" nipple deformity and hypoplasia before (A) and after (B) bilateral augmentation mammoplasty and nipple reconstruction.

3.13). Other abnormalities in shape include the cone-shaped breast (sharply tapering; Fig. 3.14) (26), the tuberous breast (resembling a tuberous root or a cylinder) (27), the "snoopy" nipple abnormality (Fig. 3.15A), and the goat udder–like breast (11). Surgical correction of these abnormalities consists of unilateral or bilateral mammaplasty with repositioning and augmentation mammoplasty if indicated (see Figs. 3.8B, 3.15B).

SUMMARY

Congenital breast anomalies are common but mostly minor in nature and often do not require surgical correction because of minimal visible deformity. Even though disfiguring breast anomalies are rare, they require a well-timed surgical correction with meticulous attention to aesthetics as well as sensitivity to the psychological impact of the deformity on the individual. Abnormalities in regression of the embryonic mammary ridge, or milk line, may lead to absence or excess of breast tissue. The precise embryonic or postnatal events leading to primary abnormalities of breast shape, symmetry, and size are not known. The nature of breast development is such that abnormalities become apparent only after the onset of puberty. As such, the primary anomalies are treatable only by surgical means if a significant deformity exists. Surgical correction poses a clinical challenge to the surgeon, even though modern developments in plastic surgery, especially the introduction of tissue expanders and new prosthetic devices, have enriched the therapeutic repertoire and helped to improve the aesthetic outcome.

References

1. Vorherr H. The breast: morphology, physiology, and lactation. New York: Academic Press, 1974.
2. Speroff L, Glass R, Kase N. Clinical gynecologic: endocrinology and infertility. 5th ed. Baltimore: Williams & Wilkins, 1994:547–550.
3. Trier WC. Complete breast absence: case report and review of the literature. Plast Reconstr Surg 1965;36:430–439.
4. Tawil HM, Najjar S. Congenital absence of breasts. J Pediatr 1968;73:752.
5. Hutchinson J. Congenital absence of hair and mammary glands. Proc R Med Chir Soc Lond 1886;69:473.

6. Haagensen CD. Diseases of the breast. 2nd ed. Philadelphia: WB Saunders, 1971.

7. McCarty KS, Glaubitz LC, Thienemann M, Riefskohl R. The breast: anatomy and physiology. In: Georgiade NG, ed. Aesthetic breast surgery. Baltimore: Williams & Wilkins, 1983:2.

8. Riefskohl R. Augmentation mammoplasty. In: McCarthy JG, ed. Plastic surgery, vol. 6. Philadelphia: WB Saunders, 1990:3879–3896.

9. Georgiade NG. Aesthetic breast surgery. Baltimore: Williams & Wilkins, 1983:24–87.

10. Argenta LC, VanderKolk C, Friedman RJ, Marks M. Refinements in reconstruction of congenital breast deformities. Plast Reconstr Surg 1985;76: 73–80.

11. Deaver JB, McFarland J. The breast: its anomalies, its diseases, and their treatment. Philadelphia: Blakiston, 1917.

12. Mimouni F, Merlob P, Reisner SH. Occurrence of supernumerary nipples in newborns. Am J Dis Child 1983;137:952–953.

13. Jojart G, Seres E. Polythelia and renal malformation. Orv Hetil 1992; 133:1755.

14. Carella A. Supernumerary breast associated with multiple vertebral malformations: case report. Acta Neurol 1971;26:136–138.

15. Mate K. Association of polythelia and aberrant ventricular conduction. Orv Hetil 1976;117:2863–2865.

16. Mehes K. Association of supernumerary nipples with other anomalies. J Pediatr 1979;95:274–275.

17. Smith DJ, Palin WE, Katch V, Bennett JE. Surgical treatment of congenital breast asymmetry. Ann Plast Surg 1986;17:92–101.

18. Georgiade NG, Georgiade GS, Riefskohl R. Esthetic breast surgery. In: McCarthy JG, ed. Plastic surgery, vol. 6. Philadelphia: WB Saunders, 1990:3839–3896.

19. Pitanguy I. Surgical treatment of breast hypertrophy. Br J Plast Surg 1967;20:78.

20. Hueston JT. Unilateral agenesis and hypoplasia: difficulties and suggestions. In: Goldwyn RM, ed. Plastic and reconstructive surgery of the breast. Boston: Little, Brown, 1976.

21. Froriep R. Beobachtung eines Falles von Mangel der Brustaruse. Notizen aus dem Bebiete der Naturund Heilkund 1839;10:

22. Poland A. A deficiency of the pectoral muscles. Guy's Hospital Report 1841;6:191.

23. Shaw WW, Aston SJ, Zide BM. Reconstruction of the trunk. In: McCarthy JG, ed. Plastic surgery, vol. 6. Philadelphia: WB Saunders, 1990:3753.

24. Amoroso PJ, Angelats J. Latissimus dorsi myocutaneous flap in Poland's syndrome. Ann Plast Surg 1981;6:287.

25. Longcare J. Correction of the hypoplastic breast with special reference to reconstruction of nipple-type breast with local dermo-fat pedicle flaps. Plast Reconstr Surg 1976;3:339.

26. Glaesmer E, Amersback R. Die pathologie der Hangebrust und ihre moderne operative behandlung. Munch Med Wochenschr 1927;74:1171.

27. Rees T, Aston S. The tuberous breast: description and surgical correction. Clin Plast Surg 1976;3:339.

Benign Tumors of the Breast

Richard E. Blackwell

The primary care physician encounters on a daily basis women who present with pain and lumpiness of the breast. Fortunately, a significant proportion of the problems represent benign processes and frequently are referred to as fibrocystic disease (Table 4.1) (1). Likewise, the conditions have been described under the terminology of benign breast disease of mammary dysplasia. Further, terms such as chronic lobular hyperplasia, cystic hyperplasia, and chronic cystic mastitis have been used. The term cystic mastitis should be discarded because inflammation is not present in this disorder. Mammary dysplasia is perhaps the most common lesion of the female breast, may be unilateral or bilateral, and most frequently occurs in the upper outer quadrants (Fig. 4.1A, B). The disorder tends to be exacerbated during the premenstrual period, and patients usually complain of pain or lumps in the breast. The breasts may be tender in many locations; however, axillary adenopathy is generally not found. The breast lumps are usually cystic, and they tend to fluctuate with the menstrual cycle and shrink after menstruation. The natural history of the disease varies, and yet it tends to resolve after menopause (2). Mammary dysplasias may be accompanied by nipple discharge and may be confused with galactorrhea. The discharge may be clear or bloody in up to 15% of individuals. The disorder may be confused with carcinoma, and a Papanicolaou smear of the discharge, mammography, and perhaps needle aspiration may be necessary to rule out a malignancy. At the time of breast aspiration, one may evacuate a cyst filled with gray, dirty, green fluid.

Anatomically, the cysts vary in size from 1 mm to many centime-

Table 4.1. *Features of mammary dysplasia*

Most common lesion in breast
Unilateral or bilateral location
Occurs in upper outer quadrants
Exacerbated during menstrual period
May persist as pain and lumps
Cysts frequently persist
Usually intermittent natural history
Nipple discharge may be present
Frequently resolve after menopause

ters (Fig. 4.2). They are usually unilocular because they probably arise as lobular lesions with dilated individual acini or terminal ducts. Whether a recruitment of other lobular units occurs is unknown. On gross histologic inspection, the cysts are lined with cells that contain a large number of mitochondria secretory granules. When stained with eosin they appear pink. The cells are columnar and may have a protuberance that appears to be bleb like (snouts). Occasionally, the large cysts will not have any evidence of epithelial

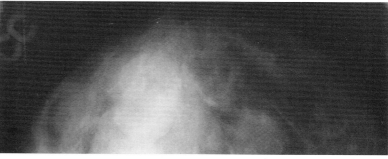

(A)

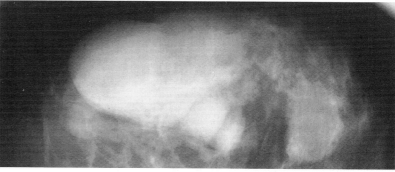

(B)

Figure 4.1. *(A, B) Mammogram showing mammary dysplasia.*

Table 4.2. Treatment of cyclic mastodynia

Discontinue caffeine
Low-dose monophasic birth control pills
Danazol (Danocrine), 100–800 mg PO every day for 6 months
Leuprolide (Lupron), 3.75 mg IM every month for 6 months

lining or may be lined with several squamous cells that are undifferentiated (3).

Because patients with mammary dysplasias present with lumpiness of the breast and pain, treatment is directed at these facets. Careful instruction in breast examination and periodic mammography should these lesions persist appear to be the most efficacious management for lumpiness. Pain at times can be relieved by avoiding methylxanthine. Further, some patients respond well to cyclic oral contraceptive use, and, in more extreme cases, danazol therapy at a daily dose of 100 mg to 800 mg/day can be used or gonadotropin-releasing hormone analogue therapy with leuprolide (Lupron) could be instituted; however, for treatment beyond 6 months, add-back therapy with estrogen and progestogen is necessary because of bone demineralization. The empiric use of bromocriptine while suppressing prolactin secretion has not been demonstrated in placebo-controlled studies to be effective in treating cyclic mastodynia (Table 4.2) (4,5).

Apocrine metaplasia (Fig. 4.3) is a readily identifiable phenomenon often associated with ductal hyperplasia. These metaplastic epithelial cells are characterized by dense eosinophilic cytoplasm, often with evident apical apocrine secretions. The metaplastic cells can also exhibit hyperplastic features. Papillary hyperplasia is particularly common in association with apocrine change. Although there are rare

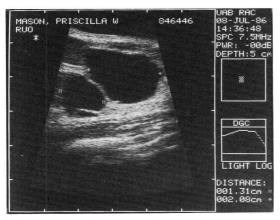

Figure 4.2. Sonogram demonstrating mammary dysplasia.

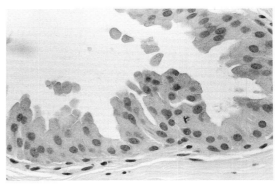

Figure 4.3. Apocrine metaplasia.

forms of mammary carcinoma with apocrine features, apocrine meta-plasia is usually considered a benign phenomenon and is seldom associated with atypical hyperplasia.

EPITHELIAL HYPERPLASIAS

Hyperplasia is defined as an increased number of cells relative to a specific basement membrane. Breast hyperplasias span a range from mild hyperplasia, which is characterized by the presence of three of more cells above the basement membrane and carries no increased risk of formation of carcinoma, to atypical ductal or lobular hyper-plasia, which contains some features of well-differentiated carcinoma and is associated with an increased risk for carcinoma in situ of 8 to 10 times. A special feature of these lobular neoplasias is their tendency to undermine normal cell populations. To complete the transition of car-cinoma in situ, one must find a uniform group of neoplastic cells populating the entire basement membrane space. Some investigators further advocate that this alteration must involve two or more spaces. It is also suggested that an intercellular pattern of rigid arches and even placement of cells must be present along with the finding of hyperchromatic nuclei (6).

Adenosis refers to increased numbers of acini within a lobular unit. Adenosis, with or without mild sclerosis, is not itself a marker of malig-nant potential. Florid sclerosing adenosis, on the other hand, has been recognized as a indicator of slightly increased cancer risk. Character-ized by both increased numbers of acini and intralobular fibrosis, sclerosing adenosis can result in marked distortion of normal archi-tecture. It can sometimes be very difficult to distinguish from inva-sive, well-differentiated carcinoma microscopically, particularly during frozen-section evaluation, and it has accounted for a large number of deferred diagnoses and occasional false-positive diagnoses during this procedure. Long-standing lesions may exhibit microcalcifications, and large complex lesions (known as complex sclerosing lesions or radical scars depending on the size) may exhibit spiculated margins on mammography, mimicking infiltrating carcinoma. The larger lesions can also resemble carcinoma on gross examination of the tissue.

Sclerosing adenosis mimics invasive carcinoma of the breast. These lesions are usually smooth and circumscribed, a double cell layer is present, the lesion is confined to the lobular units, the central spaces are most often flattened, there is rarely the finding of an atypical cytoplasmic snout, and elastic tissue masses are usually not present. These lesions are characterized by proliferation of ductal tissue, which produces a palpable lesion. These lesions are common in younger women, especially in the third and fourth decades of life, and they are

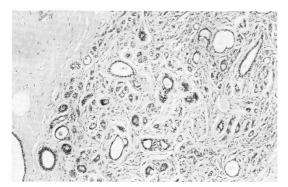 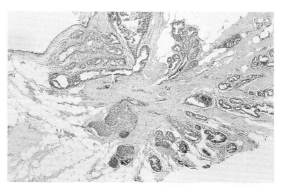

Figure 4.4. *Sclerosing adenosis. Irregular ducts and acini in dense fibrous stroma.*

Figure 4.5. *Complex sclerosing lesion (radial scar). Note distortion of both glands and stroma around a central focus. The glands show moderate hyperplasia of the usual type.*

rarely seen after menopause. Grossly, breast carcinoma is firm and gritty to palpation, whereas adenosis is usually rubbery (Figs. 4.4 and 4.5) (7).

FAT NECROSIS

Fat necrosis may present as a hard lump that may be tender and rarely enlarges. The histology of fat necrosis in the breast is no different from its appearance in other organs. One will find chronic inflammatory cells, including lymphocytes and histiocytes. Clinically, an acute phase develops approximately 1 week after the inciting event, with the findings of white cells and oily lipid material. In the acute stage, swelling, redness, and warmth are noted. In the later stage, collagenous scar, which may surround an oily cyst, is the predominant finding. Skin retraction may be seen along with irregularity of the edges, and fine stipple calcifications may be present on mammogram. About half of the patients with this history have experienced breast trauma; excisional biopsy is the treatment of choice. At biopsy, hemorrhage may be seen in fatty tissue; the greatest significance of fat necrosis is its mimicry of carcinoma (8,9).

INTRADUCTAL PAPILLOMA

Intraductal papilloma is a benign lesion of a lactiferous duct wall that occurs centrally beneath the areola in 75% of cases. Such lesions pre-

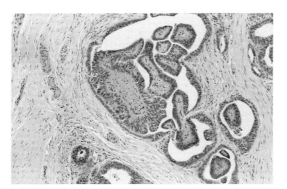

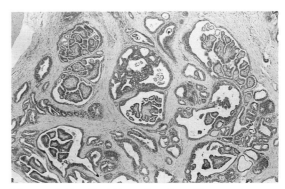

Figure 4.6. *Intraductal papilloma. Unlike papillary hyperplasia or micropapillary ductal carcinoma in situ, true papillomas are composed of projections of ductal epithelia lining fibrovascular connective tissue cores.*

Figure 4.7. *Florid intraductal papillomatosis.*

sent with pain or bloody discharge, and they are generally soft, small masses that are very difficult to palpate. The presentation of a bloody nipple discharge in association with a small, palpable mass is associated with a 75% chance of intraductal papilloma. If no mass can be palpated, Paget's disease of the nipple or carcinoma should be considered. Intraductal papilloma is not premalignant and is best managed by incision of the duct by wedge resection. Intraductal papillomas generally occur in women in the late childbearing years, although they have been reported in adolescents. In the younger patients, these lesions are found at the periphery of the breast, and multiple ducts may be involved. There may be cystic dilation, and these lesions have been called Swiss cheese disease or juvenile papillomatosis. The treatment of juvenile papillomatosis involves exicisional biopsy (Figs. 4.6 and 4.7) (10,11).

DUCT ECTASIA

Duct ectasia includes a group of entities that involve duct dilation. These lesions present clinically as lumpiness in the region of the breast under the areola, and ducts are involved in a segmental fashion. Nipple discharge is commonly found, scarring occurs, and in the majority of cases nipple inversion is noted. Periductal inflammation is the histologic hallmark of the condition and is most frequently found in the perimenopausal female. However, it can occur in younger women and can produce fissures and fistulas. Dilated ducts may be filled with pultaceous material visible on mammography and may have plaque-like calcifications occurring within the walls. At times

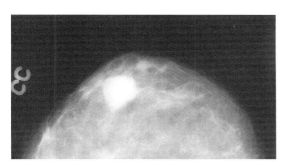

Figure 4.8. *Mammogram of patient with fibroadenoma.*

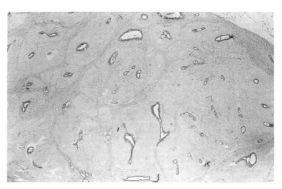

Figure 4.9. *Fibroadenoma with hypocellular, partially hyalinized stroma.*

these lesions appear as lumps fixed within scar, are inflamed, and mimic carcinoma of the comedoductal type (12).

FIBROADENOMA

One of the most common benign neoplasms of the adolescent and adult breast is the fibroadenoma (Fig. 4.8). These may be small, firm, nodular, or large, rapidly growing masses that are multiple 20% of the time (Table 4.3). The lesions may be painful. The fibroadenoma may be hormonally responsive, and rapid growth has been reported during both pregnancy and lactation. Surgically, these lesions are found to easily movable and are not fixed to the surrounding breast tissue. They are sharply circumscribed and have very smooth boundaries, and their cut surface is white and whirl like (Fig. 4.9). These lesions are not associated with an increased risk of carcinoma; however, more than 100 cases of carcinoma have been reported arising in fibroadenomas. On microscopic examination, the fibroadenoma is composed of fibrous tissue, and the stoma may be surrounded by round, duct-like epithelial

Table 4.3. *Features of fibroadenoma*

Small or large, firm, nodular lesions
Single lesion in 80% of cases
May grow rapidly
May be painful
Responds to hormone stimulation
Not associated with increased risk of breast cancer
Racial predilection; appears in blacks more frequently than whites

structures or may be arranged in a curvilinear manner. This refers to intracanalicular or pericanalicular variance. Fibroadenomas have a racial predilection; the lesions develop more commonly in blacks than in whites. Likewise, blacks are more likely to have recurrences. These lesions are best treated by excisional biopsy (13,14).

MISCELLANEOUS LESIONS

Another variance of fibroadenomas (cystosarcoma phyllodes, also known as giant fibroadenomas) has been described. These tumors are generally benign; however, a few of them have true sarcomatous potential (15).

The hamartoma of the breast is generally considered to be a tumor with a mixture of both glandular and mesenchymal components. These lesions have lobular components and are distinct. These generally present two decades after the fibroadenoma (16).

JUVENILE FIBROADENOMA

Other variants of adenomas are found in women in the young age group. About 10% of these lesions can grow rapidly and attain large size. These lesions occur around the time of menarche. Histologically, they have elements of epithelial hyperplasia as well as stromal hypercellularity.

As can be appreciated, the primary care physician is faced with a wide variety of benign tumors of the breast that have many overlapping clinical features. Many of these lesions mimic cancer of the breast or are associated with an increased risk for the disorder. Although some of these lesions occur in age ranges not generally associated with the development of cancer of the breast, special clinical and radiographic examinations, needle aspiration and biopsy, and histologic interpretation are often needed to render definitive diagnosis (17).

References

1. Ernester VL. The epidemiology of benign breast disease. Epidemiol Rev 1981;3:184.

2. Dixon JM, Scott WN, Miller WR. Natural history of cystic disease: importance of cyst type. Br J Surg 1985;72:190.

3. Wellings SR, Jensen HM, Macrum RG. An atlas of subgross pathology of the human breast with special reference to possible precancerous lesions. J Natl Cancer Inst 1975;56:231.

4. Ernster VL, Mason L, Goodson WH, et al. Effects of caffeine-free diet on benign breast disease. Surgery 1982;91:263.

5. Aksu MF, Tzingounis VA, Greenblatt RB. Treatment of benign breast disease with danazol: a follow-up report. J Reprod Med 1978;31:181.

6. Page DL, Dupont WD, Rogers LW, Rados MS. Atypical hyperplastic lesions of the female breast: a long-term follow-up study. Cancer 1985; 55:2698.

7. Jensen RA, Page DL, Dupont WD, Rogers LW. Invasive breast cancer (IBC) risk in women with sclerosing adenosis (SA). Cancer 1989;64:177.

8. Pilnik S. Clinical diagnosis of benign breast disease. J Reprod Med 1979;22:277.

9. Oberman HA. Benign breast lesions confused with carcinoma. In: McDiutt RW, Oberman HA, Ozzello L, Kaufman N, eds. International Academy of Pathology monograph: the breast. Baltimore: Williams & Wilkins, 1984:1.

10. Colman M, Mattheiem W. Imaging techniques in breast cancer: workshop report. Eur J Cancer Clin Oncol 1988;24:69.

11. Carter D. Intraductal papillary tumors of the breast: a study of 78 cases. Cancer 1977;30:1689.

12. Haagensen CD. Mammary-duct ectasia: a disease that may stimulate carcinoma. Cancer 1951;4:749.

13. Hertel B, Zaloudek C, Kemson R. Breast adenomas. Cancer 1976;37:2891.

14. Fechner RE. Fibroadenoma and related lesions. In: Page DL, Anderson TJ, eds. Diagnostic histopathology of the breast. New York: Churchill Livingstone, 1987:   .

15. Norris HJ, Taylor HB. Relationship of histologic features to behavior of cystosarcoma phyllodes—analysis of 94 cases. Cancer 1967;22:22.

16. Hessler C, Schnyer P, Ozzello L. Hamartoma of the breast: diagnostic observation of 16 cases. Radiology 1979;126:95.

17. Oberman HA. Breast lesions in the adolescent female. Ann Pathol 1979;14:175.

5

Malignant Tumors of the Breast

David Ralph Crowe and Olubunmi T. Lampejo

The use of the general term *breast cancer* belies the fact that malignant neoplasms of the breast are diverse entities with widely varying morphologic and behavioral characteristics. Clear understanding of malignant neoplasms of the breast can best be approached by briefly recalling the normal histologic anatomy of the organ. A secretory gland, the breast is composed of a group of branching ducts that connect the smallest functional unit, the acinus, to the final point of excretion, the nipple-areola unit. From the large lactiferous ducts to the acinus, the glandular system is lined by columnar to cuboidal epithelial cells, which, in turn, are surrounded by myoepithelial cells. The latter are separated from the fibrovascular stroma by a basement membrane. The most distal portion of the system, composed of an intralobular terminal ductule and its tributary acini, is the lobular unit. This is surrounded by specialized loose connective tissue stroma. The lobular units are separated by denser extralobular collagenous stroma and fat. Malignant neoplasms may arise in either the epithelial or stromal components of the breast. Malignant epithelial tumors are by far the most prevalent of the malignant breast tumors, and they are emphasized in this chapter.

NONINVASIVE EPITHELIAL BREAST DISEASE

Gynecology has provided us with two of the best characterized systems that show progression of disease from benign epithelium to malignant disease. These examples are the invasive squamous cell carcinoma of the cervix and endometrial adenocarcinoma. The accessibility of the cervix to repeated and thorough examination over time has allowed us to document sequential changes from metaplasia to dysplasia, to carcinoma in situ, and to invasive carcinoma. This model of neoplasia has proven enormously influential in directing research efforts and in spurring the search for similar models in other tumor systems. The discovery of the sequential links among endometrial hyperplasia, atypical hyperplasia, and carcinoma demonstrated the utility of this approach in neoplasms other than cervical cancer. Similar chains of events have now been described in other organs.

The breast is far less amenable to the study of preneoplastic lesions. As will be shown, the lesions associated with increased risk for the future development of carcinoma are defined by complex criteria, including architectural as well as cytologic features. An accurate diagnosis thus requires an invasive procedure that removes the aberrant tissue from the breast, thereby altering the natural history of the lesion. For this reason, although various proliferative lesions of the breast epithelium had been previously described, their relative potential for progression to or prediction for the development of invasive cancer remained largely undefined until the pioneering work of Dupont and Page (1,2). In a retrospective study of more than 10,000 women who had undergone breast biopsies for benign disease, they reviewed all available histologic material and developed reproducible criteria for the diagnosis of hyperplasia, atypical hyperplasia, lobular carcinoma in situ, and noncomedocarcinoma in situ. These diagnostic categories were tested against outcomes based on 10- to 20-year follow-up periods, and a relative risk for the future development of invasive cancer was determined for each.

Subsequent studies have demonstrated that the diagnostic criteria defined by Page et al are reproducible by other pathologists and that the risk estimates associated with those definitions are similar to those found in other studies both prospective and retrospective (Table 5.1). The main categories of Page et al's classification scheme are nonproliferative fibrocystic disease, proliferative fibrocystic disease, atypical hyperplasias, and carcinoma in situ. Entities included in the category of nonproliferative fibrocystic disease are stromal fibrosis, cystic change, apocrine metaplasia, adenosis with or without mild sclerosis, duct ectasia, fibroadenomas, inflammation, squamous metaplasia, and mild hyperplasia. These abnormalities are associated with no increase in the relative risk for the future development of invasive carcinoma. Moderate to florid ductal epithelial hyperplasia, florid sclerosing adenosis, and papillomas are included in the proliferative fibrocystic disease group. These lesions are associated with a slightly increased relative risk (1.5 to 2.0 times normal). Atypical ductal hyperplasia and atypical lobular hyperplasia are associated with a moderately increased relative risk (4 to 5 times normal). As

Table 5.1.   *Relative risk for the future development of invasive carcinoma*

Factor	Risk
Slightly increased risk	1.5–2.0 times
Moderate and florid hyperplasia	
Papilloma	
Sclerosing adenosis, well developed	
Moderately increased risk	5 times
Atypical ductal hyperplasia	
Atypical lobular hyperplasia	
Highest risk	8–10 times
Cribriform-micropapillary ductal carcinoma in situ	
Lobular carcinoma in situ	

Modified from College of American Pathologists. Relative risk for invasive breast carcinoma based on pathologic examination of benign breast tissue: policy and guidelines. Appendix DD. College of American Pathologists, Northfield, IL 1993:1–3; Page DL. Cancer risk assessment in benign breast biopsies. Hum Pathol 1986;17:871–874.

would be expected, ductal carcinoma in situ (DCIS) (noncomedo type) and lobular carcinoma in situ (LCIS) are associated with a markedly increased relative risk (8 to 10 times normal) for the future development of invasive carcinoma. The studies further demonstrate that a family history of breast cancer in a first-order relative doubles the relative risk in any category. Although subsequent series have shown some variation in outcomes, the hierarchy of increasing risk described here generally holds true to form (3–6). Most of the lesions that belong to the nonproliferative fibrocystic disease category have been described elsewhere in this book. Other proliferative epithelial lesions are described next.

EPITHELIAL HYPERPLASIA

Ductal epithelial hyperplasia of the breast can occur in an array of morphologic patterns. In its simplest form, hyperplasia is said to be present when there are three or more epithelial cell layers above the basement membrane (Fig. 5.1). Often the hyperplastic layers of epithelial cells will protrude into duct lumina, forming papillary projections. The hyperplastic epithelium may progressively expand and fill duct lumina, often with the formation of complex spaces between the crowded cells. These spaces are characteristically angulated and slit shaped but may also be compressed and indistinct. They may also appear more rounded, mimicking the punched-out, regular spaces, which are addressed later in the section on DCIS. Cytologically, ductal hyperplasia is associated with polymorphism. Hyperplastic epithelial cell nuclei often show more variation in size than those in carcinoma

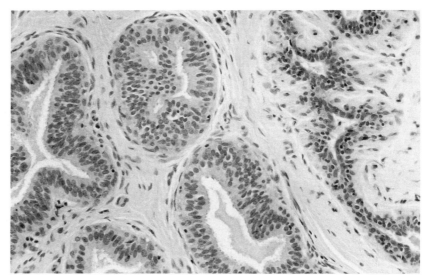

Figure 5.1. Ductal hyperplasia of the usual type with crowded, stratified epithelial cells. Compare with the relatively normal duct on the right. (Original magnification × 50.)

in situ. A myoepithelial layer composed of distinctive clear cells or lumina cells with flattened nuclei can usually be identified at the periphery of the ducts. These crowded cells often grow in swirling patterns. Small amounts of cytoplasm and indistinct cytoplasmic borders give the appearance of close nuclear contact and overlapping nuclei. Mitotic figures may be seen and are not a hallmark of either atypia or malignancy. The terms *moderate* and *florid* hyperplasia describe hyperplastic epithelium that is greater than 8 to 10 cell layers thick. In these cases, ducts are conspicuously expanded and filled with cells, sometimes to the exclusion of the irregular spaces.

Lobular hyperplasia is not a diagnostic category currently being used because it is believed that this entity cannot be reproducibly defined, and also the clinical implications of such a diagnostic category are unclear.

ATYPICAL HYPERPLASIAS

Atypical ductal hyperplasia (ADH) is most often diagnosed when only some, but not all, of the criteria for DCIS are met. The criteria of Page et al for the diagnosis of noncomedo DCIS are described more fully later; briefly, they include 1) a uniform population of cells, 2) smooth geometric spaces between the proliferating cells (sieve-like or cribriform pattern) or pseudopapillae formation (micropapillary pat-

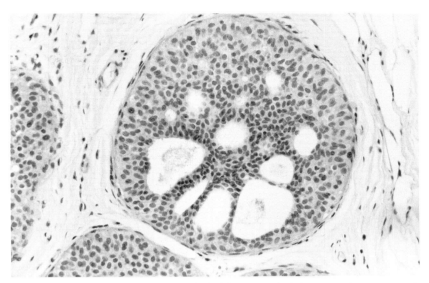

Figure 5.2.   Atypical ductal hyperplasia. The expanded duct contains two populations of cells. On the periphery a relatively monotonous population of large atypical cells with identifiable cytoplasmic borders is seen. The more normal ductal epithelium is located toward the center of the duct. In addition, some of the intraluminal spaces lack the sharply "punched-out" characteristic of cribriform ductal carcinoma in situ. (Original magnification × 50.)

ters), and 3) cytologically atypical nuclei. Both cytologically abnormal cells and either a cribriform or micropapillary architectural growth pattern must be present before the diagnosis of noncomedo DCIS can be made. In addition, the epithelium of the entire duct must be replaced by these abnormal cells (Fig. 5.2). Size criteria also exist. Even in the presence of both the cytologic and architectural features of DCIS, if the proliferation does not involve at least two duct spaces or is at least 2 mm in size (7), it is classified as ADH. Incomplete involvement of a duct by abnormal cells also qualifies a lesion as ADH.

The application of these criteria to the definition of ADH has some practical implications. The first is that the pathologist entertaining the diagnosis of ADH is obliged to sample all of the available tissue completely to exclude the possibility of DCIS. The second major consequence is that atypical hyperplasia is not a diagnosis that can be definitively established by find-needle aspiration or core needle biopsy.

In contrast to the polymorphous and often confusing lesions of ADH, atypical lobular hyperplasia (ALH) is relatively easy to define and identify in histologic sections. ALH is diagnosed when fewer than 50% of the acini within a lobular unit are filled and expanded with a monotonous population of cytologically bland cells. The cells are usually small and lack conspicuous nucleoli. The discovery of ALH in a biopsy inevitably triggers intense review of all available histologic material to exclude the possibility of occult invasion.

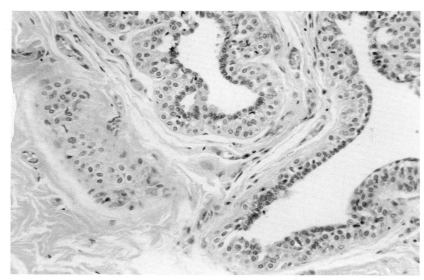

Figure 5.3. The cuboidal cells of lobular neoplasia are seen undermining the ductal epithelial cells (pagetoid spread). (Original magnification × 50.)

A phenomenon that is sometimes observed with ALH, and more often in LCIS, is the spread of these cytologically distinctive cells along ducts. These cells can occur either singly or in layered groups that undermine the normal ductal epithelial cells, separating the latter from the underlying myoepithelial layer (Fig. 5.3). Because the microscopic appearance is reminiscent of Paget's disease of the nipple, this phenomenon is called pagetoid spread of the cells of lobular neoplasia. When seen in association with ALH, pagetoid spread implies a greater relative risk for subsequently developing invasive carcinoma than does ALH alone (i.e., seven times normal rather than of four to five times normal) (8). Occasionally, pagetoid involvement of ducts by cells resembling those of lobular neoplasia is seen in biopsies in which neither ALH nor LCIS is found. This mandates a careful review of the entire specimen to ensure that ALH or LCIS has not been overlooked. If ALH and LCIS are definitely absent, the pagetoid spread phenomenon is of no established prognostic significance and may be due to local metaplastic changes mimicking the cells of lobular neoplasia.

CARCINOMA IN SITU

The emergence of carcinoma in situ as a meaningful diagnostic entity in the breast has progressed during this century roughly in parallel with its recognition in other sites. The idea of a neoplastic epithelial lesion that possesses the cytologic features of an invasive tumor but that has not yet transgressed the surrounding basement membrane and that can, therefore, be treated with a high likelihood of success is a compelling one. However, application of this model in the breast is complicated by the fact that there are at least three clinically and morphologically distinctive forms of carcinoma in situ: comedocarcinoma in situ, noncomedo DCIS, and LCIS.

Comedoductal carcinoma in situ is a variant of DCIS. The defining feature of this variant is the presence of centrally located necrotic cellular debris in ducts that are expanded and dilated by cytologically abnormal cells (Fig. 5.4). The extrusion of this gray-white, caseous, necrotic material from the cut surface of these tumors on gross examination gives this lesion its name. The epithelium lining the spaces is usually stratified and packed solid, but it may be arranged in cribriform or micropapillary patterns. The cytologic atypia is often but not always pronounced in the comedo type of DCIS. The lesions often show considerable mitotic activity. In small biopsies with extensive luminal necrosis, the paucity of viable neoplastic cells can cause diagnostic difficulty, but this can usually be resolved by more extensive sampling. The lesions in comedo DCIS are often larger than those of noncomedo DCIS, and measurements of up to 5 cm are not rare. Calcification of the necrotic debris in the ductal system often provides a distinctive mammographic appearance.

Comedo DCIS is distinguished from other forms of DCIS by its more aggressive behavior. Small foci of stromal invasion (micro-

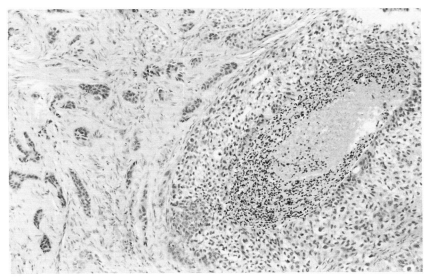

Figure 5.4. Comedoductal carcinoma in situ (right) associated with an infiltrating ductal carcinoma (left). Necrotic cellular debris is seen in the center of this markedly expanded duct. (Original magnification × 20.)

invasion) are more frequently found in association with those lesions composed primarily of comedo DCIS than in those consisting of predominantly other types. Even in those cases of comedo DCIS in which no overt invasive carcinoma can be found after extensive and careful examination, axillary lymph node metastases are observed in 1% to 2% of cases.

Noncomedo DCIS has been sorted into three main groups that essentially describe three architectural patterns. The cribriform and micropapillary patterns often occur together, hence the term cribriform-micropapillary DCIS. Cribriform-micropapillary DCIS is the most common type of noncomedo DCIS. The cribriform pattern is characterized by dilated ducts that contain a uniform population of cells that surround punched-out, sharply defined, round geometric spaces that may vary in size and distribution (Fig. 5.5). The micropapillary pattern describes ducts containing a uniform population of atypical cells that form fronds that project into the lumina, resembling the papillary fronds of a papilloma (Fig. 5.6). However, fibrovascular cores are not identified within these pseudopapillae. The third type of noncomedo DCIS has a solid growth pattern that lacks both the formation of the sieve-like spaces associated with cribriform DCIS and the formation of pseudopapillae, hence the term solid DCIS. A combination of these patterns of noncomedo DCIS may be seen in a single case, and non-comedo DCIS may coexist with comedo DCIS.

Apart from the architectural features that characterize DCIS, cytologic abnormalities are also required for this diagnosis. Two cellular

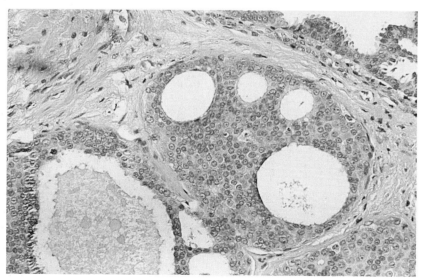

Figure 5.5. Cribriform ductal carcinoma in situ with sharply "punched-out" rigid spaces within a monotonous population of atypical cells. (Original magnification × 50.)

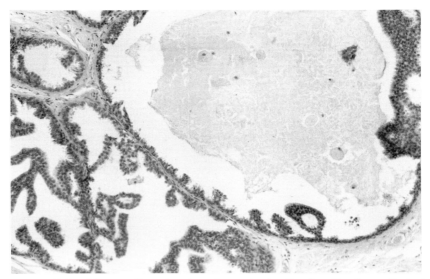

Figure 5.6. *Micropapillary ductal carcinoma in situ. The "papillary" growths lack fibrovascular cores. (Original magnification × 20.)*

patterns are often observed. In the first pattern, which is often seen in micropapillary DCIS, there are elongated cells that are compressed from side to side. They often contain hyperchromatic nuclei arranged perpendicular to the basement membrane. In the second cellular pattern, which is often seen with cribriform and solid DCIS, there are enlarged cells that have a moderate amount of pale or eosinophilic cytoplasm, sharply defined cytoplasmic borders, and enlarged nuclei that contain prominent nucleoli. A third cellular pattern, which may also be observed with any architectural pattern, consists of markedly pleomorphic, highly atypical cells that exhibit very little evidence of differentiation. As previously noted in the section on ADH, any one of these architectural patterns, when associated with appropriate cytologic features and size criteria, allows for the diagnosis of DCIS.

In some cases, apart from the obvious involvement of the larger ducts by DCIS, we also identify the same atypical cells within adjacent smaller acini. This is called cancerization of the lobules and is believed to be a retrograde spread of neoplastic cells into this region.

There are some problems associated with the diagnosis of DCIS. In some cases, there may be difficulty in differentiating between DCIS and florid duct hyperplasia. Hyperplastic cells often grow in a swirling pattern with overlapping nuclei. Nucleoli are not usually prominent, and cytologic variability can usually be observed on closer examination. The architectural criteria of DCIS are also usually lacking in cases of florid hyperplasia. Solid DCIS may resemble LCIS if the component cells are particularly small and uniform. However, the location of the cells in the larger ducts rather than in the acini suggests a diagnosis of DCIS. LCIS can also usually be identified by virtue of its association with adjacent areas of ALH. Because Page et al defined ADH as a ductal proliferative lesion showing some, but not all, of the diagnostic features of DCIS, it follows that their precise criteria for the diagnosis of DCIS must be adhered to.

The criteria used for defining DCIS in this section are among the most well established. However, they are by no means the only criteria that have been promulgated. As a result of the increasing frequency with which both pathologists and clinicians will be revisiting the issue of DCIS in the future, we discuss the salient points of two relatively newly proposed classification schemes. Lagios et al (9) proposed a four-tiered scheme that recognizes the classic comedo and the classic micropapillary types of DCIS. They also recognized two types of cribriform DCIS: one with necrosis and one with cytologic anaplasia. Their cases of cribriform DCIS with anaplasia behave in a manner similar to their cases of comedo DCIS, ultimately leaving three distinct diagnostic categories that predict for local recurrence. Holland et al proposed a three-tiered classification scheme that places the most emphasis on nuclear features and orientation. They described well-, intermediately, and poorly differentiated DCIS. Their scheme allows for a variable architectural growth pattern and variable amounts of necrosis. They have shown that this classification scheme defines three patterns of DCIS that are significantly associated with several biologic outcomes (10).

LCIS, like DCIS, has been the subject of controversy as to both the appropriate criteria for its diagnosis and its biologic significance. Epidemiologic studies have identified it as a marker for increased risk for invasive carcinoma. Paradoxically, however, the carcinomas it presages are not predictably of the invasive lobular type and they do not necessarily occur in the same breast. There is no compelling evidence for the obligate progression of LCIS to invasive lobular carcinoma. For these reasons, some authors have objected to using the term carcinoma in regard to noninvasive lobular lesions, and in the pathology literature the broad term lobular neoplasia is sometimes used to describe the lesions we refer to as ALH and LCIS.

The disease in LCIS involves the lobular units (Fig. 5.7). It is often multicentric and often accompanied by pagetoid extension of the cells of LCIS into larger ducts. The cells of LCIS are characteristically uniform with the small, round to oval nuclei that are usually only mildly hyperchromatic and often lack prominent nucleoli. Intracytoplasmic, mucin-containing vacuoles are a cytologic feature that also helps distinguish the cells of lobular neoplasia from those of ductal origin. These vacuoles may sometimes displace the nuclei peripherally, producing signet ring cells similar to those seen in gastric adenocarcinoma.

As is the case with DCIS, consistency in diagnosing LCIS can best be achieved by the careful use of well-defined criteria. Diagnosis of

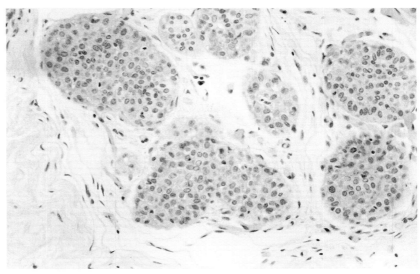

Figure 5.7. *Lobular carcinoma in situ. More than half of the acini in the lobular unit are filled and expanded by a uniform population of cuboidal cells. (Original magnification × 50.)*

LCIS in the studies of Page et al requires that each of the following criteria be fulfilled:

1. The neoplastic cells must comprise the entire population of cells within the acinus.
2. There must be filling and expansion of the acinus (i.e., intercellular spaces must not be present).
3. There must be expansion or distortion, or both, of at least one half of the acini in the lobular unit.

Although it is both customary and necessary to define and discuss hyperplasia, atypical hyperplasia, and carcinoma in situ separately, these entities are better understood as mileposts on a continuum rather than as rigid and discrete categories. It is only as markers of cancer risk that the noninvasive ductal and lobular lesions are distinctive. Thus, in a case in which an excisional biopsy shows mostly moderate ductal hyperplasia and a focal area of atypical ductal hyperplasia, the higher of the two risk estimates (i.e., the four to five times normal relative risk associated with ADH) would pertain. In addition, it should not be assumed that the presence of one entity precludes the presence of any of the others. Although atypical lobular hyperplasia and LCIS are most often seen in conjunction with each other or with invasive lobular carcinoma, they can also coexist with atypical ductal hyperplasia, DCIS, and even invasive ductal carcinoma. The reverse situation is also true. It is also important to note that the estimated relative risk associated with some of these lesions neither is location specific nor can predict the type of invasive carcinoma that may eventually develop. For example, when invasive cancer presents in a patient with a previous diagnosis of LCIS, it is equally likely to occur in the breast that had the original biopsy as it is to occur in the opposite breast. Additionally, an infiltrating ductal carcinoma might develop rather than an infiltrating lobular carcinoma.

INFILTRATING CARCINOMAS

The critical feature that differentiates invasive and in situ carcinomas of the breast is the presence of neoplastic cells outside the lobular unit, which is surrounded by the specialized loose connective tissue stroma (intralobular stroma). Extension of the neoplastic process into the interlobular dense collagenous stroma is usually, but not always, associated with a stromal response, which includes a fibroblastic proliferation and infiltration by inflammatory cells. The invading aggregates of cells usually have jagged, irregular borders rather than the smooth, rounded contours of DCIS.

The term *infiltrating carcinoma* encompasses several morphologically and behaviorally distinct entities (11). In this section, we first examine the most common and distinctive types of invasive carcinoma and then examine those features that are most useful in assessing prognosis and planning rational therapy.

Infiltrating Ductal Carcinoma

The most prevalent form of invasive carcinoma is, paradoxically, the least precisely defined. Because it is characterized in part by the absence of features seen in the more specialized forms of breast carcinoma, some authors prefer to characterize it as infiltrating carcinoma of no special type. However, infiltrating ductal carcinoma remains the most widely used diagnostic term. The principal characteristic of this tumor is the infiltration of the stroma by malignant epithelial cells that are usually arranged in nests or in cords that are two or more cell diameters wide (Fig. 5.8). The infiltrating cells often form lumina that are reminiscent of the ductal-acinar pattern of normal breast tissue. The invasive process is usually accompanied by a distinctive form of stromal fibrous proliferation known as desmoplasia (Fig. 5.9). In the early stages of this stromal response, increased amounts of mucopolysaccharide ground substance give the newly formed fibrous tissue a blue-gray appearance in hematoxylin and eosin–stained sections. The desmoplastic response is responsible for the very firm, sometimes rock-hard consistency of these tumors, and it is responsible for the

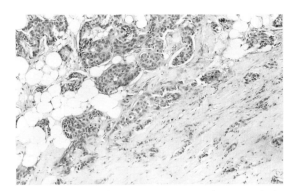

Figure 5.8. Infiltrating ductal carcinoma of the usual type. Nests and cords of atypical cells infiltrate the adipose tissue (upper left) and the dense interlobular fibrous stroma (lower right corner). (Original magnification × 50.)

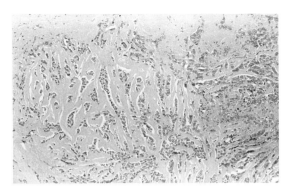

Figure 5.9. Infiltrating ductal carcinoma associated with a marked desmoplastic stromal response. (Original magnification × 20.)

older term: scirrhous carcinoma. In small lesions composed predominantly of DCIS, it is often the presence of this stromal response that first alerts the pathologist to the possibility of early stromal invasion. However, it should be noted that the stromal response may not be prominent, and situations do occur in which nests, cords, and even single malignant cells infiltrate both the interlobular stroma and adipose tissue with no fibroblastic response at all. This can result in serious underestimation of the size of invasive lesions on gross examination and is probably the most frequent cause of inadequately excised surgical margins in excisional biopsy specimens. Infiltrating ductal carcinoma is often, but not always, accompanied by focal areas of DCIS. For those invasive carcinomas in which the differentiation between invasive ductal and invasive lobular carcinoma is difficult, an intraductal component can aid in classifying the tumor as infiltrating ductal carcinoma.

Sometimes infiltrating ductal carcinomas of the breast grow in a solid or undifferentiated pattern with no special features (Fig. 5.10). When this occurs, characterizing the tumor as an infiltrating ductal carcinoma is difficult. In these cases, the best solution is to diagnose the tumor as an infiltrating carcinoma that is not otherwise specified. For all practical purposes, these tumors are best regarded as moderate- to high-grade invasive ductal carcinomas.

Infiltrating ductal carcinomas are subdivided into three categories that predict biologic behavior and potential outcomes of the disease. Of the various grading schemes that are currently in use, Elston's modification of the system that was originally proposed by Scarff, Bloom, and Richardson has been gaining in acceptance and is now widely used in this country (12). Applied to invasive ductal carcinomas, the system involves the evaluation of three features: tubule

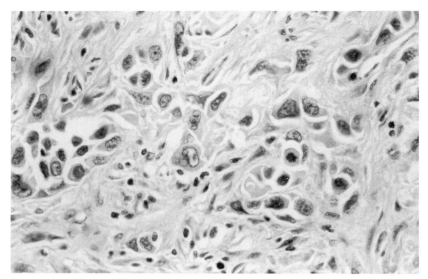

Figure 5.10. *High-grade infiltrating carcinoma with marked nuclear pleomorphism. (Original magnification × 100.)*

formation by the infiltrating neoplastic cells, the degree of nuclear pleomorphism, and the degree of mitotic activity. Each feature is scored on a scale of 1 to 3 using specific criteria. The individual scores are then added up, and the tumor's grade is allocated on the following basis:

   3 to 5 points, grade I: well differentiated
   6 to 7 points, grade II: moderately differentiated
   8 to 9 points, grade III: poorly differentiated

This grading system allows clinicians to stratify patients into three groups that have roughly 95%, 75%, and 60% 5-year survival rates, respectively, with grades II and III dropping off more sharply over longer follow-up periods.

Another grading scheme that is less commonly used in this country has been proposed by Le Doussal et al (13,14). This recognizes five grades of infiltrating ductal carcinoma, of which the first three have a good prognosis and the last two behave poorly.

Paget's Disease of the Nipple

Paget's disease of the nipple is not so much a separate type of mammary carcinoma as it is a highly specialized manifestation of ductal carcinoma. It is particularly important to clinicians because its clinical appearance may herald the presence of an otherwise occult malignancy. Because the ductal carcinomas underlying Paget's disease can be extremely inconspicuous, the obligate relationship between Paget's disease of the breast and ductal carcinoma was not always apparent. For many years, Paget's disease was thought to be merely a marker for the development of carcinoma rather than a sequela. We now understand the constancy of this association.

Grossly, the skin of the nipple and areola is frequently ulcerated and fissured. In advanced cases the nipple may be totally eroded. The surrounding skin may be indurated and hyperemic, but an underlying lump or mass is only rarely evident. Histologically, the disease is very distinctive. The epidermis is infiltrated by neoplastic cells occurring either singly or in small groups. The cells usually have somewhat paler staining cytoplasm than the adjacent keratinocytes and often show evidence of nuclear hyperchromatism and pleomorphism, although the nuclei may sometimes be quite bland. Occasionally, small groups of cells may be seen forming small acini or tubules with the epidermis. Malignant cells are also often identified in dermal lymphatics, and biopsies of sufficient depth frequently show ductal carcinoma involving lactiferous sinuses. In more subtle cases, when the malignant cells are arranged singly and their nuclei are bland, it can be difficult to distinguish the cells of Paget's disease from the glycogenated squamous cells commonly found in the nipple. In these cases, demonstration of cytoplasmic mucin by appropriate histochemical stains may be necessary to establish the diagnosis. Two unrelated lesions that may be confused histologically with Paget's disease of the nipple are squamous cell carcinoma in situ and melanoma in situ. Immunohistochemical studies may be needed to differentiate these lesions.

It is not surprising, given the frequency of involvement of the dermal lymphatics, that Paget's disease of the breast has been associated with a high incidence of nodal metastasis at the time of diagnosis.

Infiltrating Lobular Carcinoma

Infiltrating lobular carcinoma (ILC) was recognized as a distinctive variant of invasive breast cancer shortly after LCIS was defined as an entity. Unlike its in situ counterpart, ILC's ability to invade surrounding stroma, metastasize to regional lymph nodes and distant sites, and ultimately kill a patient is roughly equal to that of low- to intermediate-grade infiltrating ductal carcinomas. Invasive lobular carcinoma has been identified in different series as comprising anywhere from 3% to 4% to 14% of invasive breast cancers. Some of this variation is due to disagreement among pathologists as to precise criteria for its diagnosis.

Grossly, ILC may be indistinguishable from its infiltrating ductal counterpart. Marked stromal fibrosis may be present, causing a dis-

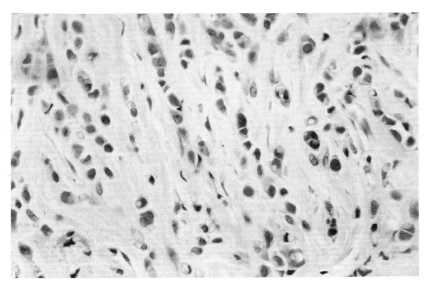

Figure 5.11. Infiltrating lobular carcinoma. The stroma is infiltrated by narrow columns of small cells. Observe the small intracytoplasmic lumina. (Original magnification × 100.)

crete, scirrhous mass. Conversely, ILC may present with very little stromal response and may be both grossly and mammographically undetectable. Cases of this type are usually discovered incidentally in biopsies for adjacent fibrocystic disease. They may also be found as the result of a painstaking search for an occult primary tumor in patients with widely disseminated metastatic disease.

The cells of ILC classically show the same cytologic features as those of ALH and LCIS. They are small and uniform with relatively little cytoplasm and regular, round to oval nuclei that show little hyperchromatism or pleomorphism. Intracytoplasmic lumina are common (Fig. 5.11). The cells characteristically infiltrate the stroma in rows that are a single cell diameter wide. These rows of cells often surround larger residual normal structures such as mammary ducts, alternating with bundles of collagen to form a concentric or "targetoid" pattern. The presence of this characteristic pattern is diagnostic of ILC even in the absence of concomitant LCIS.

Less common patterns of ILC include the solid and alveolar variants, which are characterized by a different architectural arrangement of the characteristic cells, and the pleomorphic variant of lobular carcinoma (15–17). The latter is distinguished by being composed of cells that are larger and that show considerable nuclear pleomorphism. Only the manifestation of the other features of lobular carcinoma allows this variant to be recognized. It is this form of lobular carcinoma that is most likely to be confused with an undifferentiated ductal carcinoma. Apart from the architectural and cytologic differences of these variants of infiltrating lobular carcinoma, it should also be noted that these lesions do not carry the relatively good prognosis associated with classic lobular carcinoma.

It is important to point out that ILC is also a nonspecific marker of cancer risk. To speak of cancer risk in a patient who manifestly has a carcinoma does not seem to make any sense until one recalls that lobular neoplasia is a marker for risk in both breasts, not just the one in which the lesion is found. Thus, the discovery of ILC in one breast implies an approximately 20% risk of concurrent invasive carcinoma (lobular or ductal) in the contralateral breast (18). There is also increased risk of multiple lesions in the same breast and of second primary lesions in long-term survivors. Historically, this phenomenon led to the practice of performing blind, "mirror image" biopsies of the contralateral breast when the diagnosis of ILC was made. This has been largely discontinued in favor of careful noninvasive follow-up. It should be understood that the strength of invasive lobular carcinoma as a marker of cancer risk has been established in relatively "pure" versions of the disease. When tumors have both ductal and lobular elements, the predictive value of the lobular component is much less clear.

Mucinous (Colloid) Carcinoma

Mucinous carcinoma is perhaps the most distinctive of the special types of breast carcinoma. Pure mucinous carcinomas comprise approximately 2% of invasive breast carcinomas in most series. They characteristically occur in older women and are associated with a very good prognosis in their pure form.

Grossly, mucinous carcinomas are usually 1 to 4 cm in diameter and have smooth, rounded borders. The cut surface is usually smooth and glistening, and the consistency of the tumor is usually soft. Histologically, the tumor is composed of pools of mucin in which neoplastic epithelial cells appear as floating islands (Fig. 5.12). Some tumors have such a high mucin-cell ratio that small specimens, such as core biopsies, may not initially provide adequate material for diagnosis. These clusters of cells usually have smooth, rounded borders. Smaller clusters of cells often appear solid, but larger clusters can exhibit acinar spaces and even cribriform patterns reminiscent of DCIS. The cells usually exhibit very bland cytologic features (Fig. 5.13). Necrosis is uncommon.

These tumors only rarely metastasize to axillary lymph nodes. This advantage is lost when mucinous carcinoma occurs as a component of a "mixed" invasive carcinoma, usually in conjunction with infiltrating ductal carcinoma. Studies have shown significantly poorer outcomes in patients with mixed mucinous carcinomas (19–21). When solid

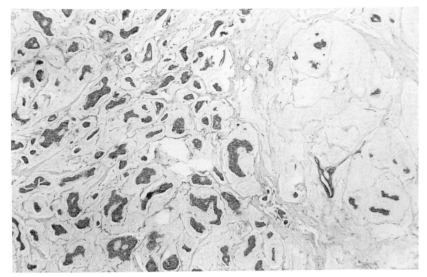

Figure 5.12. Mucinous carcinoma (colloid carcinoma). Clusters of neoplastic cells in large pools of mucin. (Original magnification × 20.)

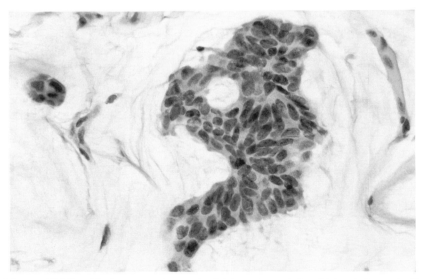

Figure 5.13. Mucinous carcinoma (colloid carcinoma). Small island of neoplastic cells that are mildly atypical. Paradoxically, these cells do not contain intracytoplasmic mucin vacuoles. (Original magnification × 100.)

areas or high-grade cytologic features are observed in tumors that appear to be mucinous carcinomas, they should probably be removed from this diagnostic category.

The one difficulty associated with the diagnosis of mucinous carcinomas is seen in those few cases in which pools of mucin without an epithelial component are identified in otherwise unremarkable tissue. In these cases, all the tissue must be thoroughly evaluated to preclude the diagnosis of benign lesions such as mucoceles or involvement of the breast by Carney's complex (22,23). Even in these cases, long-term follow-up is indicated because more recent studies suggest a continuum between benign-appearing lesions and mucinous carcinomas (24–26). In addition, follow-up is required for cases of pure mucinous carcinoma because of reported deaths from the disease many years after initial diagnosis.

Medullary Carcinoma

Nearly as uncommon as mucinous carcinoma, medullary carcinoma comprises 1% to 5% of invasive mammary carcinomas in various series. It is of considerable interest because its markedly anaplastic cytologic features belie its relatively good prognosis. The tumor usually presents in somewhat older women and is characterized grossly as a sharply circumscribed, smooth, rounded mass that is not fixed to the adjacent tissues. Histologically, the neoplastic cells are arranged in nests or islands surrounded by loose fibrovascular stroma. The tumor has pushing rather than infiltrating borders. Characteristically, the nests of cells are surrounded by a dense lymphoplasmacytic infiltrate. The inflammatory infiltrate is typically identified on the periphery of the aggregates of neoplastic cells and is not closely admixed with individual tumor cells. The cells of the tumor have large nuclei, prominent nucleoli, and abundant eosinophilic or pale cytoplasm. The nuclei are often highly pleomorphic, and bizarre shapes are not uncommon. Mitotic figures are often abundant.

The paradox of medullary carcinoma is that, in spite of the highly anaplastic cytologic appearance of its cells and despite the presence of axillary lymph node metastasis at the time of diagnosis in many cases, it is associated with a very good prognosis (27–29). Although the dense lymphoid infiltrate associated with the tumor suggests that a particularly effective host response may play a part in this phenomenon, a convincing explanation for this unusual behavior has yet to be proffered.

The accurate diagnosis of medullary carcinoma as a distinct and favorable entity requires complete sampling of the tumor and very strict adherence to diagnostic criteria. Occasionally, tumors may have some but not all of the features of medullary carcinoma. These tumors have been variably called atypical medullary carcinomas and infiltrating ductal carcinomas with medullary features. Regardless of which diagnostic term is used to label these tumors that lack all of the criteria of medullary carcinomas, their significance lies in the fact that they do not have the good prognosis associated with pure medullary carcinomas and, therefore, must be separated from that group.

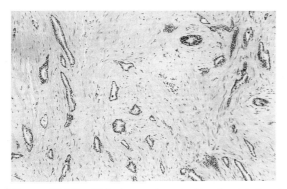

Figure 5.14. *Tubular carcinoma. Small acini, lined by a single layer of cells, in fibromyxoid stroma. Some of the tubules have the characteristic teardrop shape. (Original magnification × 20.)*

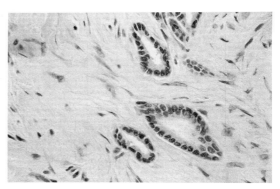

Figure 5.15. *Tubular carcinoma. The uniform, cytologically bland nuclei may cause difficulty in distinguishing these acini from benign structures. Although more than one cell layer may sometimes be observed in these tubules, a distinct myoepithelial layer is not present. (Original magnification × 100.)*

Tubular Carcinoma

Tubular carcinoma, a very well-differentiated variant of infiltrating ductal carcinoma, often presents as a small lesion that may be difficult to distinguish both clinically and histologically from a complex sclerosing lesion or radial scar. The tumor is characterized by small, gapping tubules that often have a characteristic teardrop shape (Fig. 5.14). These tubules infiltrate the surrounding dense fibrous stroma, usually spreading out from a central focus in a stellate pattern. The tubules are lined by low cuboidal cells with small, bland, round nuclei (Fig. 5.15). They are surrounded by cytoplasm that often focally protrudes in a bulbous fashion into the lumen. The tumor may be confused with and is distinguished from complex sclerosing lesions by the shape of the tubules, their invasion into adjacent adipose tissue, and the presence of a component of intraductal carcinoma. This low-grade invasive carcinoma in its pure form is usually associated with the best prognosis among the invasive breast carcinomas.

On occasion, other histologic types are observed in association with tubular carcinomas. When these make up 10% of more of the neoplastic process, they are more appropriately termed variants because they lack the excellent prognosis of pure tubular carcinomas. A close relative of the tubular carcinoma is the cribriform carcinoma (30,31). As the name implies, its features are similar to those of cribriform DCIS. However, extensive infiltration into the interlobular stroma is observed. Tubular and cribriform carcinomas are often seen in association with one another. It is generally accepted that when one encounters a mixed tubular and cribriform pattern the neoplasm is assigned to the diagnostic category of the dominant pattern.

Papillary Carcinoma

Papillary carcinomas are defined by the presence of fibrovascular cores that support the overlying abnormal epithelium. These tumors tend to occur in older women. Both the in situ (intracystic, encysted, or noninvasive) and the invasive variants share the presence of cytologically atypical cells. This finding is a major criterion when one is attempting to differentiate benign papillomas from papillary carcinomas (32). The in situ papillary carcinomas differ from their invasive counterparts in that evidence of true invasion outside the circumscribing fibrous tissue is not present in the former (Fig. 5.16).

Grossly, these tumors often present as circumscribed masses that may or may not exhibit cystic changes. The average size of these lesions varies from 1 to 3 cm. Microscopically, two types of abnormal cells are most often encountered in these lesions. They may be hyperchromatic and elongated, with side to side compression of closely packed cells. In this instance, the abnormal cells are usually observed lining the fibrovascular cores in a manner reminiscent of the epithelium in benign papillomas. The other type of atypical cells that are most often encountered have round, paler nuclei; often prominent nucleoli; and identifiable amounts of cytoplasm with sharp cytoplasmic borders. They often occur in aggregates so that they stand out against a background of relatively crowded unremarkable cells. Architecturally, these round, atypical cells may assume a growth pattern

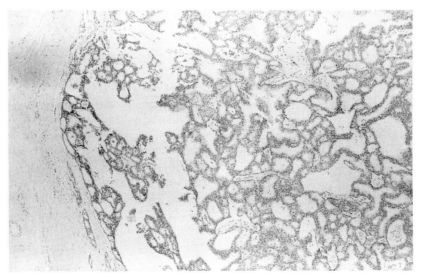

Figure 5.16. In situ papillary carcinoma. Observe the sharp demarcation of the tumor from the adjacent normal parenchyma by fibrous connective tissue. (Original magnification × 20.)

that is reminiscent of the cribriform and solid patterns that are identified in typical DCIS. It is also important to note that areas of typical DCIS may be observed in the breast parenchyma surrounding a noninvasive, well-circumscribed in situ papillary carcinoma. This is of clinical significance because in situ papillary carcinomas tend not to recur after local resection if areas of DCIS are not identified in the breast parenchyma adjacent to the main papillary lesion (33,34).

Invasive papillary carcinomas are associated with regional lymph node metastasis in about one third of the resected cases. However, on a sliding scale representing the degree of aggressive behavior associated with various types of invasive breast carcinoma, these tumors still behave in a relatively benign fashion; about 90% of patients are alive 5 years after their modified radical mastectomies (35).

Other Types of Carcinoma

Although the foregoing types of invasive carcinoma comprise the great majority of the malignant epithelial tumors of the breast, several other types can occur and are mentioned briefly.

Metaplastic carcinomas, both the sarcomatoid variants of infiltrating carcinoma and squamous cell carcinomas, usually present as larger, more aggressive neoplasms of advanced stage. Sarcomatoid variants can differentiate along various mesenchymal lines, including those with bone cartilage formation. Recognizing the sarcomatoid variants as carcinomas is important because they tend to spread to regional nodes rather than hematogenously, as is the case with true sarcomas (36,37).

Signet ring cell carcinoma is generally considered to be a variant of invasive lobular carcinoma. Intracytoplasmic lumina, which are most often seen in lobular neoplasia, are an exaggerated feature of this neoplasm. Usually of no distinctive prognostic significance, this neoplasm must be recognized as a primary breast neoplasm and not be assumed to be metastatic from the gastrointestinal tract. Its existence also needs to be documented in case metastatic disease later develops. This will preclude the need for extensive and unnecessary searches for a primary gastric carcinoma.

Neuroendocrine carcinomas, originally characterized in the gastrointestinal tract and the lungs, have been described in the breast. Their patterns vary from lesions that look like intestinal carcinoid tumors to cases of otherwise unremarkable infiltrating ductal carcinomas with focal neuroendocrine differentiation. Neuroendocrine differentiation is also commonly seen in mucinous carcinomas.

Other uncommon tumors that have been described are the salivary gland tumors like adenoid cystic carcinomas. Secretory and lipid-rich carcinomas have been described. Malignant myoepitheliomas and adenomyoepitheliomas have also been observed.

Prognostic Factors in Breast Cancer

As we have seen, the histologic type and grade of a tumor immediately provide the clinician with important prognostic information (38,39).

As expected, the size of the primary tumor also provides invaluable information (38–41). It is understood that all of the protocols for the treatment of breast carcinoma require a measurement of the tumor's size, and this information is an essential part of a pathology report. Occasionally, because of the multifocal nature of a tumor, a precise measurement is difficult to obtain, especially if invasive carcinoma is present in a re-excised margin. In these cases, the report should state this explicitly so that the best possible estimates can be made. It is important to note that it is the size of the invasive component that is critical, and this must be differentiated from the overall size of the neoplastic process.

Axillary lymph node status remains the single most powerful prognostic factor in early breast cancer (42–44).

Another prognostic factor that predicts for local recurrence after an excisional biopsy is the presence of an extensive intraductal component (EIC) in association with the infiltrating ductal carcinoma, especially in cases that are not widely excised (45–47). This is defined as an in situ component that composes 25% or more of the entire neoplastic process. A complementary phenomenon is observed in the situation in which microinvasive carcinoma is identified in an otherwise unremarkable DCIS. Although the concept of microinvasive carcinoma is familiar to practitioners who deal with squamous cell carcinoma of the cervix, its application in breast carcinoma is problematic. Although the term is widely used to suggest the earliest detectable invasive disease, there are as yet no generally accepted, precise criteria for the diagnosis of this entity. Therefore, careful communication between the pathologist and clinician is essential to avoid any misunderstanding when this term is used.

Peritumoral vascular invasion predicts for recurrence (43,48). However, the ability to consistently determine whether neoplastic cells are located within small vascular channels on routine histologic examination is fraught with difficulty and is associated with a high degree of intraobserver variability.

Another prognostic variable and, more importantly, a therapeutic decision factor is the presence or absence of estrogen and progesterone receptors in the invasive portions of the tumor (49–53). The presence of steroid receptors, determined either by biochemical assay of homogenized tumor cytosol or by immunohistochemical staining of the tumor in histologic sections, is an independent predictor of favorable prognosis as well as a predictor of tumor responsiveness to hormonal manipulation. Receptor positivity is generally related to tumor differentiation

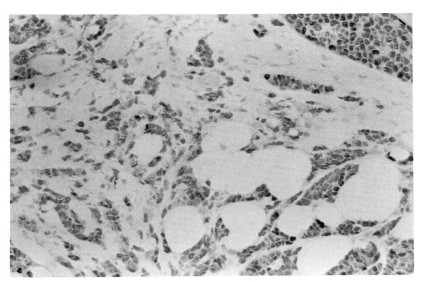

Figure 5.17. *Infiltrating ductal carcinoma. A positive immunohistochemical stain for the estrogen receptor is indicated by the brown stain of the nuclei. Antiestrogen receptor, immunoperoxidase stain; DAKO. (Original magnification × 50.)*

as reflected by histologic grade. The choice of the type of assay that is performed in a given laboratory is dependent on their practices (Fig. 5.17). Both the biochemical assays and the immunohistochemical procedures have their advantages and disadvantages (54–56).

The proliferative rate and presence of aneuploidy as measured by flow cytometry are also currently used as adjuncts in the therapeutic decision-making process. A high proportion of proliferating cells (S-phase fraction) and in some studies the presence of aneuploid populations are both predictors of poor prognosis (57–64).

Although either flow cytometric analysis or steroid receptor analysis may be performed on fresh tissue when enough material is available, it must be understood that breast masses that are smaller than 1 cm must be submitted entirely for histologic evaluation to preclude the possibility of an inadequate tissue diagnosis (65,66).

Although hormone receptor status and flow cytometric analysis are the current standard adjunct studies for mammary carcinoma, research aimed at identifying other prognostic and diagnostic tumor markers is proceeding rapidly. Oncogenes such as p53, HER-2/neu (c-*erb* B-2), Nm23, and c-*myc* have been identified as independent prognostic variables. Proteins such as the tumor growth factors, cathepsin D, and the matrix metalloproteinases are currently being investigated. Epiphenomena such as tumor-associated angiogenesis have also been identified as prognostic indicators. Although these markers are not currently being used in the day-to-day management of patients with breast carcinoma, the relative importance of such tumor markers and the role they will play in guiding therapy are rapidly evolving.

MALIGNANT STROMAL TUMORS

Although lesions like liposarcomas, malignant fibrous histiocytomas, fibrosarcomas, and osteogenic sarcomas have been described, they are extremely rare, and their discussion is beyond the scope of this very basic chapter. A discussion of slightly more common lesions follows.

Phyllodes Tumors

The tumors that belong to this category have been described under many names in the literature. These include terms like cystosarcoma phyllodes and atypical fibroadenoma. They mostly occur in middle-aged patients, although they have been described in all age groups, including children. They often present as painless masses. These neoplastic lesions range in size from tumors that are as small as 1 cm to huge masses that may occupy most of the breast. They are generally sharply demarcated from the surrounding uninvolved breast parenchyma. They may be lobulated, and cystic change or cleft formation may also be observed grossly. The diagnostic feature of these lesions is the presence of a proliferating stromal component, which may be associated with varying degrees of epithelial proliferation. Microscopic evaluation reveals the hallmark increased stromal cellularity (Fig. 5.18). This may or may not be associated with cytologic

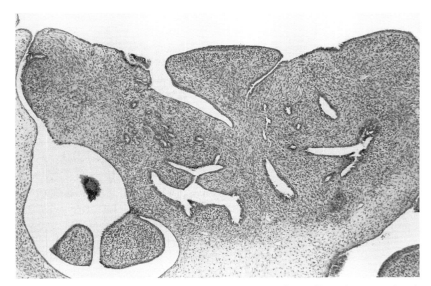

Figure 5.18. Phyllodes tumors are distinguished from fibroadenomas by the markedly increased stromal cellularity. (Original magnification × 20.)

atypia of the component cells. Also typical of these tumors are the bulbous nodular growths that extend into the cystic spaces and clefts identified within the tissue. Atypical features that are cause for concern in these neoplasms include the presence of infiltrative rather than circumscribed and pushing borders, the presence of more than three mitotic figures per 10 high-power fields, the presence of foci of stromal overgrowth that outstrips the proliferation of the adjacent epithelium, a size larger than 4 cm, and areas of tumor necrosis (67,68). Phyllodes tumors can be grouped into three main categories—benign, borderline, and malignant—that have some implications for potential biologic behavior. They represent a continuum in which an increasing number of atypical features are observed as one progresses from the benign end of the spectrum toward the malignant category. It is a combination of these atypical features that allows one to place a particular case in one of the categories that exists along this continuum.

It should be noted that all types of epithelial abnormalities may be identified in association with phyllodes tumors. These can vary from simple hyperplasia to in situ carcinoma. When a frank carcinomatous component is identified in association with a phyllodes tumor, consideration is given to other diagnostic terms such as a carcinosarcoma. Benign phyllodes tumors tend not to recur after complete local resection. In the malignant cases, recurrence usually occurs within 3 years of the initial surgical procedure. The mode of metastasis is usually through hematogenous spread, and death from the disease usually occurs within 5 years of the initial diagnosis. The biologic behavior of the borderline lesions is unpredictable although most tend not to recur.

Angiosarcoma

Although these tumors make up a minority of primary breast neoplasms, this location is the third most common site for primary angiosarcomas. They mostly occur in the third and fourth decades of life, although they have been described in the very young patients and in older patients. Many pregnant patients have been described in the literature. In addition, it has been observed that younger patients also tend to have higher grade lesions.

These tumors generally present as rapidly growing, painless masses. They are often associated with diffuse enlargement of the breast, and discoloration of the overlying skin is seen in about a third of the cases. Gross examination often shows a blue or purplish soft, multicystic mass that contains firmer gray-white areas. The size of these lesions is highly variable, and masses that measure up to 11 cm have been described. These tumors often have poorly circumscribed margins, and necrosis may be observed grossly. Microscopically, the hallmark of these tumors is the interconnecting vascular channels. These are lined by hyperchromatic endothelial cells. Other findings include the presence of endothelial tufting, the formation of papillae, the presence of solid areas with proliferating spindle cells, mitotic activity, and the presence of pools of blood called "blood lakes." Typically, these tumors dissect into fat and entrap normal breast parenchyma.

These tumors can be separated into three categories that have prognostic significance (69–71). Using one of these grading schemes, 5-year survival rates of 91%, 68%, and 14% have been described for grade I, II, and III tumors, respectively. It should be noted that rare long-time survivors of grade III lesions have been described in the literature. These tumors tend to spread hematogeneously, although occasional cases of lymph node metastases have been described. The incidence of fatal hemorrhage from these tumors and their metastatic lesions is well documented.

Angiosarcomas may arise in a breast that has been exposed to radiation as a result of therapy for a previous carcinoma (72).

Lymphomas

Primary lymphomas of the breast make up less than 1% of breast malignancies. Very strict criteria exist for establishing a diagnosis of primary breast lymphomas (73). These tumors have been described in people as young as 14 years and in women in their 80s. However, two predominant clinical patterns are observed. One pattern is seen sporadically in younger women, often around the puerperium and often with involvement of both breasts. The second pattern has a wider age range, but it is most often seen in older women and tends to be unilateral. Generally, primary breast lymphomas tend to present as rapidly growing, sharply circumscribed masses. They are often clinically thought to be carcinomas.

Microscopically and immunologically, all types of lymphomas have been described. These include various types of B-cell lymphomas and specifically T-cell lymphomas, Burkitt's lymphomas, and Hodgkin's lymphomas (74–78). However, most of the tumors belong to the non-Hodgkin's B-cell lymphoma category. Histologically, the growth patterns vary from situations in which the neoplastic cells infiltrate the lobular units and compress the ducts and acini to situations in which the normal breast parenchyma is completely destroyed and overrun by high-grade neoplastic cells, requiring the need for immunologic epithelial markers to define the underlying normal components of the lobular unit. Lymphoepithelial lesions that have been observed in lymphomas arising in mucosa-associated lymphoid tissue (MALT lymphomas) have also been described in primary lymphomas of the breast. Other findings that have been described in association with primary breast lymphomas include the expression of immunoglobulin

M and immunoglobulin A monoclonality by the neoplastic lymphoid cells, and the presence of serum protein abnormalities. An association with lymphocytic mastopathy has also been described (79).

There is an ongoing debate over the inclusion of primary breast lymphomas in the MALT lymphoma category. Arguments that support the contention include the presence of lymphoepithelial lesions, immunoglobulin A monoclonality, the tendency of spreading to other MALT areas before or without nodal dissemination, plasma cell differentiation of the cells in some of these tumors, and the tendency toward an absence of bone marrow involvement in the early stages of the disease. Arguments against classifying these tumors with the MALT lymphomas include the clinical and histologic observations that most primary breast lymphomas are of the intermediate- or high-grade category. Survival statistics have significantly improved in recent times; 5-year survival rates of greater than 80% are reported in the literature.

References

1. Dupont WD, Page DL. Risk factors for breast cancer in women with proliferative breast disease. N Engl J Med 1985;312:146–151.
2. Page DL. Cancer risk assessment in benign breast biopsies. Hum Pathol 1986;17:871–874.
3. Jensen, et al. Invasive breast cancer risk in women with sclerosing adenosis. Cancer 1989;64:1977–1983.
4. London SJ, et al. A prospective study of benign breast disease and the risk of breast cancer. JAMA 1992;267:7, 941–944.
5. Dupont WD, et al. Breast cancer risk associated with proliferative breast disease and atypical hyperplasia. Cancer 1993;71(4):1258–1265.
6. College of American Pathologists. Updated consensus statement. Relative risk for invasive breast carcinoma based on pathologic examination of benign breast tissue: policy and guidelines. Appendix DD. College of American Pathologists, Northfield, IL 1993:1–3.
7. Tavassoli FA, Norris HJ. A comparison of the results of long-term follow-up for atypical intraductal hyperplasia and intraductal hyperplasia of the breast. Cancer 1990;65:518–529.
8. Page DL, et al. Ductal involvement by cells of atypical lobular hyperplasia in the breast: a long-term follow-up study of cancer risk. Hum Pathol 1988;19:201–207.
9. Lagios MD, et al. Mammographically detected duct carcinoma in situ: frequency of local recurrence following tylectomy and prognostic effect of nuclear grade on local recurrence. Cancer 1989;63:618–624.
10. Millis RR, Eusebi V, eds. Semin Diagn Pathol 1994;11:165–235.

11. Page DL, Anderson TJ. Diagnostic histopathology of the breast. Edinburgh: Churchill Livingstone, 1987.

12. Elston CW, et al. The cancer research campaign (Kings/Cambridge) trial for early breast cancer—pathological aspects. 1982;45:655–669.

13. Le Doussal V, et al. Prognostic value of histologic grade nuclear components of Scarff-Bloom-Richardson (SBR): an improved score modification based on a multivariate analysis of 1262 invasive ductal breast carcinomas. Cancer 1989;64:1914–1921.

14. Le Doussal V, et al. Nuclear characteristics as indicators of prognosis in node negative breast cancer patients. Breast Cancer Res Treat 1989;14:207–216.

15. Martinez V, Azzopardi JG. Invasive lobular carcinoma of the breast: incidence and variants. Histopathology 1979;3:467–488.

16. Dixon JM, et al. Infiltrating lobular carcinoma of the breast. Histopathology 1982;6:149–161.

17. Weidner N, Semple JP. Pleomorphic variant of invasive lobular carcinoma of the breast. Hum Pathol 1992;23:1167–1171.

18. Dixon JM, et al. Infiltrating lobular carcinoma of the breast: an evaluation of the incidence and consequence of bilateral disease. Br J Surg 1983;70:513–516.

19. Silverberg SG, et al. Colloid carcinoma of the breast. Am J Clin Pathol 1971;55:355–363.

20. Toikkanen S, Kujari H. Pure and mixed mucinous carcinomas of the breast: a clinicopathologic analysis of 61 cases with long-term follow-up. Hum Pathol 1989;20:758–764.

21. Andre S, et al. Mucinous carcinoma of the breast: a pathologic study of 82 cases. J Surg Oncol 1995;58:162–167.

22. Rosen PP. Mucocele-like tumors of the breast. Am J Surg Pathol 1986;10:464–469.

23. Carney JA, et al. Dominant inheritance of the complex of myxomas, spotty pigmentation, and endocrine overactivity. Mayo Clin Proc 1986;61:165–172.

24. Ro JY, et al. Mucocelelike tumor of the breast associated with atypical ductal hyperplasia or mucinous carcinoma: a clinicopathologic study of seven cases. Arch Pathol Lab Med 1991;115:137–140.

25. Fisher CJ, Millis RR. A mucocele-like tumour of the breast associated with both atypical ductal hyperplasia and mucoid carcinoma. Histopathology 1992;21:69–71.

26. Weaver MG, et al. Mucinous lesions of the breast: a pathological continuum. Pathol Res Pract 1993;189:873–876.

27. Ridolfi RL, et al. Medullary carcinoma of the breast: a clinical pathological study with 10 year follow-up. Cancer 1977;40:1365–1385.

28. Pedersen L, et al. Medullary carcinoma of the breast, proposal for a new simplified histopathological definition: based on prognostic observations and observations on inter- and intraobserver variability of 11 histopathological characteristics in 131 breast carcinomas with medullary features. Br J Cancer 1991;63:591–595.

29. Pedersen L, et al. Medullary carcinoma of the breast, prognostic importance of characteristic histopathological features evaluated in a multivariate Cox analysis. Eur J Cancer 1994;30A:1792–1797.

30. Page DL, et al. Invasive cribriform carcinoma of the breast. Histopathology 1983;7:525–536.

31. Venable JG, et al. Infiltrating cribriform carcinoma of the breast: a distinctive clinicopathologic entity. Hum Pathol 1990;21:333–338.

32. Kraus FT, Neubecker RD. The differential diagnosis of papillary tumors of the breast. Cancer 1962;15:444–455.

33. Carter D, et al. Intracystic papillary carcinoma of the breast: after mastectomy, radiotherapy or excisional biopsy alone. Cancer 1983;52:14–19.

34. Lefkowitz M, et al. Intraductal (intracystic) papillary carcinoma of the breast and its variants: a clinicopathological study of 77 cases. Hum. Pathol 1994;25:802–809.

35. Fisher ER, et al. Pathologic findings from the National Surgical Adjuvant Breast Project (protocol no. 4): VI. Invasive papillary cancer. Am J Clin Pathol 1980;73:313–322.

36. Pitts WC, et al. Carcinomas with mataplasia and sarcomas of the breast. Am J Clin Pathol 1991;95:623–632.

37. Banerjee SS, et al. Pseudoangiosarcomatous carcinoma: a clinicopathological study of seven cases. Histopathology 1992;21:13–23.

38. Rosen PP, et al. Prognosis in T2N0M0 stage I breast carcinoma: a 20-year follow-up study. J Clin Oncol 1991;9:1650–1661.

39. Rosen PP, et al. Factors influencing prognosis in node-negative breast carcinoma: analysis of 767 T1N0M0/T2N0M0 patients with long-term follow-up. J Clin Oncol 1993;11:2090–2100.

40. Collan YU, et al. Prognostic studies in breast cancer: multivariate combination of nodal status, proliferation index, tumor size and DNA ploidy. Acta Oncol 1994;33:873–878.

41. Mansour EG, et al. Prognostic factors in early breast carcinoma. Cancer 1994;71(suppl 1):381–400.

42. Fisher B, et al. Relation of number of positive axillary nodes to the prognosis of patients with primary breast cancer. Cancer 1983;52:1551–1557.

43. Fisher E, et al. Pathologic findings from the National Surgical Adjuvant Project for Breast Cancers X Discriminants for tenth year failure. Cancer 1984;53:712–723.

44. Fisher E, et al. Pathologic findings from the National Surgical Adjuvant Breast and Bowel Projects (NSABBP). Cancer 1990;65:2121–2128.

45. Schnitt SJ, et al. Pathologic predictors of early local recurrence in stage I and stage II breast cancer treated by primary radiation therapy. Cancer 1984;53:1049–1057.

46. Schnitt SJ, et al. Breast relapse following primary radiation therapy for early breast cancer: II. Detection, pathologic features and prognostic significance. Int J Radiat Oncol Biol Phys 1985;11:1277–1284.

47. Borger JH. The impact of surgical and pathological findings on radiotherapy of early breast cancer. Radiother Oncol 1991;22:230–236.

48. Lee AKC, et al. Lymphatic and blood vessel invasion in breast carcinoma: a useful prognostic indicator? Hum Pathol 1986;17:984–987.

49. Osborne CK, et al. The value of estrogen and progesterone receptors in the treatment of breast cancer. Cancer 1980;46:2884–2888.

50. Allegra JC, et al. Estrogen receptor status: an important variable in predicting response to endocrine therapy in metastatic breast cancer. Eur J Cancer 1980;16:323–331.

51. McGuire WL, et al. Role of steroid hormone receptors as prognostic factors in primary breast cancer. Natl Cancer Inst Monogr 1986;1:19–23.

52. Spyratos F, et al. Prognostic value of estrogen and progesterone receptors in primary infiltrating ductal breast cancer: a sequential multivariate analysis of 1262 patients. Eur J Cancer Clin Oncol 1989;25:1233–1240.

53. Maass H, et al. New trends in the endocrine treatment of breast cancer. Recent Results Cancer Res 1990;118:225–232.
54. Stegner HE, Jonat W. Breast carcinoma. Curr Top Pathol 1991;83:459–474.
55. Snead DRJ, et al. Methodology of immunohistological detection of oestrogen receptor in human breast carcinoma in formalin-fixed, paraffin-embedded tissue: a comparison with frozen section methodology. Histopathology 1993;23:233–238.
56. Battifora H, et al. Estrogen receptor immunohistochemical assay in paraffin-embedded issue: a better gold standard? App Immunohistochem 1993;1:39–45.
57. Kallioniemi OP, et al. Improving the prognostic value of DNA flow cytometry in breast cancer by combining DNA index and S-phase fraction: a proposed classification of DNA histograms in breast cancer. Cancer 1988;62:2183–2190.
58. Clark GM, et al. Prediction of relapse or survival in patients with node negative breast cancer by DNA flow cytometry. N Engl J Med 1989; 320:627–633.
59. Lewis WE. Prognostic significance of flow cytometric DNA analysis in node-negative breast cancer patients. Cancer 1990;65:2315–2320.
60. O'Reilly SM, et al. Proliferative activity, histologic grade and benefit from adjuvant chemotherapy in node-positive breast cancer. Eur J Cancer 1990;26:1035–1038.
61. O'Reilly SM, et al. Node-negative breast cancer: prognostic subgroups defined by tumor size and flow cytometry. J Clin Oncol 1990;8:2040–2046.
62. Frierson HF Jr. Ploidy analysis and S-phase fraction determination by flow cytometry of invasive adenocarcinomas of the breast. Am J Surg Pathol 1991;15:358–367.
63. Frierson HF Jr. Grade and flow cytometric analysis of ploidy for infiltrating ductal carcinomas. Hum Pathol 1993;24:24–29.
64. Hedley DW, et al. Consensus review of the clinical utility of DNA cytometry in carcinoma of the breast. Cytometry 1993;14:482–485.
65. Recommendations of the Association of Directors of Anatomic and Surgical Pathology: Part I. Immediate management of mammographically detected breast lesions. Hum Pathol 1993;24:689–690.
66. Immediate management of mammographically detected breast lesions. Association of Directors of Anatomic and Surgical Pathology 1993;17:850–851.
67. Pietruszka M, Barnes L. Cystosarcoma phyllodes. A clinicopathologic analysis of 42 cases. Cancer 1978;41:1974–1983.
68. Ward RM, Evans HL. Cytosarcoma phyllodes. A clinicopathologic study of 26 cases. Cancer 1986;58:2282–2289.
69. Merino MJ, et al. Angiosarcoma of the breast. Am J Surg Pathol 1983; 7:53–60.
70. Donnell RM, et al. Angiosarcoma and other vascular tumors of the breast. Pathologic analysis as a guide to prognosis. Am J Surg Pathol 1981;5:629–642.
71. Rosen PP, et al. Mammary angiosarcoma. The prognostic significance of tumor differentiation. Cancer 1988;62:2145–2151.
72. Fineberg S, Rosen PP. Cutaneous angiosarcoma and atypical vascular lesions of the skin and breast after radiation therapy for breast carcinoma. Am J Clin Pathol 1994;102:757–763.
73. Wiseman C, Liao KT. Primary lymphoma of the breast. Cancer 1972; 29:1705–1712.

74. Dixon JM, et al. Primary lymphoma of the breast. Br J Surg 1987;74:214–216.

75. Lamovec J, Jancar J. Primary malignant lymphoma of the breast: lymphoma of the mucosa-associated lymphoid tissue. Cancer 1987;60:3033–3041.

76. Hugh JC, et al. Primary breast lymphoma: an immunohistologic study of 20 new cases. Cancer 1990;66:2602–2611.

77. Cohen PL, Brooks JJ. Lymphomas of the breast: a clinicopathologic and immunohistochemical study of primary and secondary cases. Cancer 1991;67:1359–1369.

78. Kosaka M, et al. Primary adult T-cell lymphoma of the breast. Acta Haematol 1992;87:202–205.

79. Katsuyki A, et al. Malignant lymphoma of the breast: immunologic type and association with lymphocytic mastopathy. Am J Clin Pathol 1992;97:699–704.

6

Epidemiology of Breast Cancer

Richard E. Blackwell

Nearly 25 years ago, Ronald Grant described breast cancer as the foremost of cancers. He justified this by saying that "breast cancer was the most fatal cancer in women in the United States, the most feared cancer, "the most self-discovered cancer, the cancer that has given rise to the largest number of articles in medical journals, the cancer for which most biopsies are performed, the cancer for which more x-ray examinations are performed, the cancer whose treatment is perhaps the most controversial, the cancer whose treatment is extremely radical, the cancer for which the most surgical operations are performed, the cancer for which the most radiation therapy is given, the cancer for which the most chemotherapy is administered, the cancer for which the most hormonal therapy is administered, the most costly cancer in terms of cost to society, and the most prolific cancer." These observations are true today (1,2).

The national cancer data base, which is a joint project of the Commission on Cancer for the American College of Surgeons and the American Cancer Society, derives data from cancers diagnosed and treated in more than 1000 hospitals throughout the United States (3). In 1991, reports were submitted from 937 hospitals, including 507,203 cases. More than 50% of overall cancers were reported in individuals aged 60 to 79 years; 85% are non-Hispanic whites; the majority are derived from the South Atlantic, East, North-central, and Pacific regions; 52% of the individuals have incomes between $32,000 and $53,000; and the majority live in urban regions. Highlights from the data base suggest a marked increase in the percentage of patients being staged by the American Joint Committee on Cancer/International Union Against

Cancer criteria and that the percentage of patients diagnosed with stage II and III disease decreased; however, the percentage of patients with stage IV disease remained constant. The stage of presentation was related to income; a large percentage of high-income patients presented with a lower stage disease. The data base also suggests a relationship to ethnicity; a larger percentage of white women present with lower stage disease. This finding is further amplified by the racial difference in survival from breast cancer; 75% of the difference may be accounted for by the sociodemographic variables rather than race (4). This is further reflected by the finding that, when one compares the stage of the disease by census region, there are some minor variations; patients living in the South-central regions, both East and West, show less early-stage disease than patients in other regions. The youngest and oldest cohorts present with a higher stage, that is, stage III or IV disease.

Finally, it is suggested that there are marked regional variations in the use of partial mastectomy, the highest being in the New England region and the lowest in the East, South-central regions. This is confirmed by reports suggesting that breast-conserving surgery with radiation therapy is not performed on the majority of women with stage I or II disease as recommended by the National Institutes of Health. Further, against this background, when one evaluates cohorts from 1973 through 1987, cardiovascular disease was found to decrease among the populations in both the United States and Sweden, whereas cancers among whites increased, and this increase could not be linked to either age or smoking (5).

Breast cancer, because it strikes 180,000 women in the United States, kills 46,000 annually, and leaves in its wake a survivor group of 1.5 million, is a political disease (6). The National Breast Cancer Coalition (NBCC), through lobbying efforts has persuaded Congress to double the amount of money spent on breast cancer research. The National Cancer Institute's (NCI) budget for breast cancer research was increased from $133,000,000 to $197,000,000; however, $210,000,000 went to the Department of Defense to be administered by the Department of the Army. For NCI alone, this represents a 177% increase in commitment to breast cancer research over the recent years, whereas the overall NCI budget has grown by 35%. As a result of the increase in funding, the NCI has established Specialized Programs for Research Excellence (SPORES), which is aimed at the transfer of basic science into clinical trials and treatment as rapidly as possible.

Despite the investment that has been made in breast cancer over the last 20 years, little headway has been made in explaining the relentless increase in this disease (Table 6.1). Women living in the United States have a risk of 1 in 8, which is twice that in 1940. At age 25 years, a woman has a 1 in 19,608 risk of developing breast cancer;

Table 6.1.   Risk factors for breast cancer

Established factors	Possible risk factors
Family history	Exposure to diethylstilbestrol
Diet	History of mammary dysplasia
Obesity	Caffeine consumption
Smoking	
Ethyl alcohol consumption	
Nulliparity	
Age at parity	
Age at menarche and menopause	

by age 40 this increases to 1 in 217; by age 50, 1 in 50; by age 70, 1 in 14; and by age 85, 1 in 9. Genetics appears to be clearly responsible for some women's breast cancer; the idea that a high-fat diet is responsible has faded from fashion (7). Epidemiologic risk factors are beginning to suggest that perhaps hormones, particularly estrogen, may play an important role in allowing the expression of breast cancer. The origin of the estrogen may be endogenous or exogenous, as demonstrated by the following observations: Breast cancer occurs more frequently in older women versus younger women, it occurs more frequently in northern Europe and North America than in Asia or Africa, upper socioeconomic women are at greater risk than women in lower classes, women who have never been married are at higher risk than those who have ever been married, women who delay childbearing past the age of 30 years have a much higher incidence than women who conceive at age 20 years or younger, obese women have a higher incidence of breast cancer than thin women, women who undergo early menarche are at higher risk than those whose menstrual periods begin later, and women who have delayed menopause are at higher risk than those who have earlier menopause. In addition, a family history of premenopausal breast cancer increases a woman's risk for this disorder, as does having cancer in one breast. Further, having a first-degree relative with breast cancer increases a woman's risk, as does a history of primary cancer of the ovary or endometrium.

ROLE OF FAMILY HISTORY AND THE CAUSE OF BREAST CANCER

There appears to be a two- to threefold increased risk in the incidence of breast cancer in women who have a female relative with the disease. For the patient with an affected mother or sister, there is a 2.3 relative risk; with an affected aunt or grandmother, a 1.5 relative risk;

and with both affected mother and affected sister, a 14% relative risk. Hereditary forms of breast cancer appear to make up about 8% of the disease; and in women with a strong family history, breast cancer tends to develop at a younger age. Studies examining a Utah population data base suggest a threefold increased risk as estimated by odds ratio (8). This analysis indicates that women are at increased risk if they have not only a first- or second-degree relative with the disease, a ratio of 1.3 (95%) confidence level, but also if they have a third-degree relative (ratio ranging from 1.07 to 1.64). From these estimates it appears that between 17% and 19% of breast cancers in this population could be attributed to family history. It was found that women who have a first-degree relative with colon cancer had a 30% increased risk of breast cancer.

In addition to family history, it appears that drug exposure during pregnancy may increase the risk of breast cancer (9). In 1984, a cohort of 6000 women, half of whom received diethylstilbestrol (DES) during pregnancy, were monitored for an average of 29 years. There were a total of 198 breast cancers recorded, and this was interpreted as a moderate increase in breast cancer incidence in the mothers given DES during pregnancy. Preliminary data suggested that this risk became greater over time, no increase was apparent for the first 20 years, but there was an increase between 20 and 29 years of age. The relative risk after 30 years was estimated to be 2.5. However, further evaluation of a larger sample from this cohort suggests a modest but statistically significant increased risk of breast cancer with DES exposure; however, the risk does not appear to increase over time.

Further, there appears to be a fourfold increase in the risk of breast cancer in women with a history of proliferative or atypical forms of fibrocystic change. It is important to remember that only approximately 5% of women with breast cancer have a history of benign breast disease. Women with atypical hyperplasia have a relative risk of 3.5, whereas those with atypia have a relative risk of approximately 1.1 compared with risks in women as a whole.

If a woman develops breast cancer in one breast, a number of factors contribute to the development of a bilateral lesion (10). Women with bilateral breast cancer, on average, are younger at the time of diagnosis of the first cancer. The overall distribution of tumor spread at the diagnosis of the second breast cancer is similar to that of the first; however, there is a less favorable distribution of secondary breast cancers if developed in women younger than 50 years. The survival rates after diagnosis of the second breast cancers are worse than those after the first.

Perhaps one of the most exciting events to have occurred in breast cancer research is the identification of one gene that predisposes to breast cancer and the first genetic mapping of another (Table 6.2) (11–14). These findings appeared in three papers published in the Septem-

Table 6.2. Genetics of breast cancer

BRCA1
  Located on chromosome 17q
  Responsible for 33% of breast cancer cases
  Possession of gene is associated with a 60% risk by age 50 years and an
    overall risk of 90%
  Isolated by Skolnick of Myrad Genetics, Inc., and University of Utah
BRCA2
  Located on chromosome 13q12.13
  Mapped by International Breast Cancer Linkage Consortium

ber 30 and October 7 issues of *Science.* These two genes called BRCA1 and BRCA2 together account for about two thirds of familial breast cancer, or roughly 5% of all cases. It also appears that BRCA1 is associated with the predisposition to ovarian cancer. BRCA1 is located on a locus on chromosome 17q. An analysis of 200 families has shown that BRCA1 is responsible for multiple cases of breast cancer in about 33% of families but more than 80% of families in which there is both breast cancer and epithelial ovarian cancer. Women who inherit the BRCA1 gene have a 60% risk of acquiring breast cancer by age 50 years and a 90% overall lifetime risk. Linkage mapping refined the chromosomal location of BRCA1 to the 1-2 mega-base pair region of chromosome 17q12-21q. The final sequencing was carried out by Mark Skolnick of Myrad Genetics, Inc., and the University of Utah. The gene consists of 21 exons distributed over 100 kilobases of genomic deoxyribonucleic acid adjacent to locus D17S855 encoding a protein of 1863 amino acids. Northern blot shows there is a single 7.8-kilobase transcript that is expressed in a number of tissues, including the breast and ovary. The amino terminal region of the protein contains a C3HC4 zinc finger domain, and the rest of the protein, especially the carboxy terminus, contains an excess of acidic residues, suggesting that the protein is a transcription factor. Mutations of BRCA1 have been identified that involve a stop codon, a frame shift, and a missense substitution, which results in the substitution of methionine with arginine. The mutations are compatible with a loss of function or domain-negative effect, and it may be that the transcript for one of the BRCA1 alleles is absent, consistent with the idea that this may function as a tumor suppressor.

A second gene, BRCA2, was mapped by International Breast Cancer Linkage Consortium. The predisposing gene apparently lies within a 6-centimorgan interval on chromosome 13q12.13 centered on D13S260. The loss of this gene may also result in elimination of suppressor function.

These discoveries open the way for the possibility of genetic testing. The BRCA1 gene is large, and the mutations may be widely distributed. The development of a large-scale screening process will be difficult but may occur in the near future.

Role of Cigarettes, Coffee, Alcohol, and Diet in the Development of Breast Cancer

Tobacco accounts for approximately 400,000 deaths in the United States each year. Tobacco-related cancers appear in the lung, esophagus, oral cavity, pancreas, kidney, bladder, and breast. Therefore, smoking remains the chief preventable cause of death and illness in the United States. It is responsible for approximately 17% of all deaths, and although smoking decreased from 40% in 1965 to 29% in 1987, more than 50 million Americans continue to smoke, and the incidence of smoking in women has risen at an alarming rate. This rate nearly parallels the increased occurrence of lung cancer in women, and the impact on breast cancer is not known as yet. Further, there has been an abrupt increase in smoking in girls aged 11 to 17 years, and this coincided with the 1967 launch of cigarette brands aimed specifically at female consumers (15).

The consumption of methylxanthine-containing compounds has been implicated as a causative factor in the development of fibrocystic disease of the breast and cancer. The Boston Collaborative Drug Surveillance Program evaluated some 16,000 patients and involved 210 women with fibrocystic disease and 204 women with breast cancer treated with mastectomy. An increased risk was detected in women who drank between one and three cups of coffee or tea per day (16).

Several studies have evaluated the role of alcohol and its association with an increased risk of cancer. Women who consume more than three drinks per day have been reported to have a 40% increase in the risk of breast cancer. Consumption of one alcoholic drink per day is associated with the relative risk of 1.6. The National Health and Nutrition Examination Survey cohort study revealed a 40% to 50% increased risk in breast cancer in women who drank fewer than three alcoholic drinks per week; however, the greatest risk appeared to be associated with women who drank more than 5 grains of alcohol per day. The mechanism by which alcohol increases the risk of breast cancer is unclear; however, given its hepatotoxic effects, one could postulate that this may be secondary to altered estrogen metabolism (17,18).

Diet, particularly the intake of dietary fat, has been thought to be associated with altering the risk of breast cancer. It was noted that postmenopausal women in the United States are at much higher risk for breast cancer than are Oriental women. This does not appear to be geographic, because the movement of Oriental women to either the Hawaiian Islands or the Pacific coast of the United States seems to eradicate the difference in incidence. However, the expression of the disease usually required one to two generations to demonstrate significance. It was assumed that these changes occurred because of the high animal fat in American diet, including hamburgers, french fries, potato chips, bacon, and red meats. Other populations with high fat intake but relatively low risk of breast cancer, such as Greece or Spain, use monounsaturated fats composed primarily of oleic acid. Likewise, fish oil, which is rich in n-3 fatty acids, has been associated with a lower incidence of breast cancer in countries ranging from Greenland to Japan. Walter Willett at the Harvard University School of Public Health began the analysis of the Harvard Nurses Health Study in 1978 (7). This study was launched in 1976 and included 120,000 women who in successive years were asked questions about many health-related issues, including diet, use of birth control pills, estrogen supplement, and smoking. After a decade of follow-up, no association has been demonstrated between fat intake in the adult diet and breast cancer. It has been suggested that women with extremely high-fat diets, that is, greater than 15% energy intake, are at little or no more risk than those who adhere to lean diets (less than 29% fat). These studies are all the more credible because of Willett's demonstration that fatty diets are linked to colon cancer. Studies carried out by Brinton at the NCI in the 1980s tend to confirm Willett's findings. A 12 case data analysis published in 1990 by Howe suggests a weak association between fat intake in the adult and breast cancer. Therefore, it appears that even a large reduction in fat intake, as much as 25%, would have minimum impact on the incidence of breast cancer.

ASSOCIATION BETWEEN STEROID HORMONES AND BREAST CANCER

As mentioned previously, the risk of breast cancer increases with the age at which a woman bears her first full-term child. A woman who has a child before the age of 18 years has about one third the risk of a woman who delivers after the age of 35 years. However, pregnancy must occur before the age of 30 to be protective, and, in fact, a woman who gives birth after the age of 30 appears to be at greater risk than a woman who has never been pregnant (19,20). Although the cause of these changes and risks is unknown, it appears that pregnancy produces some subtle changes in the hormonal environment. For instance, there is a decrease in dehydroepiandrosterone (DHEA) and its sulfate (DHEAS), as well as in prolactin levels, after delivery (21). There is a 70% risk reduction in the incidence of breast cancer in women who undergo oophorectomy before the age of 35 years (22). There also appears to be a small increased risk in patients who experience early menarche as well as late menopause (23). In addition, there appears to be a sixfold increase in the incidence of breast cancer in women excreting less than 0.4 mg of etiocholanolone, a metabolic by-product of androstenedione, which is produced by the adrenal and ovary. Likewise, it has been suggested that estriol, which is produced in high concentrations in pregnancy, may be protective against the possible cancer-inducing effects of the more potent estrogens. Further, women with progesterone deficiency appear to have a 4.5 times increased relative risk of breast cancer during the premenopausal years, and women with anovulation have a three to four times increased risk of cancer after the age of 50 (24,25).

Korenman has suggested that the endocrine milieu influences the susceptibility of the breast environmental carcinogens. This is the so-called estrogen window hypothesis, which suggests that unopposed estrogen stimulation at certain periods of life favors tumor induction. The longer unopposed estrogen stimulation acts on the breast, the greater is the risk factor. Pregnancy, with its high progesterone state, is thought to "close the window." It is known that progesterone downregulates estrogen receptors in the endometrium and is protective against the development of endometrial cancer. Although the data appear inconclusive at present, one might speculate that a similar mechanism might be active at the level of the breast (26).

CHEMOPREVENTION OF CANCER IN WOMEN

The information regarding increased or decreased incidence of cancer in women on the basis of parity, age at the time of birth of the first child, age of menarche and menopause, and the occurrence of surgical menopause suggests that hormones play a major role in the cause of human cancers. A number of agents have been shown either to be chemoprotective or to cause remission in certain endocrine active cancers (Table 6.3) (27). Oral contraceptive agents clearly reduce the incidence of endometrial and ovarian cancer through an antiestrogenic effect and through inhibiting ovulation. Gonadotropin-releasing hor-

Table 6.3. *Relationship of hormone agents to breast cancer*

Agent	Effect
Birth control pills	No increased risk of cancer
Gonadotropin-releasing hormone analogues	Decreased estrogen production
Tamoxifen	Is antiestrogen
Estrogens	Genetic reactive metabolites that may stimulate tumorigenesis
Progestogens	Regulates estrogen expression but can induce significant mitosis of both epithelium and stroma

mone (GnRH) agonists can be used to treat cancer of the breast, endometrium, and ovary by both inhibiting ovulation and inhibiting ovarian steroidogenesis and hormonal production. Various progestogens have an antiestrogenic effect on the endometrium. Tamoxifen, an antiestrogen, is used as an adjunct to the treatment of breast cancer, and finasteride, a 5α-reductase inhibitor, is used to treat prostate cancer. In view of those observations, one might suspect that oral contraceptive pills might decrease the incidence of breast cancer. Three major prospective studies, the Oxford Family Planning Association Study, the American Walnut Creek Study, and the Royal College of General Practitioners Oral Contraceptive Study, demonstrated no significant difference in the incidence of breast cancer between women who do and women who do not use oral contraceptive pills (28–30). Reports from the Centers for Disease Control showed no increased risk of breast cancer in women using oral contraceptive agents before the age of 20 years, with a duration of more than 4 years, or before the age of 25 years, with a duration of more than 6 years. Furthermore, their analysis indicated that there is no increase in breast cancer risk relative to the type of oral contraceptive agent used.

Despite this reassurance, controversy continues to exist over the long-term risk of oral contraceptive use in young women. An analysis by the Royal College study showed that women diagnosed with breast cancer between the ages of 30 and 34 years were more likely to have used oral contraceptives. An analysis of data from the Contraceptive Steroid Hormone Study indicated that women who were younger than 13 years at menarche and who remain nulliparous increase their risk for breast cancer if they used oral contraceptive agents for 8 or more years.

Not all studies have found evidence of an increased risk of breast cancer among young women who use oral contraceptives. Because there is no increased risk overall; however, some investigators suggested that oral contraceptives may accelerate the development of breast cancer in a small group of women so destined. At present, it is believed that women who use birth control pills have a relative risk of 1 for the development of breast cancer. Whether further studies will demonstrate that these agents have a protective effect, as they do in ovarian and endometrial cancer, remains to be answered (31).

ROLE OF REPLACEMENT SEX STEROIDS IN BREAST CANCER

At least 30 epidemiologic studies designed to identify an association between hormone replacement therapy in the postmenopausal woman and breast cancer have been published since 1974. Four large meta-analyses have been published since 1988; two concluded that estrogen replacement therapy does not increase the risk of breast cancer, and two concluded that it does. Therefore, it is not clear whether estrogen replacement therapy increases the risk of breast cancer (32,33). However, it appears that progestogen therapy neither increases nor decreases the risk of breast cancer.

ROLE OF ESTROGENS AND PROGESTERONES IN CARCINOGENESIS

A number of mammalian species, including primates, will form neoplasms, both benign and malignant, in various organs after exposure to sex steroids, including both estrogens and progestogens. One of the most commonly studied experimental models in carcinogenesis involves the use of estrogen-induced tumors in hamster kidneys and livers (34). It has been proposed that neoplastic transformation in these animal organs occurs via both hormonal and metabolic activities operating in concert. Estrogens generate the production of reactive metabolites and bind to cellular macromolecules. A number of studies suggest that estrogen metabolism generates reactive estrogen metabolites that stimulate tumorigenesis. In the hamster kidney, estrogen will induce the formation of estrogen receptors as well as increase its number. Estrogen-induced renal progesterone receptors can be significantly inhibited by antiestrogens, androgens, and to some extent synthetic progestogens.

Renal cytotoxicity has been seen as an initial event in estrogen-induced kidney tumorigenesis. Further, it has been observed that extensive liver damage in Armenian hamsters is elicited by chronic exposure to estrogens, and this can be reversed by concomitant tamoxifen treatment (35). Likewise, the culture of normal diploid Syrian hamster embryo fibroblasts in vitro with either estradiol-17 or DES resulted in aneuploidy in cell transformation. Therefore, this suggests that estrogen-induced aneuploidy may be a key event in cell transformation in carcinogenesis. DES has further been shown to affect microtubal preliminarization and depreliminarization. This is dose dependent, and the molecule covalently binds to brain β-tubulin at the carboxy terminal domain. It is suspected that chromosome imbalance as a consequence of the aneuploidy condition plays a significant role in the development of estrogen-induced malignancies.

All of this information suggests that a hormone, particularly estrogen, is a nongenotoxic carcinogen. A nongenotoxic carcinogen is defined as a carcinogen that does not directly or indirectly interact with genetic material and yet results in hereditary changes with other mechanisms. The end result ultimately causes hereditary change in the structure at the level of nucleic acids or genes.

Likewise, progestogens have been shown to regulate cell proliferation (36). Cell proliferation is the delicate balance among hormones, various regulatory molecules, and growth factors (37). Studies using breast cancer cells illustrate how estrogens control via autocrine and paracrine mechanism growth factor production. Progesterone appears to be a regulator of estrogen expression. It does not always function in an antiproliferative role. In fact, stroma proliferates within the uterus, and lobular-alveolar proliferation occurs in the mammary gland. For example, in the mouse uterus, progesterone administration significantly alters the proliferative response to estradiol. Pretreatment for 3 days with progesterone inhibits epithelial cell proliferation while sensitizing stromal cells to respond to estradiol with increased mitosis. Progesterone alone is capable of inducing significant mitosis in both the epithelium and stroma.

ROLE OF ESTROGEN REPLACEMENT THERAPY IN THE WOMAN WITH A HISTORY OF BREAST CANCER

Fifty epidemiologic studies have failed to demonstrate an increased risk in the incidence of breast cancer in postmenopausal women treated with various forms of estrogen replacement therapy. Whether the risk of breast cancer is increased in the postmenopausal woman administered estrogen at recommended doses is unknown. Several indirect lines of evidence suggest its safety. For instance, the morbidity and mortality statistics in pregnant women who develop breast cancer do not show a decreased survival rate or greater incidence of node involvement. Likewise, a subsequent pregnancy does not appear to increase the risk of recurrence of breast cancer. Short-term studies using continuous estrogen-progestogen protocols have not demonstrated an increased recurrence rate. That women with prior breast cancer have an increased risk of a secondary primary lesion and those with even the best prognosis have a 30% recurrence rate in 10 years is disconcerting. Likewise, bilateral oophorectomy as an adjunct for the treatment of breast cancer has fallen into disfavor because it produced no improvement in survival rates. However, evidence from the early breast cancer trial of a collaborative group indicates that ovarian ablation significantly affects the recurrence-free survival rate and mortality rates. Further, there is a significant improvement in the survival of node-positive patients treated with bilateral oophorectomy, although this effect disappears after 50 years of age.

Costa Rican women observed for 6 years were reported to have an increased risk if they used depo-medroxyprogesterone acetate. A case-control study from New Zealand, however, failed to demonstrate an overall increased risk, and a third study conducted by the

World Health Organization for more than 9 years showed that the relative risk of disease was not increased in the treated group compared with controls. Therefore, a committee opinion rendered by the American College of Obstetricians and Gynecologists in April 1994 suggested that there are "no data to indicate an increased risk of recurrent breast cancer in postmenopausal women receiving estrogen replacement therapy" (32).

References

1. Hollet AI. Breast cancer: change and challenge. Cancer 1991;41:69. Editorial.
2. Grant RM. The foremost cancer. Cancer 1969;19:72. Editorial.
3. Steele GD, Osteen RT, Winchester DP, et al. Clinical highlights from the National Cancer Data Base: 1994. Cancer 1994;44:71.
4. Eley JW, Hill HA, Chen VW, et al. Racial differences in survival from breast cancer. JAMA 1994;272:947.
5. Davis DL, Dinse GE, Hoel DG. Decreasing cardiovascular disease and increasing cancer among whites in the United States from 1973 through 1987. JAMA 1994;271:431.
6. Marshall E. The politics of breast cancer. Science 1993;259:616.
7. Marshall E. Search for a killer: focus shifts from fat to hormones. Science 1993;259:618.
8. Slattery ML, Kerber RA. A comprehensive evaluation of family history and breast cancer risk. JAMA 1993;270:1563.
9. Colton T, Greenberg ER, Noller K, et al. Breast cancer in mothers prescribed diethylstilbestrol in pregnancy. JAMA 1993;269:2096.
10. Brenner H, Engelsmann B, Stegmaier C, Ziegler H. Clinical epidemiology of bilateral breast cancer. Cancer 1993;72:3629.
11. Futreal PA, Liu Q, Shattuck-Eldens D, et al. BRCA1 mutations in primary breast and ovarian carcinomas. Science 1994;266:120.
12. Miki Y, Swensen J, Shattuck-Eldens D, et al. A strong candidate for the breast and ovarian cancer susceptibility gene BRCA1. Science 1994; 266:66.
13. Nowak R. Breast cancer gene offers surprises. Science 1994;265:1796.
14. Wooster R, Neuhausen SL, Mangion J, et al. Localization of a breast cancer susceptibility gene, BRCA2 to chromosome 13q12-13. Science 1994; 265:2088.
15. Rosenbert L, Schwingi PA. Breast cancer and cigarette smoking. N Engl J Med 1984;310:92.
16. Welsch CW. Caffeine and the development of the normal and neoplastic mammary gland. Proc Soc Exp Biol 1994;207:1.
17. Schotzkin A, Jones DY, Hoover RN, et al. Alcohol consumption and breast cancer in the epidemiologic followup study of the first national health and nutrition examination survey. N Engl J Med 1987;316:1169.

18. Willett WC, Colditz G, Stampfer MJ, et al. A prospective study of alcohol intake and risk of breast cancer. Am J Epidemiol 1986;124:540.

19. Bland KI. Risk factors as an indicator for breast cancer screening in asymptomatic patients. Maturitas 1987;9:135.

20. Pathak D, Speizer FE, Willett WC, et al. Parity and breast cancer risk: possible effect on age at diagnosis. Int J Cancer 1986;37:21.

21. Musey VC, Collings DC, Musey PI, et al. Long-term effects of a first pregnancy on the secretion of prolactin. N Engl J Med 1987;316:219.

22. Henderson BE, Pike MC, Casagrande JT. Breast cancer and the effect of the estrogen window hypothesis. Cancer 1981;2:363.

23. Trichopolous D, MacMahon B, Cole P, et al. The menopause and breast cancer risk. J Natl Cancer Inst 1984;48:605.

24. Cowan LD, Gordin L, Tonascia JA, Jones GS. Breast cancer incidence in women with a history of progesterone deficiency. Am J Epidemiol 1981; 114:209.

25. Gonzalez ER. Chronic anovulation may increase postmenopausal breast cancer risk. JAMA 1983;249:445.

26. Korenmann SC. Estrogen window hypothesis of the etiology of breast cancer. Lancet 1980;1:700.

27. Henderson BE, Ross RK, Pike MC. Hormonal chemoprevention of cancer in women. Science 1993;259:633.

28. Ramcharan S, Pellegrin FA, Ray RM, Hsu J-P. The Walnut Creek Contraceptive Drug Study: a prospective study of the side-effects of oral contraceptives. J Reprod Med 1980;25:366.

29. Royal College of General Practitioners Oral Contraceptive Study. Further analysis of mortality in oral contraceptive users. Lancet 1981;1:541.

30. Kay CR, Hannaford PC. Breast cancer and the pill—a further report from the Royal College of General Practitioners; oral contraceptive study. Br J Cancer 1988;58:675.

31. Peterson HB, Wingo PA. Oral contraceptives and breast cancer: any relationship? Contemp Obstet Gynecol 1992;37:31.

32. Committee on Gynecologic Practice. Estrogen replacement therapy in women with previously treated breast cancer. ACOG Committee Opinion 1994:135.

33. Speroff L. HRT for the woman who has had breast Ca? Contemp Obstet Gynecol 1993:33.

34. Li JJ, Li SA. Estrogen carcinogenesis in hamster tissues: a critical review. Endocrinol Rev Monograph 1. Endocrine Aspects of Cancer 1993,1:86.

35. Li JJ. Estrogen carcinogenesis in hamster tissues: update. Endocrinol Rev Monograph 1. Endocrine Aspects of Cancer 1993,1:94.

36. Clarke CL, Sutherland RL. Progestin regulation of cellular proliferation. Endocrinol Rev Monograph 1. Endocrine Aspects of Cancer 1993,1:96.

37. Klijn JGM, Berns PMJJ, Schmitz PIM, Foekens JA. The clinical significance of epidermal growth factor receptor (EGF-R) in human breast cancer: a review on 5232 patients. Endocrinol Rev Monograph 1. Endocrine Aspects of Cancer 1993,1:156.

Breast Imaging

Nancy S. Pile, Wanda K. Bernreuter,
and Eva Rubin

A mammogram is an x-ray examination of the breast performed on specialized equipment designed to specifically image breast tissue. Mammograms may be performed on women (and occasionally men) with signs or symptoms of breast disease, in which case they are designated as *diagnostic* mammograms, or on asymptomatic patients for the purpose of screening for breast cancer, in which case they are designated as *screening* mammograms. Because of the large number of potential screening mammograms in women at risk for breast cancer, the disagreements regarding risk-benefit ratios, particularly in women younger than 50 years, and the cost of performing large numbers of screening examinations in this country, mammograms have been subject to more scrutiny and controversy than any other x-ray examination currently being performed. As of October 1994, all facilities performing mammography require certification by the Food and Drug Administration.

SCREENING MAMMOGRAPHY

Most screening examinations can be expected to be normal. Because of this, one can easily be lulled into a false sense of security about the difficulties inherent in the interpretation of mammograms. Screening of women older than 40 years in the United States should yield approximately six to eight cases of breast cancer per 1000 women screened (prevalence screen). If screening of these same women were to continue, the rate of detection would approach that of newly emerging cancers (i.e., one to two cases per 1000 women [incidence screen]). At these rates, if all screening mammograms were to be interpreted as normal, the error rate would be less than 0.5%.

Although the risk of an individual woman having breast cancer at the time of a single screening examination is low, the risk over a lifetime is relatively high. The lifetime risk for an American woman who reaches age 85 is presently 1 in 9. In the United States, breast cancer accounts for nearly 33% of female cancers (excluding non-melanoma skin cancer and carcinoma in situ) and is responsible for 18% of cancer deaths, exceeded only by lung cancer. It is now estimated that 12.5% of women in the United States will be diagnosed with breast cancer and that 3.5% will die from it. Deaths from breast cancer exceed the combined total deaths for all gynecologic cancers.

Because of the perception of high risk both on the part of patients and their physicians and the high expectations raised by the promise of early detection with screening mammography, the missed or delayed diagnosis of breast cancer is a source of significant medicolegal risk for physicians. It currently represents the most common medical misdiagnosis claim and produces the greatest overall expense in litigation of any medical malpractice claim. The frequency of litigation for breast cancer is more than twice the frequency of breast cancer in the general population. Of all physicians sued in breast cancer–related actions, almost one third are gynecologists.

Performance of optimal screening mammography requires sophisticated equipment, meticulous attention to technique, expert and certified radiologic technologists, sensitivity to patient factors that influence compliance, the detection of often subtle abnormalities, and accuracy in the interpretation of these abnormalities.

The Equipment

Mammograms are performed on specialized x-ray units that are designed to deliver radiation at low kilovoltages to optimize the differences between the fatty and soft tissue (fibroglandular) components of the breast and allow detection of tiny calcifications, which may be the first indicators of malignant disease in the breast. Most mammograms are performed in the 25- to 28-kilovolt (peak) range, which is several orders of magnitude lower than the kilovoltage used to produce radiographs of the chest or abdomen. The high contrast and spatial resolution required for mammography cannot be achieved with standard equipment used to image other body areas.

Modern mammographic units incorporate photodetectors, which set exposure on the basis of an estimate of the density of the breast tissue underlying the area of the detector (phototiming). These exposures are typically very short, 100 to 300 milliseconds, resulting in radiation doses that are considered to produce negligible risk of induction of radiogenic cancers.

Mammographic units also are equipped with compression paddles or plates. A good quality mammogram requires the use of a moderate degree of firm compression of the breast. The compression not only immobilizes the breast but also decreases its thickness and makes the thickness penetrated by the x-ray beam more even. This allows a more uniform exposure to be obtained at considerably less dose than would be required if the breast were uncompressed. The compression is only applied for a few seconds. Many modern mammographic units have automated compression devices that allow the technologist to release compression as soon as the exposure is terminated.

Risk

The risk of breast cancer is increased from exposure to radiation at high levels, such as occurred in women exposed to the fallout from the atomic bombings of Hiroshima and Nagasaki. This risk is strongly age dependent, the highest risks occur in women younger than 40 years at the time of exposure. The risk begins 5 to 10 years after exposure, and the mortality risk peaks at about 20 years after exposure. This is one reason why asymptomatic women without unusual risk factors are discouraged from beginning mammographic screening before the age of 40 years.

For a woman with breasts of average size and density, a two-view mammogram results in an average radiation dose of 2.0 to 4.0 mGy. It is estimated that a single two-view mammogram at an average dose of 3.0 mGy might result in an excess of 1.3 deaths per 100,000 women exposed; annual screening beginning at age 40 years might result in an excess of 13.8 deaths per 100,000 women screened. These risks must be compared with the estimated lifetime risk of breast cancer for the average woman, which is about 3000 per 100,000 women, a risk that is 200 to 1000 times higher than the estimated risk of mortality from radiation-induced cancer. Thus, even if benefit from screening mammography was as low as 1%, a positive risk-benefit ratio would result from beginning annual screening at age 40.

Technique

Screening mammograms in the United States consist of two views of each breast. Although it is possible to screen with a single view of each breast, and this has been done in some of the randomized, controlled trials of screening mammography performed in Europe, it is estimated that 15% to 20% of cancers that would otherwise be detectable will not be seen if only a single-view screen is performed. In addition, many more patients would require callback for additional views if only one projection were obtained, resulting in increased cost, inconvenience, and anxiety.

The standard screening projections are the mediolateral oblique (MLO) and the craniocaudal (CC), both performed with the patient upright whenever possible. This combination maximizes the volume of breast tissue imaged and optimizes visualization of those areas where breast cancer is most likely to occur, notably the upper outer quadrants and axillary tails.

On the MLO view, the lateral side of the breast is placed against the film holder, and the x-ray beam penetrates the breast from its medial to its lateral aspect. Because the lateral part of the breast is closest to the film, laterally located lesions will be imaged better than those in the medial part. The oblique orientation allows visualization of breast tissue in the axillary tail, which is not imaged in true lateral projection. The degree of obliquity is determined by the angle of the patient's pectoral muscle, which may range from 30 to 60 degrees depending on body habitus.

On a properly performed MLO view, the pectoral muscle is visible to the plane of the patient's nipple, the breast is pulled up and forward as much as possible away from the chest wall, allowing visualization of fat in the retromammary area; the breast does not sag; the inframammary folds are displayed; and no fibroglandular tissue reaches the edge of the film (Fig. 7.1A). If possible, the nipple should be placed in profile but not if this requires sacrifice of the amount of breast tissue that can be imaged. By convention, a marker indicating left or right and the projection is placed on the film adjacent to the upper part of the breast. The oblique projection has some minor disadvantages; it is less reproducible than true lateral projections and may make accurate assessment of superior or inferior location of lesions more difficult.

The CC projection is performed with the inferior part of the breast against the film with the x-ray beam traversing the breast from its superior to its inferior aspect (Fig. 7.1B). The breast is pulled forward, away from the chest wall as much as possible. A small amount of pectoral muscle is imaged in the minority of patients on the CC projection and should not be mistaken for a mass lesion. The medial area of the breast is emphasized on this view because it is the area seen least well in the MLO projection. Retromammary fat should be seen posterior to all of the medial fibroglandular tissue with no medial tissue extending to the edge of the film, and there should be no medial fibroglandular tissue reaching the edge of the film. If possible, the nipple is placed in profile. By convention, a radiopaque marker is placed adjacent to the lateral side of the breast to designate left or right and the projection.

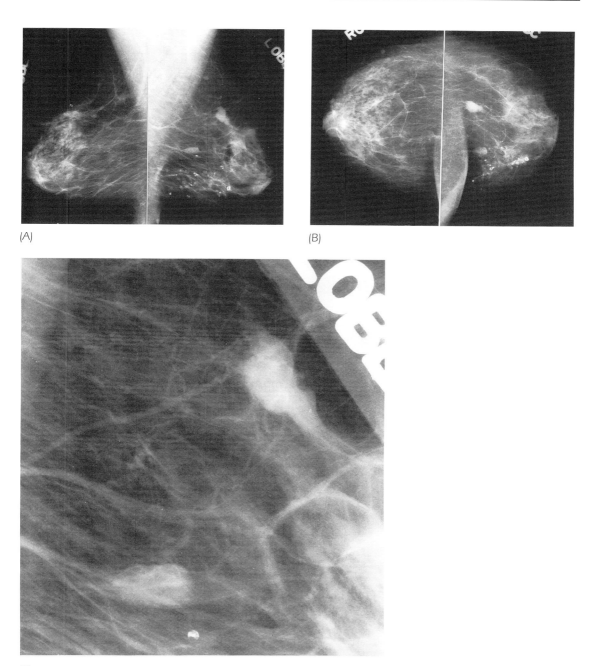

(A)

(B)

(C)

Figure 7.1.   (A) Mediolateral oblique views demonstrate good positioning on the left. The right pectoral muscle has a concave border, indicating that it is not relaxed. As a result, less of the lateral breast tissue is imaged. (B) Craniocaudal views emphasize the medial breast, and the pectoralis muscle can be seen bilaterally. There is a small amount of residual glandular tissue. In the left breast, there are two nodules as well as coarse, benign-appearing calcifications. (C) Magnified view of the nodules shows some smooth margins, but some of the borders are more indistinct, particularly in the superior lesion. The decision of how far to go with the diagnostic procedure should be based on the most malignant findings. Core needle biopsy was performed and medullary carcinoma was found.

The Technologist

To be accredited, mammograms must be performed by radiologic technologists certified by the American Registry of Radiologic Technologists (ARRT). It is also recommended that radiologic technologists performing mammography pass the advanced qualification examination in mammography administered by the ARRT. There are few radiologic examinations that require more on the part of the technologist than the mammogram. Although technologic innovations such as automatic exposure controls and compression release devices have significantly improved the technologist's ability to obtain a technically good quality mammogram, the ability to put the patient at ease to obtain good positioning and cooperation is a skill that is not universal. The time of the mammography examination is often one of high anxiety, and patients may not behave well in such high-stress situations. This requires high dedication and commitment on the part of the technologist in addition to technical expertise. Some otherwise well-trained technologists are not suited to performing mammography.

The compression required to perform good mammography may be uncomfortable for some women. Because the expectation of pain is one of the leading determinants of the experience of pain, educating women about the need for compression is critical. Ideally, mammograms should be scheduled at times when the breast is likely to be least tender. For premenopausal women, it is advisable not to schedule a mammogram for the week before menstruation. Sensitivity to these issues on the part of the scheduler and the technologist will ensure a better examination and improve compliance.

Detection of Abnormalities on the Mammogram

Like most paired organs in the body, the breasts have a tendency to symmetry. Most radiologists display mammograms on the view box such that the corresponding oblique and CC views are mounted side by side. If comparison examinations are available, these are also displayed. The first task of the interpreter is to determine whether an asymmetric area is present and then to analyze its cause. Minor degrees of asymmetry are common and, unless new or associated with a palpable finding, are usually not cause for concern (Fig. 7.2). In some patients, a cause for the asymmetry, such as a history of biopsy, may be known; in others, there will be no apparent cause. The differentiation of innocuous areas of asymmetric density from potentially malignant mass lesions is often one of the most difficult tasks for the mammographer. The lack of invariable anatomic landmarks in the breast, the variations in the amount and distribution of soft tissue densities in the breast, and the inherent lack of contrast between some malignant masses and the normal soft tissue constituents of the

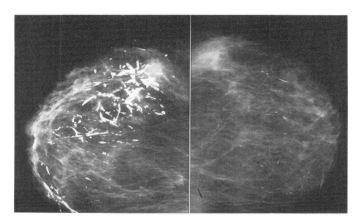

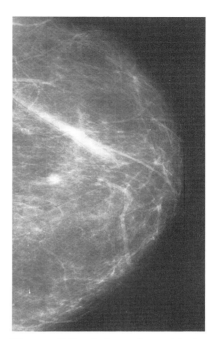

Figure 7.2. Right craniocaudal and left craniocaudal views. Benign intraductal calcifications. There are fine, linear, nonbranching calcifications in the left breast oriented toward the nipple that are in normal-sized ducts. On the right, the calcifications are much larger and are contained in ectatic ducts. Their borders are smooth, and many demonstrate a central lucency. Both are examples of calcifications that do not require biopsy. Note also that there is a mild asymmetry of the breast tissue, with more density on the right. This asymmetry was present on previous years' examinations and is unchanged.

Figure 7.3. Left craniocaudal view of a predominately fatty replaced breast with an 8-mm spiculated density seen in the subareolar region. Biopsy showed this to be an invasive ductal carcinoma. Note also the skinfold in the medial portion of the breast. This can be seen when there is skin retraction or when there is deformity of the breast from prior surgery. In this patient, it was due to improper positioning and was not present on a repeat film.

breast contribute to difficulties in detecting lesions and a significant error rate for mammography, which may range from 5% to 69%.

Physicians unfamiliar with mammographic interpretation may labor under the misimpression that mammograms are among the easiest radiographs to read. Indeed, some are. Even a very tiny spiculated cancer is easily perceived in a fatty breast (Fig. 7.3), and the calcifications most distinctive for malignancy (i.e., those of comedocarcinoma) are often not difficult to see (Fig. 7.4). In fact, one could ask a reasonably intelligent 6-year-old to look for "stars" and "spilled salt," and the child would likely be able to detect some very tiny cancers. The tiniest star may be readily seen on a clear night, but bring on the clouds and even the full moon disappears. The highly variable nature of the breast and the often subtle differences between benign and malignant disease are what make many mammographic interpre-

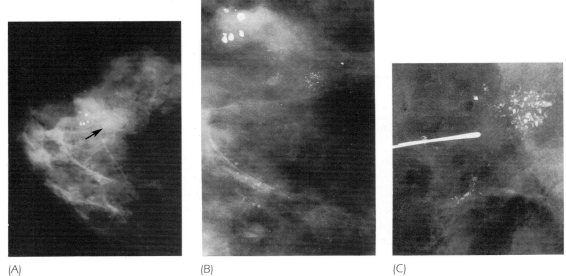

(A)   (B)   (C)

Figure 7.4. (A) Right craniocaudal view of dense breast parenchyma. There are dense, clearly benign calcifications in the outer portion of the breast and scattered, fine calcifications throughout the breast. There is also a focal cluster of calcifications that have a third morphology (*black arrow*). All of these cacifications can easily be seen despite the density of the glandular tissue. (B) Magnified view of this area shows a cluster of microcalcifications with varying density and shape. (C) Specimen radiograph confirms the removal of the suspicious cluster and more clearly demonstrates the malignant characteristics. Localization wire can also be seen in the specimen. Pathologic diagnosis was ductal carcinoma in situ, comedo type.

tations difficult. Very large malignancies may be inapparent when surrounded by dense tissue, and microcalcifications of significance may be difficult to appreciate when multifocal or extensive calcification is present.

Mammographic detection of malignancy is not as size dependent as other radiographic methods of tumor detection. With optimal technique, microcalcifications will be visible on mammography and primarily present problems of interpretation. Mass, on the other hand, may present problems of perception as well as interpretation. As a general rule, if one misses a cancer manifest by a tiny cluster of microcalcification without mass for 1 year, the consequences are likely to be less dire than if one misses a cancer that has already formed a mass. Presently, the greatest hope for reduction of breast cancer mortality lies in recognition of invasive breast cancer before it has exceeded 1 cm in size.

Although the mammographic identification of larger cancers is important and the ability of a mammographer to detect palpable breast cancer enhances the credibility of the technique to the referring physician (and patient), the major focus of the mammographer should be detection of invasive cancer at the smallest possible size. The increasing recognition of breast cancers of ductal type in their noninvasive stage is likely to have mortality benefit. However, the magnitude of reduction of breast cancer mortality as a result of the detection of noninvasive cancer is unknown, primarily because we do not know what proportion of mammographically detected noninvasive cancers is destined to become invasive.

Mammographic Interpretation

Analysis of Mass Lesions

Is it in the breast? The first question to be answered in analyzing a mass visible on mammography is whether the mass is truly in the breast. The most common nonbreast mass to cause problems is a skin lesion; moles are the most frequently encountered. Some moles and other skin lesions are readily recognizable because of their surface irregularities or because of the lucency (produced by entrapped air) visible at their margins. Some mammographers have their technologists place radiopaque markers on all visible skin lesions. Alternatively, one may have the technologist mark the location of visible abnormalities—skin lesions, scars, tattoos, and so on—on a diagram of the breast and reserve the use of markers for those instances in which there is still some question.

Another anatomic structure that may cause problems is the sternal insertion of the pectoral muscle. This may be visualized in the medial posterior breast on well-positioned CC views. Its triangular shape, bilaterality, and continuity with the pectoral muscle usually allow it to be recognized as a normal variant. Occasionally, the patient's chin, ear, abdomen, or fingers may project into the imaged field and simulate a mass. Likewise, any object interposed between the x-ray tube and breast or the breast and the image receptor may produce mass-mimicking artifacts.

Is it a real mass? The next question to be answered is whether the perceived mass is real. Pseudotumors may be produced by isolated islands of normal glandular tissue, asymmetric densities that are normal variants, nodular asymmetries related to previous breast surgery, or simply overlap of normal fibroglandular elements. Both pseudotumors and real tumors may be seen on only one view of the mammogram. The analysis of lesions that are seen on only one view is one of the most difficult tasks of the mammographer.

Analysis of Lesions Seen on Only One Projection

As stated previously, the standard screening mammogram consists of two projections; the MLO and the CC. There is some difference of opinion among expert mammographers as to which of the many additional projections is most helpful. The leading contenders are the true lateral (TL) view and the laterally extended (exaggerated) CC view (LECC). The TL view corrects the geometric distortion produced by

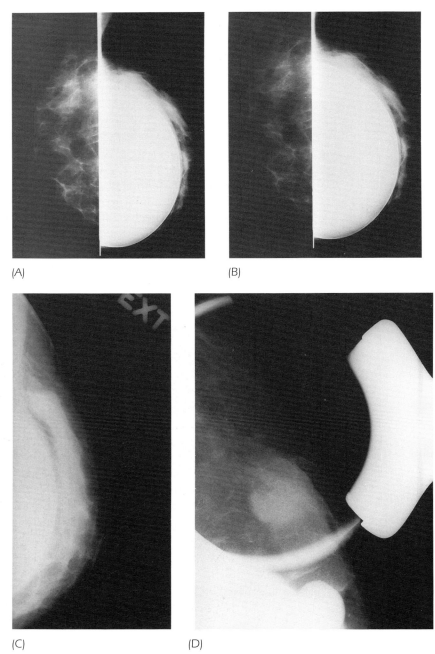

(A)   (B)

(C)   (D)

Figure 7.5. (A) LOBL, push-back and implant views. (B) Left craniocaudal push-back and implant views. The push-back views allow for imaging of the greatest amount of tissue. The implant view allows for evaluation for implant integrity and can include some tissue not seen on the push-back view. There is a nodule, seen in the upper portion of the LOBL implant view that is not seen in any of the other standard views of the left breast. (C) A laterally extended craniocaudal implant view establishes that the nodule is in the lateral portion of the breast. (D) The nodule is further characterized with a magnified, spot-compressed view that shows that the borders are ill defined, particularly along the superior and anterior margins. This underwent biopsy, and invasive ductal carcinoma was found.

imaging the breast obliquely; the LECC not only orients the tissue differently but also often images tissue not seen of the standard views. Even in the absence of questionable mass, this view may be indicated as part of the routine examination in women in whom the most lateral portions of breast tissue are not imaged on standard CC views (Fig. 7.5).

For lesions that are visible on MLO only, an LECC view is often the first requested additional view. This is reasonable because the lateral breast is the most frequent site for breast masses and some lateral breast tissue is commonly not imaged on the standard CC. Alternatively, one may use parallax to identify whether an abnormality seen on MLO is located medially or laterally (Fig. 7.6). As one goes from MLO to TL projection, a lateral lesion will move down and a medial lesion will move up (mnemonic: LDMU, or lovely dependable mammography unit). Centrally located lesions will maintain approxi-

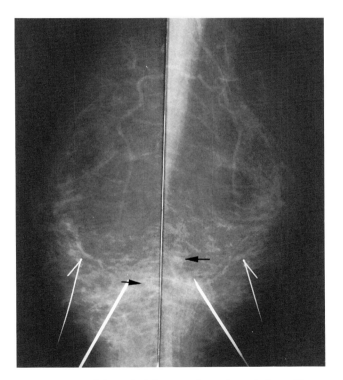

Figure 7.6. *Right mediolateral oblique and true lateral views. The anterior wire marking a tiny cluster of calcifications has already been deployed. They are located in the 6 o'clock position and, therefore, would not be expected to move up or down with a change in the degree of obliquity. The posterior needle is also at the 6 o'clock position. The cluster of microcalcifications (black arrows) could not be imaged on a craniocaudal projection. Because they move up relative to the needle and wire as the projection is changed from mediolateral oblique to true lateral, they must be located in the medial portion of the breast.*

mately the same position. Similarly, rolled views allow one to determine whether a lesion seen only on CC is in the upper or lower portion of the breast. For example, assume a nodule is visible in the medial area on CC view. If one rolls the top of the breast medially and the bottom laterally, the lesion must be in the upper breast if it remains medial on the rolled view.

What if one has done an additional view (LECC, TL, tangential) and the "lesion" is still not visible? Does this prove without a doubt that one is dealing with a pseudotumor? The answer is no. What, if anything, is done next depends on the level of suspicion, which is based on what was perceived on the projection that initially appeared abnormal. If the abnormality was simply a contour deformity (rounded area of glandular tissue or convexity of a breast margin) that did not persist on the additional view and appeared compressible, this may be sufficient evidence that one is dealing with benign asymmetry. If some doubt persists, a compression spot film performed in the original projection that appeared abnormal or altering the breast position slightly with a rolled view or one performed at a slightly different angle will usually suffice to assure that a mass is not present.

However, if concern was raised because of an area of architectural distortion or spiculation in a patient who had not had a biopsy, magnification views should be performed in two projections, including the one that appeared abnormal. If no abnormality is seen, no further views are necessary. However, if mass or distortion is verified on one of the magnified views, the exact location of the abnormality must then be determined. This may require views that place the lesion closer to the film such as the lateromedial view for medially located lesions or the caudocranial view for superiorly located lesions, magnification views in orthogonal projection focusing on areas where overlap of tissue is most likely to have obscured a lesion, or ultrasonography. Some cancers may be readily identifiable on ultrasonogram when x-ray mammograms reveal subtle or indeterminate findings (Fig. 7.7).

Should a short-term follow-up be obtained for lesions that after evaluation are thought to be pseudotumors? In most cases, this should be unnecessary. However, if one's confidence level is lowered because of the presence of very dense or nodular tissue, a 6-month follow-up may be reassuring, particularly when no comparison mammograms are available.

Characteristics To Be Defined

Once a mass is established to be real, the following characteristics must be defined: 1) size; 2) location; 3) single or multiple, unilateral or bilateral; 4) margin characteristics; 5) density; 6) presence and type of calcifications in or around the mass; 7) presence of distortion; and 8) presence of secondary signs of breast cancer (nipple or skin retraction, skin thickening, increased vascularity).

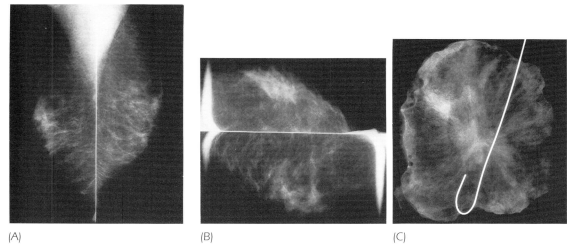

(A)   (B)   (C)

Figure 7.7.   *(A) Right and left mediolateral oblique (MLO) views showing an asymmetric density in the right subareolar area. (B) Spot compression with magnified views (MLO and craniocaudal) shows some subtle distortion but no discrete mass. An ultrasonogram clearly delineated a solid mass and biopsy was performed. (C) Specimen radiograph confirms the removal of the mass, and its highly suspicious, spiculated margins are easily seen. Diagnosis was invasive lobular carcinoma.*

Size and location are important descriptors that should always be included in the mammogram report but have relatively little differential diagnostic value. Some important exceptions are that very large masses in the breasts of younger women are likely to be phyllodes tumors, and uniform density nodules in the lower, inner, or anterior breast are unlikely to be intramammary lymph nodes. Multiple, bilateral breast masses, none with individually suspicious characteristics, can safely be presumed to be benign (Fig. 7.8). Ultrasonography may be helpful to verify that the majority of masses are cysts or as a guide to aspirate larger masses, either to relieve symptoms or to facilitate clinical or mammographic follow-up. When one or more of the masses appear suspicious, ultrasonography (and ultrasonogram-guided aspiration) is often the simplest way to increase one's confidence that biopsy is, or is not, indicated. Multiple masses in one breast only may be multifocal carcinomas, and each should be evaluated individually. Bilateral multifocal primary cancers can occur but are unlikely to be manifest as numerous "benign-appearing" nodules.

Among the features listed, margin characteristics are the most useful predictors of malignancy. Spiculated (stellate) margins in association with a palpable mass in a woman who has not had a recent biopsy, trauma, or breast infection are virtually certain indicators of breast cancer (see Fig. 7.3). Even when a mass is nonpalpable, the presence of spiculated margins carries a 70% to 80% likelihood of malignancy. The predictive value of nodular, multilobulated, fading, or indistinct margins for the presence of breast cancer is considerably

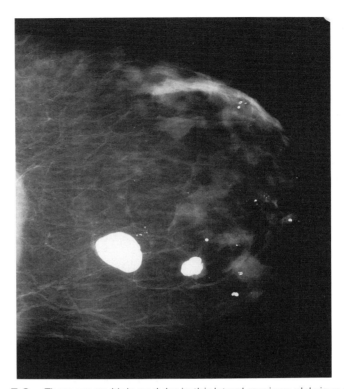

Figure 7.8. *There are multiple nodules in this lateral craniocaudal view, some of soft tissue density and some entirely of the density of calcium. The calcified nodules have a classic appearance if hyalinized fibroadenomas. Ultrasonogram showed all the nodules of soft tissue density to be solid, consistent with noncalcified fibroadenomas. The multiplicity of the nodules lends confidence to the benign diagnosis. Biopsy is not necessary unless one of these nodules changes over time.*

less, on the order of 20%. Nonpalpable masses 2 cm in size or smaller with perfectly well-circumscribed margins have a predictive value for breast cancer very close to 0.

High density of a lesion relative to its size favors the diagnosis of malignancy; however, high density per se has lost much of its significance because mammographic techniques have improved and the size of detected lesions has decreased. An encapsulated fatty lesion (lipoma, oil cyst, galactocele) is always benign (Fig. 7.9). Well-circumscribed nodules with central (hilar) fat can be diagnosed with certainty as intramammary lymph nodes. Encapsulated masses containing fat and soft tissue elements (hamartomas, fibroadenolipomas) are also distinctively benign lesions (Fig. 7.10). Heavily calcified (hyalinized) fibroadenomas are also pathognomonically benign (Fig. 7.11). The presence of fat streaming into an area of architectural distortion was at one time thought to strongly support a benign process. Biopsy scars, radial scars (complex sclerosing lesions), and fat necrosis often manifest this finding. However, it has since become apparent

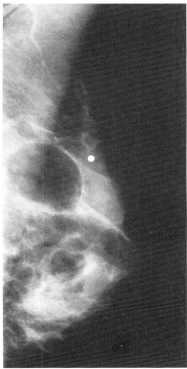

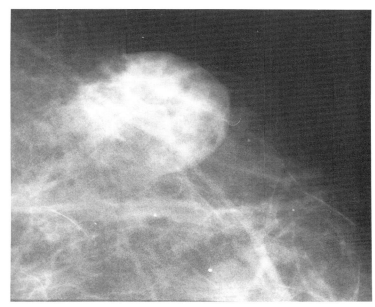

Figure 7.9. Left oblique view with a metallic marker over a palpable nodule. There is a well-circumscribed nodule of fat density that corresponds to the palpable abnormality. This is a lipoma and does not require biopsy.

Figure 7.10. Magnification view of a nonpalpable mass. It contains both soft tissue and fat density. This is pathognomonic for a fibroadenolipoma (hamartoma). These lesions can contain varying amounts of each component. If any fat at all can be demonstrated within the lesion, it can be considered benign and does not require biopsy.

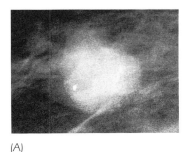

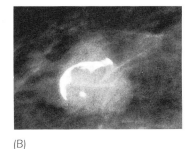

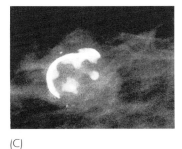

(A)   (B)   (C)

Figure 7.11. (A) Magnification view of a poorly circumscribed nodule containing a coarse, benign-appearing calcification. Because the nodule was indeterminate in appearance, a core needle biopsy was performed, and the diagnosis was hyalinized fibroadenoma. (B) One year and (C) 2 years later further calcification of this benign lesion is seen.

that invasive lobular cancers and even some invasive ductal cancers may appear to have fat within them. Thus, spiculation, in the absence of a history of biopsy or trauma in the area, is almost always an indication for biopsy regardless of whether there is central density or lucency.

Breast cancers may contain any type of calcification. The presence of malignant-type calcifications in a mass that appears otherwise benign is an indication for biopsy. However, benign-appearing calcifications in a malignant-appearing or indeterminate mass do not ensure a benign mass.

The circumstances in which cancers may contain benign-appearing calcifications are 1) incorporation of preexisting benign calcifications, 2) formation of dystrophic calcification in necrotic areas of tumor, and 3) development of fat necrosis in or near regions of tumor.

Architectural distortion may be visible in the absence of appreciable mass. This may occur when cancer is present in dense tissue. Ultrasonography will usually show the mass or shadowing in these cases. Architectural distortion in the absence of mass occurring in fatty regions of the breast has a high likelihood of benignity if the converging lines radiate to a point and if the distortion is inapparent on orthogonal views. This is commonly the case with maturing biopsy scars or areas of fat necrosis; if this clinical history is available, followup rather than biopsy is indicated.

Secondary signs of breast cancer such as skin retraction or thickening are rarely present with small cancers unless they are very superficially located. These signs should, however, be sought whenever the breast is either dense or nodular, because they may be the only indicators of breast cancer in such cases. Increased vascularity, usually resulting from a prominent draining vein, is often a feature of large breast cancers. Localized increased vascularity in the absence of localized breast abnormality may be due to 1) normal variation, 2) asymmetric compression, 3) venous obstruction outside the breast, or 4) congestive heart failure. Further diagnostic evaluation of the breast is not warranted.

Pathognomonically Benign, Likely Malignant, and Indeterminate Masses

Breast masses may be categorized into those that are pathognomonically benign, those that are virtually surely malignant, and those that are indeterminate. Indeterminate masses may be further subdivided into those with high and low levels of suspicion for malignancy. Optimal interpretation involves avoiding biopsy in the first instance, ensuring it in the second, and assigning the third category to biopsy or follow-up in such a way as to ensure that malignant lesions are identified with the minimum number of unnecessary (benign) biopsies.

Pathognomonically Benign Breast Masses
Pathognomonically benign breast masses include the following:

1. Intramammary lymph nodes
2. Lipomas
3. Oil cysts with or without rim calcification
4. Galactoceles
5. Hyalinized fibroadenomas
6. Foreign bodies
7. Nodules with sedimented calcium (milk of calcium in microcysts)
8. Cysts (when documented by calcification ultrasonography)

These lesions need not undergo biopsy even when palpable.

Masses Highly Likely To Be Malignant
As mentioned earlier, spiculated masses or masses with malignant-appearing calcifications should undergo biopsy except in very specific instances such as recent biopsy or trauma, hemorrhage associated with a bleeding diathesis, or presence of overt signs of infection. Some biopsied spiculated masses will prove to be benign and are listed next.

1. Radial scar
2. Sclerosing adenosis
3. Papilloma(tosis)
4. Granular cell myoblastoma
5. Biopsy scar
6. Fat necrosis
7. Pseudotumor

Lesions 1 to 4 require biopsy for confirmation of benignity. Biopsy is often avoidable for lesions 5 to 7 (Table 7.1).

Additional Mammographic Views

The use of altered positioning and views with radiopaque markers has been covered in the early part of this discussion. Spot compression views are helpful in the separation of overlapping structures and in imaging lesions located near the chest wall. These views allow better compression of specific areas of breast tissue and may be preferable to magnification views for lesions in very dense or very thick breasts when detail is likely to be compromised by patient motion because of the long exposure time required for magnification in such cases. Coning down to a smaller area of the breast minimizes scatter and improves detail.

Table 7.1. Techniques available for the evaluation of indeterminate masses

Additional mammographic views
  Altered positioning
    Laterally (medially) extended craniocaudal
    True lateral
    Lateromedial or caudocranial views
    Cleavage view
    Rolled or tangential views
  Addition of radiopaque markers
  Spot compression views
  Magnification views and spot magnification views
Ultrasonography
Computed tomography
Magnetic resonance imaging
Aspiration or core biopsy
  X-ray guided with or without stereotactic equipment
  Ultrasonography guided

Magnification views are most helpful in the assessment of margin characteristics of masses and in defining the characteristics of calcifications (see Fig. 7.4). The combination of magnification and spot compression may provide the most ideal detail but is difficult to achieve in the absence of an identifying marker for the lesion in question, such as focal skin retraction or a lumpectomy scar.

Ultrasonography

Mass

Ultrasonography should be performed in the evaluation of any solitary mass, other than those deemed sufficiently suspicious on x-ray mammography so that biopsy will be recommended regardless. The identification of a simple cyst concludes the investigation (Fig. 7.12). If a fluid-containing mass is identified that does not fulfill criteria for a simple cyst (for example, if it has thick walls, contains debris levels or intracystic nodules) in a patient who has no reason to have a hematoma, ultrasonogram-guided aspiration is the simplest guide when deciding whether open biopsy is necessary. If the lesion resolves with aspiration, biopsy is unnecessary. If pus is encountered, antibiotic therapy or drainage, or both, are indicated. If neither of these scenarios apply, open biopsy may be indicated. Opinion is divided as to whether a solid nodule with so-called classic features of fibroadenoma on ultrasonography (smooth, well-circumscribed margins, homogeneous internal echoes, axis parallel to skin, and long axis two times greater than anteroposterior [AP] dimension) can be safely followed (Fig. 7.13). Ultrasonography does not allow definitive differentiation of benign from malignant solid masses. However, it is probably safe

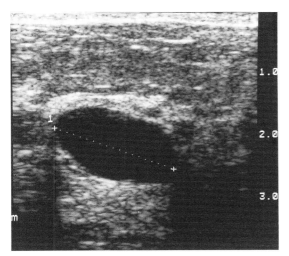

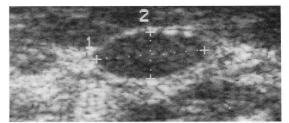

Figure 7.12. Simple cyst. This is a well-circumscribed, thin-walled, anechoic structure. There is a sharp back wall and enhanced posterior sound transmission.

Figure 7.13. Ultrasonogram of a typical fibroadenoma. This hypoechoic nodule is well circumscribed with a homogeneous echo texture. This is enhanced through sound transmission. The long axis of the nodule is oriented parallel to the skin surface. This nodule underwent biopsy at the patient's request, and the diagnosis was fibroadenoma.

to follow lesions with "classic" features of fibroadenoma in certain circumstances, including 1) patient age less than 20 years, 2) presence of multiple lesions, 3) history of biopsies for fibroadenoma, and 4) nonpalpable lesions identified on the ultrasonogram only.

The most important noncystic mass seen on ultrasonography examination is breast carcinoma. Although carcinoma can have variable appearances on ultrasonography, including features similar to benign lesions, several characteristics raise the suspicion of malignancy (Fig. 7.14). Classically, carcinoma is markedly hypoechoic, sometimes appearing nearly anechoic, on ultrasonography but with irregular or angular margins, unlike simple cysts. Compared with the thin, well-circumscribed, and continuous rim seen surrounding a benign lesion such as a fibroadenoma, the rim of a cancer is often thick and highly echogenic. In the early experience with breast ultrasonography, it was thought that demonstration of acoustic shadowing posterior to a lesion was a strong indication of malignancy. As further experience has been gained, it has become apparent that some benign lesions can also demonstrate this finding and many malignant masses do not. Just as on x-ray mammography, the most important feature of a mass that suggests a malignant nature is its morphology.

Although fibroadenomas typically have an oblong shape with the long axis parallel to the skin surface, breast cancers tend to have an AP diameter at least equal to their transverse diameter and appear more rounded. This may be the only clue that a lesion is malignant

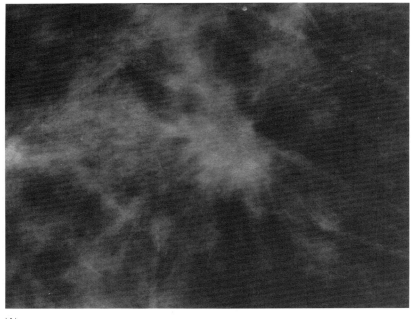

(A)

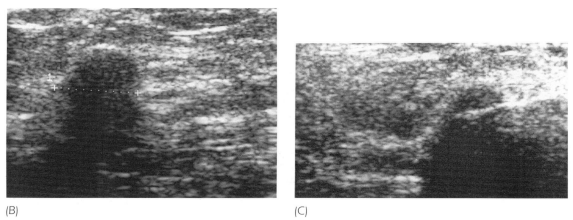

(B)   (C)

Figure 7.14. (A) Magnified view of a spiculated mass. (B) Ultrasonogram demonstrates a poorly circum-scribed, hypoechoic mass with posterior shadowing. (C) An ultrasonogram-guided core needle biopsy was performed with a 14-gauge biopsy needle. The needle can be seen in its entirety perpendicular to the ultrasound beam; the tip is within the mass.

when its borders are well circumscribed and its internal echo texture is homogeneous, as with many medullary and mucinous cancers.

Breast ultrasonography can play a crucial role in evaluating patients who have a normal mammogram and a palpable mass. It is well recognized that very large malignancies that do not produce distortion or do not contain calcification may be undetectable in dense breast tissue. This fact is largely responsible for the significant false-negative rate in the identification of some clinically apparent breast cancers. Few, if any, such cancers will fail to be recognized on ultrasonography, although for various reasons ultrasonography continues to be underused in this setting.

Some cancers may also be mammographically undetectable because of their manner of growth. These include diffuse uncalcified in situ carcinomas, which may occur without evident ductal dilatation on mammography, and invasive lobular carcinomas, which tend to spread by forming sheets of cells along normal breast structures rather than by formation of a distinct mass (Fig. 7.15). Both of these may be manifest clinically as indeterminate areas of thickening that simulate fibrocystic change. Ultrasonography may be helpful in both of these by confirming the presence of abnormal ducts or a mass and thus ensuring prompt intervention rather than follow-up.

Secondary signs of malignancy, such as skin thickening and parenchymal distortion, can be seen with ultrasonography and may be helpful in confirming one's suspicion that an associated mass is likely malignant. Such signs, however, are not diagnostic because they may also be seen with inflammatory and infectious processes. A more useful function of ultrasonography in the diagnostic evaluation of suspected breast cancers is in the identification of satellite lesions, multicentric foci of disease, and chest wall invasion and in the evaluation of the axilla. Disruption of the normal, linear echo-

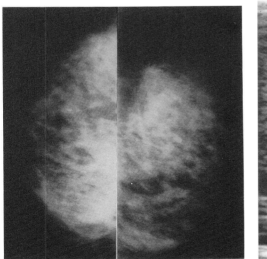 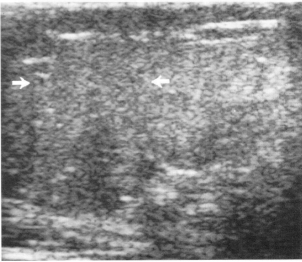

(A)   (B)

Figure 7.15.   (A) This patient presented with a palpable mass in the right upper outer quadrant. Craniocaudal and mediolateral oblique views of the right breast show scattered, fine calcifications and dense glandular tissue. No mass could be seen. (B) Ultrasonography over the palpable abnormality revealed a subtle, poorly circumscribed area of low echogenicity (*arrows*). Ultrasonogram-guided core needle biopsy yielded a diagnosis of invasive lobular carcinoma.

genic lines of the pectoralis muscles adjacent to a suspicious mass may be found in cancers that involve the pectoral muscle. Enlarged, rounded uniformly hypoechoic lymph nodes suggest metastatic involvement.

Fibrocystic Changes

There are findings on ultrasonography that are best classified by the generic term *fibrocystic changes,* given an appropriate clinical history. Ultrasonography is usually performed in these women because of a history of cyclic tenderness, often localized to a particular area in one breast, or because of a focal area of palpable thickening. Rarely is a discrete mass visible unless it corresponds to a cyst. Less often, ultrasonography is performed to add to the level of confidence in the negative interpretation of an extremely dense mammogram. Fibrocystic changes include areas of highly echogenic fibroglandular tissue (fibrosis) containing mildly to moderately ectatic ducts (basket weave pattern). Cysts of varying size can also be seen, ranging from "microcysts" of fewer than 5 mm in diameter to macrocysts 5 to 6 cm in diameter.

Implants

Until the relatively recent advent of specific magnetic resonance techniques for implant imaging, mammography combined with ultrasonography was the only method for the evaluation of breast implants for evidence of leakage or rupture. On routine mammographic views, the implants are included on the film, and their overall contour can be seen. The pushback or Eklund mammographic views are done purposely to exclude the implant from the imaging field to better visualize the breast tissue itself (Fig. 7.16A). Still, portions of the implant and a variable percentage of the breast tissue are invariably excluded from the images. In symptomatic patients or in patients who have concern about the integrity of their implants, ultrasonography can add considerable information. Implants should be evaluated at two transducer depth settings. First, the transducer should be focused near the superficial margin of the implant so that the envelope and the breast tissue anterior to it can be examined. Next, a deeper focal plane should be selected to visualize the contents of the implant itself as well as its posterior margin.

A normal, intact implant has a double echogenic line corresponding to the implant envelope. This line should be continuous in all imaging planes. The appearance of the implant envelope may have some variability, depending on the type of envelope (smooth or textured surface) and whether or not it is a single- or double-lumen implant. Silicone contained within an intact implant should be largely echo free, although a few freely floating echogenic specks

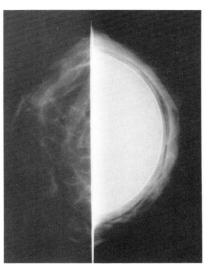
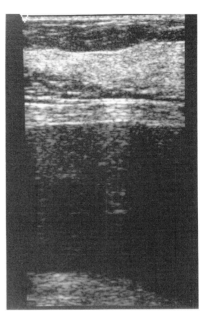

(A)   (B)

Figure 7.16. (A) Right craniocaudal "push-back" and implant views in a patient with subpectoral implants. The contour of the implant is smooth and continuous. The pectoralis muscle can be seen as a density adjacent to the implant. (B) Ultrasonogram of an intact, subpectoral implant. The implant contents are essentially anechoic. (Echoes in the more superficial portion are due to artifact.) The envelope is continuous, and there were no deformities of contour. The pectoralis muscle can be seen as a linear structure just anterior to the implant, and echogenic glandular tissue can be seen just anterior to that.

should not be considered abnormal (Fig. 7.16B). Focal changes in the contour of the implant are compatible with encapsulation of the implant and should not be mistaken for rupture.

Ultrasonography can detect both intra- and extracapsular implant rupture. In the case of an intracapsular leak, the normally echo-free silicone within the confines of the implant shell becomes echogenic. Lucencies within these echogenic areas may represent silicone trapped within the collapsed envelope, but infolding of implants that are not taut may produce the same appearance, and often the distinction cannot be made. Certainly, if the double echogenic line representing the envelope cannot be continuously imaged, rupture should be strongly suspected (Fig. 7.17B). A stair-step pattern of the outer envelope is also strongly suggestive of rupture. As opposed to the normal implant, in which the posterior wall can be seen, an intracapsular rupture will cause posterior acoustic shadowing, and visualization of the deep breast tissue will be precluded. Unfortunately, coarse calcifications surrounding the implant shell, which are often present in long-standing implants possibly because of the phenomenon of gel bleed, may also

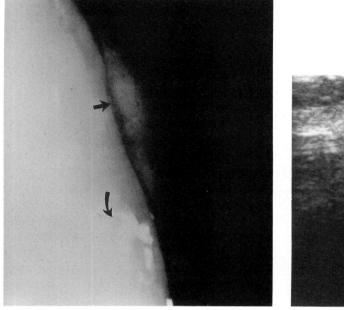
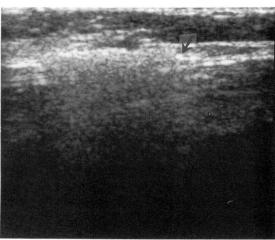

(A)   (B)

Figure 7.17.   (A) A collection of silicone outside the envelope of the implant indicates rupture (*arrow*). There is also dense calcification about the implant (*curved arrow*). (B) Ultrasonogram shows disruption of the double echogenic line of the envelope (*arrow*) and echogenicity within the implant substance consistent with rupture.

produce apparent irregularities and discontinuities of the implant surface simulating the findings of rupture (Fig. 7.17A).

Extracapsular rupture of implants has findings similar to intracapsular rupture with the additional finding of free silicone in the breast parenchyma. The axilla and the medial and lateral chest walls may also be involved. Free silicone is highly echogenic on ultrasonography and demonstrates acoustic shadowing, often producing complete obliteration of the underlying structures, called a "snowstorm" appearance (Fig. 7.18). Echogenic silicone can also be seen in the axillary lymph nodes, which are otherwise hypoechoic. Ultrasonography is more sensitive than mammography alone in detecting free silicone; however, magnetic resonance imaging is more sensitive than both for detecting implant rupture and free silicone and has become the imaging modality of choice when the less expensive methods, x-ray mammography and ultrasonography are not diagnostic.

Computed Tomography

Computed tomography currently has relatively few indications in the investigation of breast lesions. In addition to its expense, a number of technical factors make computed tomography unsuitable for screening. The limited spatial resolution of computed tomography does not

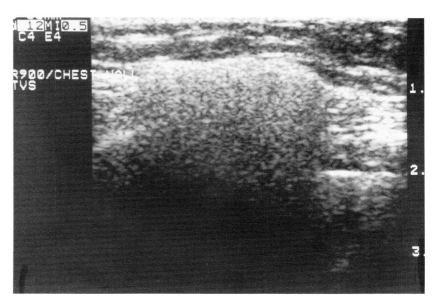

Figure 7.18. Ultrasonogram of free silicone in the soft tissues of the chest wall in a patient whose silicone implants ruptured and were removed. Note the "snow-storm" appearance, obliterating all detail posterior to the silicone.

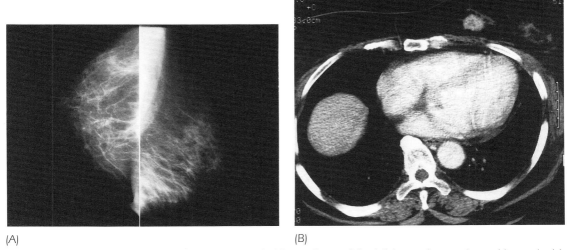

(A)   (B)

Figure 7.19. (A) Craniocaudal and mediolateral oblique views of the left breast in a patient with a palpable mass. Because of its posterior location, the mass slipped off the cassette every time compression was applied. (B) A computed tomographic scan of the chest clearly demonstrates a spiculated mass in the medial aspect of the left breast.

allow identification of potentially important breast microcalcifications. In addition, intravenous contrast is required to allow identification of most breast masses. Computed tomography may have some utility in imaging lesions in areas that are difficult to image on x-ray mammography (e.g., very high, very medial or lateral, or very posterior lesions)

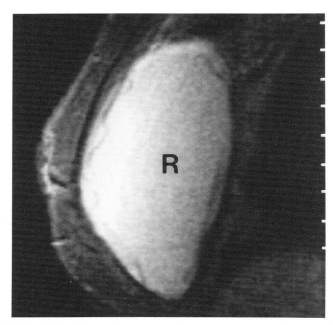

Figure 7.20. T2-weighted, fat-saturated magnetic resonance image of a silicone implant rupture, showing the "linguine sign": the wavy black line extending to the edges of the implant in at least two spots. This line is the collapsed envelope.

(Fig. 7.19) and may occasionally be useful in the evaluation of lesions in patients who will not or cannot be imaged with x-ray mammography, such as some patients with breast prostheses, pacemakers implanted in breast tissue, and so on.

Magnetic Resonance Imaging

Magnetic resonance imaging (MRI) also has limitations that prevent its use as a screening method. These, as for computed tomography, include expense and inability to identify lesions manifest as calcification only. Identification of malignant masses on MRI of the breast is facilitated by the use of gadolinium contrast. A number of studies suggest that MRI may be more sensitive than x-ray mammography for the detection of breast cancer, particularly in dense breasts. Further studies will be necessary to define its utility and indications. Currently, the only widely accepted use for breast MRI is in the patient with strong suspicion of implant rupture that cannot be visualized with x-ray mammography or ultrasonography (Fig. 7.20).

Imaging-guided Biopsies

Fine-needle aspiration and core biopsy of mammographically detected nonpalpable lesions are rapidly gaining acceptability and can significantly improve the yield in surgical biopsies recommended for such lesions. In this country, the ratio of biopsies performed for each cancer detected ranges from 3 to more than 10. Unless other diagnostic methods, such as fine-needle aspiration and core biopsy, are used, it is difficult to exceed a true positive rate of 30% to 40% without missing the smallest occult cancers. Although fine-needle aspiration has a long history of usage for evaluation of palpable breast lesions, its use for nonpalpable lesions is not as well established. Its use in this setting is also limited by the lack of well-trained cytopathologists and by the high percentage of inadequate samples obtained from aspiration of small, nonpalpable lesions. Core biopsy techniques provide histologic samples that can be interpreted by most general pathologists. With appropriate selection of cases, both fine-needle aspiration and core biopsy techniques can improve the true positive yield of x-ray mammography more than 50%, such that one or fewer benign biopsies are performed for each malignancy detected.

X-Ray–guided Procedures

Fine-needle aspiration and core biopsy can be performed with standard mammographic units equipped with add-on stereotactic devices or with stand-alone stereotactic equipment. Some of the newer stereotactic units are now equipped with digital mammography, which significantly increases the ease and speed with which these procedures can be done. Nonetheless, the equipment remains expensive and its cost effectiveness, except in practices in which large numbers of procedures can be done, is questionable. The principle of stereotactic equipment is that one can calculate accurate depth by performing two views of an area angled similarly from opposite directions. With available stereotactic units, the abnormality is positioned within a small rectangular area, and views are obtained angled 15 degrees to each side. The equipment then calculates the appropriate depth of placement of the biopsy needle, and multiple tissue fragments are obtained with a biopsy device as described in the section on ultrasonography-guided procedures. For biopsy of calcified lesions unassociated with mass, some type of stereotactic equipment is required; most true mass lesions can undergo biopsy with ultrasound guidance, and this has been the preferred method at our institution.

Ultrasonography-guided Procedures

The most common breast interventional procedure performed under ultrasound guidance is ultrasonography-guided cyst aspiration. There are three indications for cyst drainage: patient discomfort or anxiety, cystic lesions that do not fulfill the criteria for simple cysts on ultrasonogram, and cysts that are so large as to obscure significant volumes of breast parenchyma.

Cysts may become exquisitely tender, and aspiration can provide prompt relief. Large cysts close to the skin surface may become visible, deforming the contour of the breast. Patients are usually quite grateful to have such cysts aspirated even knowing that they pose no threat. For some women, the knowledge that they have "something" in their breast, even if it is not palpable, is so distressing that they will constantly worry that it might "turn into something." Cyst aspiration can provide enormous relief of anxiety in these women. A nodule that is seen on mammography or that is palpable and that demonstrates the classic findings of a simple cyst on ultrasonogram does not need to be aspirated for diagnosis.

Ultrasonography-guided cyst aspiration may be performed by marking the skin over the site corresponding to the center of the lesion and inserting the needle directly into the lesion to a predetermined depth or by approaching the lesion obliquely with the transducer held over the lesion. The former approach is advantageous for lesions that are large and relatively deep but has the disadvantage that the needle axis is not directly visible (Fig. 7.21). The latter approach is most useful for small, superficially located lesions and has the advantage that the entire needle is visible as it enters the lesion. The skin is prepared with alcohol or povidone-iodine (Betadine). We, as well as our patients, prefer to use local anesthesia for all breast interventions, al-

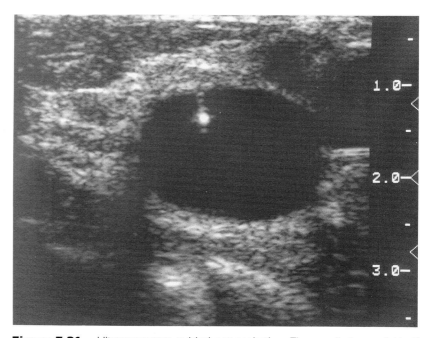

Figure 7.21. Ultrasonogram-guided cyst aspiration. The needle is parallel to the ultrasound beam, and only the tip is visualized within the cyst.

though we recognize that many physicians forgo its use for breast cyst aspirations. A 21-gauge needle attached to a 5- to 10-mL syringe (larger is the cyst is extremely large) is used for aspiration. Often the cyst wall will be quite firm, and a moderate amount of pressure will be required to puncture it. Once as much fluid as possible has been aspirated, with the needle still in place, the area is scanned again to confirm resolution of the cyst. If some fluid remains, the cyst will probably reaccumulate, so it is worthwhile to reposition the needle and try to draw off all fluid that remains. Occasionally, it will not be possible to aspirate any fluid even though the ultrasonogram clearly shows the needle to be properly positioned. In these cases, for example, when aspirating an abscess, it can be helpful to switch to a larger needle; a 20-gauge or larger needle can be used to aspirate very thick fluid.

Sending fluid off for cytologic evaluation is an extremely low-yield procedure, and in most instances it is appropriate to discard the fluid after noting its amount and color. Exceptions include a bloody aspirate in what was believed to be a nontraumatic procedure, and when features of the lesion put it in a high index of suspicion category. Even then, the diagnostic yield is low and if there is a high index of suspicion for malignancy, negative cytology should not preclude further investigation. If the fluid appears to be infected, it may be sent for the appropriate cultures.

The technique for fine-needle aspiration biopsy is essentially the same as for cyst aspiration. Ideally, the cytotechnologist should be in the room, prepared to smear the aspirate on slides immediately. It is also optimal if the cytologist is also present to view the material aspirated under the microscope immediately and advise if more aspirate is needed. A 21-gauge needle is positioned in the lesion and the location confirmed sonographically. If there is any question that the sonographic abnormality corresponds to a mammographic abnormality, a CC and lateral mammogram can be performed at this point to confirm needle placement in the lesion. Negative pressure is applied with an attached syringe as the needle is gently moved about slightly within the lesion. The suction is carefully released and the needle withdrawn. Multiple passes can be made to ensure that adequate material is obtained. A few seconds of firm pressure at the skin entrance site will control any bleeding.

The technique for core needle biopsy differs substantially from cyst aspiration or fine-needle aspiration biopsy. Essential equipment is a large-bore needle cannulated with a cutting device attached to a biopsy gun. The lesions are approached in an oblique horizontal plane such that the length of the biopsy needle can be imaged along the transducer's linear array and can actually be seen to enter the lesion when the biopsy gun is fired (see Fig. 7.14C). If the position of the lesion will allow it, choosing an entrance site for the needle in a radial location from the lesion will facilitate moving the needle through the breast tissue, presumably because fewer of the "support" structures like Cooper's ligaments have to be crossed. After appropriate skin preparation, the entire anticipated path of the needle should be anesthetized. Lidocaine (1%), with a small amount of epinephrine (1:10,000), is used to reduce bleeding. (The epinephrine is not necessary with any other procedure.) A small nick is made in the skin with a No. 11 surgical blade. The transducer is positioned over the lesion with the long axis parallel to the needle.

The needle is ideally positioned parallel to the chest wall, with the tip just at the proximal edge of the lesion. The throw distance of the cutting device varies by manufacturer. If the core needle tip is too close to a small lesion, the cutting device may go through the lesion and take a sample beyond it. That the cutting device indeed passes through the lesion can be confirmed by ultrasonogram and then the needle is withdrawn. Most of the time a visible needle tract remains in the lesion marking each pass. Four to five passes that are clearly within the lesion are generally adequate for a diagnosis. After the biopsy, the patient holds firm pressure with an ice pack over the biopsy site for 15 minutes.

Timing and Length of Follow-up Examinations

Short-term follow-up is not indicated for any lesion characterized as pathognomonically benign or any lesion with a high likelihood of malignancy. For lesions in the indeterminate category, follow-up may be elected after all appropriate evaluations have been completed. Considerations in recommending follow-up rather than biopsy for a solitary mass that appears solid on ultrasonographic examination include the following:

1. Palpable or nonpalpable (biopsy more likely if palpable)
2. Size (biopsy more likely if larger than 1.5 cm)
3. Margin characteristics (biopsy more likely if margins irregular)
4. History of biopsy for similar lesion
5. Patient age (biopsy more likely for older patient)
6. Patient preference (family history, anxiety make biopsy more likely)
7. Medicolegal considerations
8. Available data on breast cancer growth rates
9. Reliability of benign diagnoses made on the basis of fine-needle aspiration cytology or core biopsy in a given institution

If mammographic follow-up is elected, a mammogram consisting of at least two views of the abnormal breast should be performed at 6 months. Doubling times for breast cancers are highly variable, but doubling times of 30 days or less are exceedingly rare (Table 7.2).

Except for the most rapidly growing cancers—note: volume doubling times of fewer than 30 days have not been observed for primary

Table 7.2. Expected change in diameter of a 5-mm breast cancer followed for 6 months at various doubling times*

Volume doubling time (days)	Tumor diameter after 6 months (mm)
30	20.0
60	10.0
120	7.0
240	6.0
1000	5.2

*Exponential growth of a single focus is assumed.

breast cancers in vivo—tumor size should not exceed 1 cm with a 6-month follow-up interval. In fact, rapid growth of a mass (e.g., from 5 mm to 5 cm in fewer than 6 months) is highly likely to be due to a benign process (expanding cyst, hematoma, seroma, abscess). Thus, follow-up intervals of less than 6 months are likely to be helpful only to follow resolution of benign disease.

How long should short-term follow-up be continued if the mass appears stable at the 6-month follow-up? Although it is recognized that stability of a mammographic mass over several years does not guarantee benignity, it is probably safe to assume that a cancer that does not grow or that grows very slowly is not a threat to life at that stage of its development. Accordingly, 6-month follow-ups for 2 to 3 years should be sufficient to identify most potentially life-threatening lesions.

ANALYSIS OF CALCIFICATION

Is it in the breast? There are many causes of artifactual calcification on mammograms. Improper screen maintenance, processing artifacts, dust, fingerprints, and so on can all produce confusing specks that mimic microcalcification. Optimum mammography requires meticulous attention to detail. Lotions, powder, ointments, deodorant, tattoos, and other material applied to the skin may also mimic calcification. Projection of some of the patient's hair into the x-ray beam will also produce opacities that look like calcification.

Once potentially significant calcifications have been identified, the following characteristics must be described:

1. Location
2. Size of focus or foci and extent
3. Morphology
4. Distribution

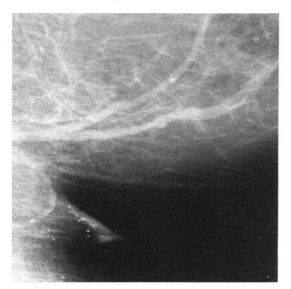

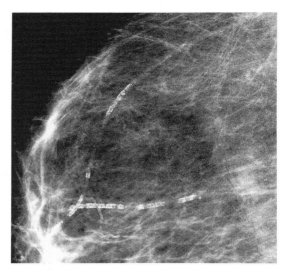

Figure 7.22. *Skin calcifications. These are small, round calcifications with lucent centers that represent calcifications in skin pores. They are typically seen in the medial inferior portion of the breast, although they can be seen anywhere. If there is any question of the nature of these calcifications, tangential views can establish their location in the skin. These calcifications do not require biopsy.*

Figure 7.23. *Typical vascular calcifications of the breast. The soft tissue density of the blood vessel itself cannot always be seen. These calcifications do not require biopsy.*

Location, size, and extent are important descriptors but have relatively little differential diagnostic value. Extent alone is a poor indicator of benignity. Malignant calcifications may involve all or most of a breast or even both breasts. Unfortunately, too often it is assumed that extensive fine calcification occupying a large volume of breast tissue is benign and that stability of calcifications over time indicates a benign process. Neither of these features is a reliable determinant. The absolute number of calcifications present in a focus is used by many mammographers as a determinant of biopsy. Five is a popular number, but again this is of relatively limited utility. Ten uniform punctate calcifications have a high likelihood of being benign, whereas one or two thin rods may well be malignant.

Morphology and distribution are the most important characteristics of calcifications to be considered. In combination, these allow some calcifications to be dismissed as pathognomonically benign and others to be recognized as almost assuredly malignant.

Pathognomonically benign calcifications (Figs. 7.2, 7.8, 7.11, 7.22–7.24) include the following:

1. Artifacts
2. Skin calcifications

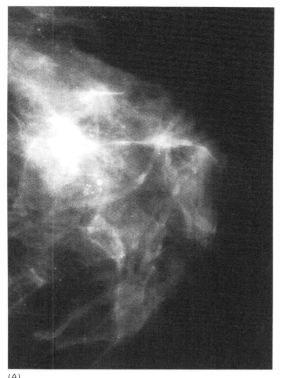 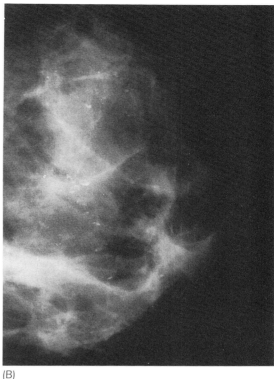

(A)   (B)

Figure 7.24. (A) Lateral craniocaudal view and (B) left oblique view. There are rounded, "smudgy" calcifications scattered throughout the breast. These change in configuration on the oblique view, seen as curvilinear densities. These are classic "teacup" calcifications or "milk of calcium" that is found in microcysts. The ease with which the change in configuration of the calcifications can be seen on the oblique view varies with the amount of obliquity. If there is any question, a true lateral view can confirm the presence of milk of calcium. These calcifications do not require biopsy.

3. Vascular calcifications
4. Benign intraductal calcifications
5. Foreign bodies
6. Spheric calcifications, particularly with lucent centers
7. Milk of calcium
8. Dystrophic or popcorn calcification

Artifacts are common but are unlikely to cause great concern unless they appear on both projections. If this is the case, a repeat film should be performed once the likely cause has been identified and, it is hoped, corrected. Skin calcifications are also common. They are usually small and round with lucent centers and are most commonly seen near the chest wall medially and inferiorly. Vascular calcifications have a distinctive parallel track appearance when larger vessels are involved. When the calcifications are in smaller vessels, the two individual wall calcifications may not be resolved. Fortunately, this most often occurs in settings in which extensive large-vessel calcification is also present. The serpiginous, branching nature of vascular calcifications is also a helpful distinguishing characteristic.

Duct ectasia may be associated with calcification. In most cases, the calcification is intraductal, either associated with inspissated material within the duct lumen, which is uniformly calcified or associated with calcification around debris, resulting in a lucent center. Periductal calcification also occurs, most commonly with plasma cell mastitis, and may also produce rounded or tubular calcifications with lucent centers. Most commonly, duct ecstasia (so-called secretory disease) is characterized by relatively long and relatively thick (>0.5 mm) calcifications, some of which may branch. When the rod-like calcifications are very fine, they cannot be reliably differentiated from malignant calcifications, although typically in such instances both fine and coarse rods will be present and will be present in both breasts.

Foreign substances injected into the breast for augmentation, such as paraffin and silicone, may cause formation of granulomas, which often calcify. Numerous rounded or ovoid nodules with rim calcification are the result. Sutures may calcify. The calcifications are usually curvilinear or tubular, and knots may be readily apparent. Cyst wall calcification may occur in fluid-filled cysts of fibrocystic disease, or oil cysts resulting from fat necrosis may calcify. Uniform, round or oval rim ("eggshell") calcification is the usual appearance. Occasionally, a dilated duct will calcify; however, ductal calcification is usually elongated on at least one projection. When numerous, round, uniform size, tiny (<0.5 mm) calcifications are present, widely distributed in both breasts, they are most often due to benign proliferative disease in the breast, often sclerosing adenosis or papillomatosis. Identifying malignant calcification in such breasts may be quite challenging.

Microcysts occurring in cases of cystic hyperplasia may contain calcific debris. When imaged in an upright true lateral projection, the calcification will conform to the dependent portion of the cyst, producing a "teacup" or meniscal shape. In the orthogonal projection, such calcification is often less apparent and appears fuzzy or indistinct.

Dystrophic calcifications may occur in any traumatized area and are often found in irradiated breasts. The calcifications are usually relatively large and irregular in shape and may have lucent centers. Hyalinized fibroadenomas that have been present for many years may develop distinctive coarse clumps of calcification. If most or all of the tumor calcifies, a distinctive "popcorn" configuration of calcification is seen.

Regarding indeterminate or malignant calcification, individual calcifications in a cluster that are amorphous or indistinct on both orthogonal projections cannot be characterized as definitively benign. Although most such calcifications will be associated with benign disease, biopsy is usually indicated. Pleomorphic granular-type calcifications carry an even higher risk of being malignant, and their identification will usually result in a recommendation for biopsy. If malignancy is found in cases of amorphous or granular calcification without associated mass, it is more likely to be of the small cell, or noncomedo variety of ductal carcinoma in situ. The calcifications in such instances are not readily distinguishable from benign processes such as sclerosing adenosis, and distribution may be the most important discriminant (Fig. 7.25).

The most distinctively malignant calcifications are fine linear ("casting") calcifications (Figs. 7.4 and 7.26). The calcifications conform to a duct lumen that is irregularly filled with carcinoma. Because of this, the outer surface of the calcification is usually more irregular than in duct ectasia, the calcifications are often discontinuous, and they may branch. These calcifications are often seen in association with other pleomorphic calcifications in a so-called shattered glass pattern: variable size, variable shape, jagged (Table 7.3).

It is important to remember that none of the determinants listed in Table 7.3 is absolute. Cancers may contain macrocalcifications, and the number of calcifications in them may be few. Extensive scattered calcification may be malignant, and breasts may contain both benign

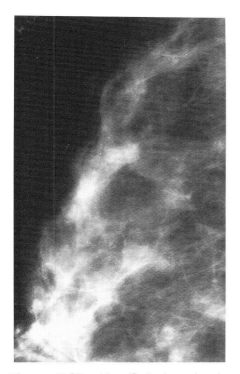

Figure 7.25. *Magnified view showing scattered fine calcifications of sclerosing adenosis. These can be virtually indistinguishable from noncomedo types of ductal carcinoma in situ.*

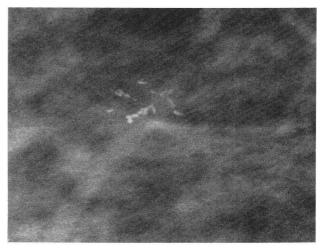

Figure 7.26. *Magnified view of typical casting-type calcifications associated with comedo-type ductal carcinoma in situ. They are irregular in size and density. There were no other calcifications elsewhere in either breast.*

Table 7.3. Factors affecting predilection to malignancy and benignity

Factor	Favor malignancy	Favor benignity
Number	Many	Few
Size	Micro (<0.5 mm)	Macro
Focality	Clustered	Scattered
Morphology	Irregular, pleomorphic	Uniform
Stability	Changing	Unchanging

and malignant calcifications. New calcifications may occur with benign disease and malignant calcifications may resorb. Lesions should always be judged by their worst features (e.g., a malignant-appearing mass with benign calcification in a patient without clinical history to support trauma or infection should be presumed malignant). Conversely, a benign-appearing mass with suspicious calcifications should not be presumed benign. It is also important to recognize the importance of direct correlation of mammographic and histologic findings, to avoid the trap that any calcific focus, no matter how benign appearing, may be an indicator of breast cancer. Biopsy of benign calcifications may lead to detection of coincidental cancers or high-risk lesions, such as lobular carcinoma in situ and atypical hyperplasia. This does not mean that one should perform a biopsy of every cluster of calcification regardless of its appearance any more than surgeons should perform a biopsy on every area of thickening because occasionally they also find coincidental occult cancer.

Histologically detectable calcifications may not be mammographically apparent; radiographically detected calcifications may not be apparent on the histologic specimens. In the first instance, the calcifications are too small to resolve on radiographs; in the second, there are several possible explanations. Larger calcifications may be shattered by the microtome; smaller calcifications may be leached out by acid fixatives used in processing of the histologic sections. The radiographic calcifications may be at a deeper level of the paraffin block than was used for the slides interpreted, or they may only be visible microscopically using polarized light.

Results of Screening Studies

The first randomized, controlled trial of breast cancer screening was begun 30 years ago under the auspices of the Health Insurance Plan (HIP) of New York. This trial showed a 20% reduction in breast cancer mortality through 18 years of follow-up for the women allocated to the screening arm. Screening in the HIP trial involved annual physical examination and mammography for 5 years. Compliance was relatively poor compared to later trials, the mammography used was that available in the 1960s, and comparatively few cancers diagnosed were so-called minimal breast cancers (invasive cancer smaller than 1 cm or in situ ductal cancer). Nonetheless, the trial was important for demonstrating that breast cancer death rates could be reduced by screening.

Two randomized, controlled trials performed in Sweden in the early 1970s, the Swedish W-E (two county) trial and the Malmo trial, demonstrated that similar reductions in breast cancer mortality were achievable with use of mammography alone. Compliance was better than in the HIP trial, mammography was that available in the early 1970s, and only a single-view mammogram was performed at 2- to 3-year intervals. At 12 years of follow-up, the Swedish two-county trial showed a 30% reduction in mortality among the women invited to undergo screening.

Several other randomized, controlled trials, as well as case-control studies, have been performed (Table 7.4). The trials are not equivalent in many ways, differing in study design, type and quality of mammography, compliance rates, screening intervals, and length of follow-up. There has been a regrettable tendency to regard all the trials as equivalent, leading to projections regarding the efficacy of current-day mammography, which cannot be justified on the basis of the available data. The data from the randomized, controlled trials are too disparate to be suitable for a meta-analysis. Unfortunately, there is no available trial that indicates what is achievable with state-of-the-art mammography of the 1990s performed at yearly intervals. Still, despite the flaws in the trials performed to date, it is possible to conclude that significant mortality reductions can be expected from mammographic screening of women aged 50 to 65 years.

Table 7.4. Breast cancer screening trials

Trial	Interval	No. rounds	PE	Patient age range (yr)	N	RR	Follow-up
Randomized controlled trials							
HIP	1	4	Y	40–64	61,000	8	0.79
Swedish W-E	2–3	3	N	40–74	133,000	8	0.79
Malmo	1–2	5	N	45–69	42,000	11	0.83
Edinburgh	2	4	Y	45–64	45,000	7	0.84
Canada	1	5	Y	40–49	50,430	7	1.36
Canada	1	5	Y	50–59	39,405	7	0.97
Case-control studies							
BCDDP	1	5	Y	35–74	55,000	9	0.80
Nijmegen	2	4	Y	35+	52,000	7	0.48
Utrecht	1–2	4	Y	50–64	36,000	7	0.30
Florence	2.5	6	N	40–70	40,000	7	0.53

PE = physical examination included; RR = relative risk; HIP = Health Insurance Plan of New York; BCDDP = Breast Cancer Detection Demonstration Project.

The available data are less compelling for women younger than 50 years. Although breast cancer is a major cause of mortality in this age group, the prevalence of the disease is considerably lower than in older women; thus, the necessity for a more "perfect" test. The results of the National Breast Screening Study (NBSS), often referred to as the Canadian trial, have been interpreted as demonstrating that screening mammography is ineffective in younger women. This trial included women in the early 1980s to be screened with annual mammography and physical examination. Quality control of mammography, particularly in the early years of patient accrual, was considerably less than ideal. In addition, for reasons still poorly explained, a disproportionate number of women with advanced-stage breast cancer were allocated to the screening arm of the trial. This fact, along with significant contamination of the control arm resulting from a 26% rate of mammography among the women allocated to the control group, makes interpretation of the early mortality data hazardous.

Insufficient numbers of women were screened in the Canadian trial to make up for the selection bias and contamination that occurred. The impact of screening is delayed in younger women because breast cancer deaths, other than those resulting from advanced-stage disease on which screening has no impact, take longer to occur and accumulate; therefore, it is possible that benefit, even if it occurred under the suboptimal conditions of the NBSS trial, will not be demonstrable for several more years.

THE DIAGNOSTIC MAMMOGRAM

Until recently, most breast cancers were self-detected as a result of the presence of a palpable mass. Currently, more than 50% of breast cancers are mammographically detected. A very small percentage are detected because of nipple discharge, Paget's disease, axillary adenopathy, or the appearance of distant metastases. The remaining are still detected because of a palpable abnormality, and most are detected by the woman herself rather than by a physician.

Although both self-examination and physical examination are capable of detecting breast cancers, for the most part neither of these detects breast cancer at an early curable stage. The threshold for physical detection of breast cancer by skilled examiners appears to be about 6 mm. Even up to 1.5 cm in size, the majority of cancers are not detectable by palpation. Once breast cancers exceed this size, most are detectable both by palpation and mammography. Nonetheless, it should be emphasized that the greatest potential for cure occurs when tumors are detected before they attain this size, which can only be reliably achieved by screening mammography.

This does not suggest that self-examination and physical examination of the breasts have no role in breast cancer identification. The false-negative rates for mammography cover a broad range from a low of 5% to a high of 69%. Self-examination has some desirable features in that, aside from the anxiety it induces in some women and the time involved in its performance, it has no cost. Some studies have shown that women who routinely perform self-examination detect their cancers at a more favorable stage than those who do not.

It is probably desirable to encourage self-examination and annual physical examination of the breasts by a physician for those women whose mammograms are most likely to result in a false-negative result (i.e., any woman with dense breast tissue). Whether there is significant benefit to be derived by physical examination of the breasts in women whose breasts are fatty replaced and who are having annual mammography of high quality can be questioned. The current American Cancer Society guidelines recommend that women begin breast self-examination at the age of 20 years and have annual physical examinations of their breasts by a physician beginning at age 40 years.

The detection rate of breast cancer by mammography is highly correlated with the mammographic density of the breast. Assuming optimal technique and positioning, nearly all cancers arising in breasts composed of predominantly adipose tissue should be detectable. The detection rate of cancer in a breast composed of predominantly fibrous or glandular tissue may be a low as 50% or 60%. Cancers manifest by microcalcifications are still detectable in such breasts, but cancers developing as nondescript soft tissue densities will fail to be appreciated until they either distort the surrounding parenchyma or are large enough or superficial enough to produce an abnormality in contour or secondary sign such as skin thickening or retraction.

Patients Presenting with Palpable Abnormalities

There is a wide range of possibilities when one is dealing with "palpable" areas in the breast. These may represent anything from normal tissue to advanced malignant lesions. For patients with true three-dimensional mass lesions on palpation, the likelihood of malignancy is about 20%. A number of factors increase the likelihood that a palpated mass will be malignant. These include the age of the patient, her risk profile, whether her mammogram is also abnormal, and the presence of associated secondary signs of malignancy or palpable lymph nodes.

In the patient with clinically apparent breast cancer, an x-ray mammogram is still mandatory. The mammogram is particularly important for evaluation of the contralateral breast and is also useful for assessing the extent of involvement of the ipsilateral breast.

Patients with palpable breast masses who do not have either definitively benign or malignant corresponding masses on mammography require further diagnostic evaluation. This includes a full mammographic workup, which may include any of the additional views listed in the section on workup of screen-detected abnormalities. If mammographic workup is completed and the mass remains indeterminate, further evaluation is indicated. This may include ultrasonography, fine-needle aspiration, or core biopsy or some combination of these.

Ultrasonography, as described previously, may be particularly helpful in the evaluation of mass lesions obscured by surrounding dense tissue. Breast cancer masses are virtually always hypoechoic lesions. Because the fibrous and glandular elements of the breast are echogenic, these masses are readily appreciable on ultrasonogram and they may be totally inapparent on x-ray mammography. In our experience, palpable breast cancer is virtually always detectable on high-quality breast ultrasonograms even and perhaps particularly if undetectable on x-ray mammography (see Fig. 7.15).

Needle Localization Biopsy

Surgical excision of a suspicious mammographic abnormality requires special techniques to ensure that the appropriate area is removed without sacrifice of large amounts of uninvolved breast tissue. Various methods of preoperative localization have been developed for this purpose. In the United States, needle localization methods are the most popular; localization with vital dyes and inert carbon is used somewhat more frequently in Europe.

Two critical steps are involved in localization methods: 1) placement of a marker (e.g., needle, wire, dye, carbon) in or near the lesion to be removed using x-ray mammographic, ultrasonographic, or stereotactic guidance, and 2) performance of a specimen radiograph of the excised tissue, preferably at the time of surgery. Specimen radiographs should be performed in *all* breast biopsies requiring localization to ensure that the appropriate tissue has been excised (see Figs. 7.4 and 7.7). Both masses and foci of calcification are well depicted in properly performed specimen radiographs, and information may be derived regarding multifocality and the presence or absence of an intraductal component.

The successful needle localization is a cooperative effort involving the patient, radiologist, surgeon, and pathologist. For needle localizations performed with x-ray mammographic guidance, the needle is inserted in the projection that provides the shortest distance to the lesion. Although this can be performed freehand, estimating distance and position from preliminary orthogonal views, most American radiologists prefer to use a localizing grid and an approach that parallels the chest wall. The skin over the chosen needle entry site is prepared, and local anesthesia may be administered. A needle containing a thin wire is then inserted into the breast through an opening in the plastic compression plate, immobilizing the breast. The needle is then advanced fully or until a lesion is encountered. (Although lesions requiring needle localization for biopsy are by definition nonpalpable, they may provide a different resistance to the needle tip if they are actually traversed by the needle.) A mammogram in the appropriate projection, lateral for CC approaches or CC for lateral approaches, is then obtained to assess depth of the needle relative to the area being localized. Adjustment is made, if necessary, and the wire is extruded from the needle. In most cases, the needle is then withdrawn. A final set of mammograms in lateral and CC projections is obtained to show the position of the tip of the wire relative to the lesion. More than one wire may be placed to bracket an extensive area of involvement or to localize multiple lesions.

Localization of lesions for surgical biopsy can also be performed with ultrasound guidance. It is quicker and easier than with x-ray methods, and has the advantage that the needle enters the breast along the axis closest to that which will be used for surgical access. We prefer the use of retractable needle-wire assemblies for ultrasonogram-guided needle localizations. Once the needle is placed in the suspicious lesion, the wire is deployed and lateral and CC mammograms are performed, both to confirm that the proper area is localized and for the surgeon to refer to in the operating room. The deployed wire prevents migration of the needle during the manipulation of the breast during the mammogram. If the mammogram shows that the needle is not properly located, the wire can be retracted and the needle repositioned. Either of the techniques described for ultrasonogram-guided cyst aspiration, direct or oblique approaches, can be used. To ensure that the needle does not penetrate the chest wall when the direct approach is chosen, it may be helpful to pull the breast tissue forward manually as the needle is introduced and then advance it further if necessary under ultrasonogram guidance. This is particularly helpful in patients with very thick skin (a skin nick may solve this problem as well) or in those with very fibrous breast tissue or very firm lesions. As with biopsies localized with x-ray mammography, a radiograph of the surgical specimen is mandatory.

An understanding of the various methods available for breast imaging and diagnosis is essential for all those involved in health care for women. Tremendous advances have been made in the last few decades both in our ability to identify significant breast disease and to diagnose it with minimal anxiety, trauma, and cost. It is an area that remains in evolution, and one can confidently anticipate that the coming years will see further progress and better methods to ensure that more and more breast cancers are identified at a curable stage. Eventually, one can hope that the ultimate goal—prevention—will be achieved, making most of the foregoing chapter of historic interest only.

BIBLIOGRAPHY

Basic Texts

Bassett LW, ed. Breast imaging: current status and future directions. Philadelphia: WB Saunders, 1992.

Kopans DB. Breast imaging. Philadelphia: JB Lippincott, 1989.

NCRP. Mammography: a user's guide, report no. 85. Bethesda, MD: National Commission on Radiological Protection, 1986.

Page DL, Anderson TJ. Diagnostic histopathology of the breast. New York: Churchill Livingstone, 1989.

Tabar L, Dean PB. Teaching atlas of mammography. New York: Thieme-Stratton, 1983.

Supplementary Texts

Bland KI, Copeland EM III. The breast: comprehensive management of benign and malignant diseases. Philadelphia: WB Saunders, 1991.

Haagensen CD. Diseases of the breast. Philadelphia: WB Saunders, 1986.

Harris JR, Hellman S, Henderson IC, Kinne DW. Breast diseases. 2nd ed. Philadelphia: JB Lippincott, 1991.

Lanyi M. Diagnosis and differential diagnosis of breast calcifications. Berlin: Springer-Verlag, 1986.

Parker SH, Jobe WE. Percutaneous breast biopsy. New York: Raven Press, 1993.

Svane G, Potchen EJ, Sierra A, Azavedo E. Screening mammography: breast cancer diagnosis in asymptomatic women. St. Louis: CV Mosby, 1993.

Journal Articles

Bird RE. Low-cost screening mammography: report on finances and review of 21,716 consecutive cases. Radiology 1989;171:87–90.

Bird RE, Wallace TW, Yankaskas BC. Analysis of cancers missed at screening mammography. Radiology 1992;184:613–617.

Caskey CI, Berg WA, Anderson ND, et al. Breast implant rupture: diagnosis with US. Radiology 1994;190:819–823.

Chu KC, Smart CR, Tarone RE. Analysis of breast cancer mortality and stage distribution by age for the Health Insurance Plan clinical trial. J Natl Cancer Inst 1988;80:1125–1132.

Dodd GD. American Cancer Society guidelines on screening for breast cancer: an overview. CA Cancer J Clin 1992;42:177–180.

Dupont WD, Page DL. Risk factors for breast cancer in women with proliferative breast disease. N Engl J Med 1985;312:156–161.

Egan RL, McSweeney MB, Sewell CW. Intramammary calcifications without an associated mass in benign and malignant diseases. Radiology 1980; 131:1–7.

Eklund GW, Busby RC, Miller SH, Job JS. Improved imaging of the augmented breast. AJR 1988;151:469–473.

Feig SA, Shaber GS, Patchefsky A, et al. Analysis of clinically occult and mammographically occult breast tumors. AJR 1977;128:403–408.

Fisher B, Redmond C, Poisson R, et al. Eight-year results of a randomized clinical trial comparing total mastectomy and lumpectomy with or without irradiation in the treatment of breast cancer. N Engl J Med 1989;320:822–828.

Gorczyca DP, DeBruhl ND, Ahn CY, et al. Silicone breast implant ruptures in an animal model: comparison of mammography, MR imaging, US, and CT. Radiology 1994;190:227–232.

Haus AG, Feig SA, Ehrlich SM, et al. Mammography screening: technology, radiation dose and risk, quality control and benefits to society. Radiology 1990;174:627–656.

Martin JE, Moskowitz M, Milbrath JR. Breast cancer missed by mammography. AJR 1979;132:737–739.

Mendelson EB. Evaluation of the postoperative breast. Radiol Clin North Am 1992;30:281–312.

Mendelson EB, Harris KM, Doshi N, Tobon H. Infiltrating lobular carcinoma: mammographic patterns with pathologic correlation. AJR 1989;153:265–271.

Parker SH, Lovin JD, Jobe WE, et al. Nonpalpable breast lesions: stereotactic automated large-core biopsies. Radiology 1991;180:403–407.

Rubin E, Dempsey PJ, Pile NS, et al. Needle-localization biopsy of the breast: impact of a selective core needle biopsy program on yield. Radiology 1995;195:627–631.

Schnitt S, Silen W, Sadowsky N, et al. Ductal carcinoma in situ. N Engl J Med 1988;318:898–903.

Seidman H, Stellman SD, Mushinski MH. A different perspective on breast cancer risk factors: some implications of the nonattributable risk. CA Cancer J Clin 1982;32:301–313.

Sickles EA. Periodic mammographic follow-up of probably benign lesions: results in 3,184 consecutive cases. Radiology 1991;179:463–468.

Sickles EA, Kopans DB. Deficiencies in the analysis of breast cancer screening data. J Natl Cancer Inst 1993;85:1621–1624.

Sigfusson BF, Andersson I, Aspoegren E, et al. Clustered breast calcifications. Acta Radiol 1983;24:273–281.

Tabår L, Dean PB, Pentek Z. Galactography: the procedure of choice for nipple discharge. Radiology 1983;149:31–38.

Tabår L, Fagerberg G, Duffy SW, et al. Update of the Swedish two-county program of mammographic screening for breast cancer. Radiol Clin North Am 1992;30:187–210.

Wellings SR, Alpers CA. Subgross pathologic features and incidence of radial scars in the breast. Hum Pathol 1984;15:475–479.

Wolfe JN. Breast patterns as an index of risk for developing breast cancer. AJR 1976;126:1130–1139.

8

Magnetic Resonance Imaging of the Female Breast

Philip J. Kenney

It has been some 15 years since the first report of magnetic resonance imaging (MRI) of breast carcinoma (1). The initial stimulus for use of MRI was largely curiosity concerning this newest of imaging methods. MRI should be worth investigating in this area because it has inherent sensitivity to differences in normal and pathologic tissues and it does not present the same concern of potential carcinogenesis as do diagnostic x-ray methods. In addition, there are deficiencies in standard methods both for detection of breast cancer and breast implant disorders. Considerable work has been done with MRI, and this work has confirmed that MRI does have great potential as a diagnostic imaging method for detection of disorders of the female breast. In particular, MRI has been shown to be the best imaging procedure for evaluation of breast implants (2). Several authors have reported impressive results for detection of breast cancer with MRI (3,4).

Nevertheless, the role of MRI in female breast disease remains uncertain, particularly with regard to breast tumors. MRI is a very expensive procedure with limited availability. Except for evaluation of suspected implant rupture, there have been no studies that document cost-effective superiority of MRI over other methods of diagnosis. In addition, there is considerable variation in the capabilities of different instruments and radiologists. Many of the published studies were done using specialized techniques not available in general practice. Further technical developments can be expected, and the usefulness of MRI will probably increase with both technical evolution and more clinical studies.

GENERAL TECHNICAL ASPECTS

Many years of experience have shown that critical attention to the quality of image production (as well as interpretation) is needed to optimize the value of x-ray mammography. In the same way, the method used to produce images will greatly affect the accuracy of MRI for diagnosis of breast disease. In some regards, the breast should be easy to image well with MRI: It is superficial, relatively small, is composed of a limited number of tissues, and is prone to a relatively limited number of diseases. With a specialized coil designed to image the breast, it should be possible to achieve images with both high spatial resolution and good contrast between the different tissues (i.e., fat, water, silicone, cancer). Because MRI is a cross-sectional technique, there is no need to compress the breast, which can produce discomfort. However, imaging the breast also presents some challenges. Without a specialized coil, images of the breast using the standard body coil will have low spatial resolution (such that small tumors or small leaks of silicone would not be detectable). Not all MRI manufacturers have produced specialized breast coils, and, because of the expense, not all imaging centers have obtained these even if available. The superficiality of the breast also presents a difficulty because of the air interface and the nonuniform shape, which can contribute to artifacts. Although there are a limited number of tissues in the breast, the architecture is not regularly organized as in the brain or kidney (where distortion of the normal architecture is a sign of disease). In the breast, there is an unpredictable mixture of fat and glandular tissue with many interfaces between fat- and water-predominant tissues (Fig. 8.1). This produces many chemical shift artifacts on T2-weighted images. In addition, if looking for a small, bright spot of enhancement on a postcontrast study (believed by most to be the best sign of tumor), one must literally look for a "needle in the haystack" among all the bright spots produced by fat.

In general, MRI of the female breast is best done with a specialized coil designed for imaging the breast. These allow good image quality as well as reliable, relatively comfortable patient positioning. The patient is usually placed prone, with the breasts not compressed and dependent on openings in the device, with the receiving coils around the breasts. Some devices allow imaging of only one breast at a time, some image both at the same time, some allow selection of one or both. There is no inherent advantage of high field strength, although much of the published work has been done at 1.5 T. Good coils and imaging sequences are more important than field strength.

Although normal and abnormal structures in the breast, including masses, can sometimes be seen on the standard T1- and T2-weighted sequences used for most parts of the body, most investigators have found that these sequences are not optimal for differentiation of abnor-

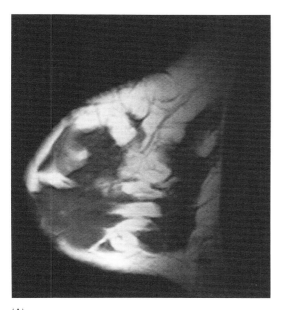
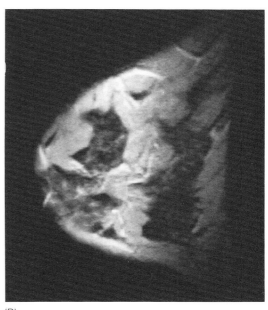

(A)   (B)

Figure 8.1.   Sagittal (chest wall to the right) views of a normal breast in a young woman with (A) T1- and (B) T2-weighted spin echo technique in a specialized breast imaging coil. Note the glandular breast tissue is relatively low signal on both scans and is interspersed with high-signal fat.

malities. For implants, methods that highlight (or suppress) silicone, suppress fat, and enhance differences between silicone and saline are most useful.

A large variety of imaging techniques have been advocated for the detection of breast tumors. It has been noted that "the use of contrast agents is mandatory for distinguishing benign from malignant breast disease, and there is unanimous agreement that early enhancement is an important feature of breast carcinoma" (5). Other than this, there is no consensus regarding the preferred imaging technique for breast cancer. The optimal dose of contrast, imaging time, type of imaging sequence, and method for documentation of enhancement are all controversial. The decisions partly relate to the role for which MRI is being used: primarily for detection of an abnormality or primarily for diagnosis of a known lesion. In part, the decision is difficult because of the current limits of MRI scanners. It is not currently possible to repeatedly image the entire breast (certainly not both breasts simultaneously) with the thin slices needed (<5 mm) in the short time period (<60 seconds) that would seem optimal. One must choose rapid, repetitive imaging of a limited volume of tissue or less rapid imaging of a large volume of tissue.

Further investigation will likely lead to further technical developments. However, developments by the manufacturers will be limited until consensus develops regarding the acceptable role for MRI, so the proper methods to attain that goal can be designed. This development will occur only if it is likely the research investment is sound to the manufacturer.

MRI OF BREAST IMPLANTS

It has been estimated that some 2 million women in the United States have had breast implants either for reconstruction after mastectomy or trauma, or for cosmetic reasons. Because of both the actual incidence of significant complications of these implants and the emotional concern surrounding the issue, there has been a need for a definitive, noninvasive diagnostic method. Many implant ruptures will be signaled by symptoms and physical signs, but some ruptures are asymptomatic, and some patients with suggestive symptoms or signs do not have rupture. Both x-ray mammography and sonography have limitations in detection of implant complications. Mammography is often especially uncomfortable for patients with implants. Both mammography and sonography are poor at demonstrating abnormalities deep within or posterior to an implant. A better diagnostic method could help properly select patients for surgical removal.

MRI should be capable of evaluating implants. Not only should MRI be capable of imaging the breast well, when using proper technique as discussed previously, but MRI can take advantage of the differences among silicone, water, and fat. All of these tissue types have different MRI characteristics. Silicone implant rupture is the greatest concern, and technique is selected to optimize detection of this. Methods that highlight (or suppress) signal from silicone, suppress fat signal, and enhance differences between silicone and saline- or water-containing tissues (glandular tissue, cysts, or serous fluid) are most useful. Fast inversion recovery (STIR) or fast-spin echo T2-weighted sequences (with or without water suppression) have been most widely used with good results (6). Although some specialized sequences have been advocated for detection of silicone (7,8), they are not widely available. Also the factors of time of acquisition and spatial resolution may predominate over tissue contrast (9).

With these fat-suppressed methods, both saline and silicone are very bright. Fibrous scar and implant envelope usually can be seen as relatively low signal structures compared with silicone. Methods that selectively suppress silicone and methods that show saline as brighter than silicone can also be useful in certain circumstances. At our institution we routinely use a dedicated breast coil and image both breasts in patients with breast implants. A fat-suppressed fast inversion recovery dual-echo sequence (Turbo STIR with inversion time [TI] of 100 mseconds, repetition time [TR] of 5000 mseconds, and echo times [TE] of 19 and 93 mseconds) is done in transverse, coronal, and sagittal planes. All three planes are done to optimize detection of abnormalities in any area in or around the implant as well as to avoid missing an abnormality that may be obscured by artifact (often produced by cardiac pulsation) on one of the planes. A T2*-weighted gradient recalled echo (GRE) sequence in which saline is brighter than silicone (three-dimensional PSIF coronal) is also done. This has a higher spatial resolution than the STIR sequence and is especially useful with saline or double-lumen implants. A silicone-suppressed sequence (STIR with TI of 400 mseconds) can be useful when it is unclear whether a certain collection is silicone or some other substance. Total imaging time is about 45 minutes.

Many different types of implants have been manufactured and implanted over the years (Fig. 8.2) (10). Most have a silicone gel within a silicone polymer envelope. There may be differences in the exact constitution of the silicone of the gel and envelope in different implants. Some envelopes have been made of other substances, including polyethylene. Saline within a silicone envelope is the next most common type. Double-lumen implants (most have saline in the outer segment and silicone in the inner segment, but some have saline centrally and silicone in the outer shell), and various composite implants have been placed. Patients are not always aware of the exact type of implant they have received.

Although there may be some variability depending on the exact makeup of the implant, there is generally development of a fibrous capsule around a silicone implant, apparently a foreign body–type reaction. This may produce hardening, deformity, and folding of the implant. Thirty percent to 50% of patients with silicone implants develop contractures, although the incidence is less with newer low-bleed and textured envelopes; about 10% will require surgery (11). Some implants will eventually rupture. In most cases, because rupture occurs well after development of the fibrous capsule, silicone gel may extrude out of the envelope but will remain confined within the fibrous capsule (confined, or intracapsular, rupture) (Figs. 8.3 and 8.4). In an occasional case, the silicone may extend through a deficiency in the fibrous capsule and track further into the chest wall tissues (extracapsular rupture) (Fig. 8.5). There is some controversy regarding permeation of silicone through an intact (nonruptured) envelope. Most of the silicone envelopes are not impermeable (although the degree of permeability is variable, with more recent manufactures less so) (11). Thus, small amounts of silicone may be found outside the implant in the absence of a true rupture. Whether this is of clinical significance is not defined. Although uncommon with most implants, some reactive fluid may develop around the implant or in the site of a previously removed implant. Again, the clinical significance of this is not certain. From an imager's viewpoint, the important factor is to recognize whether such collections are fluid (water-type signal) or silicone, because only silicone external to the envelope is definitive evidence of a rupture.

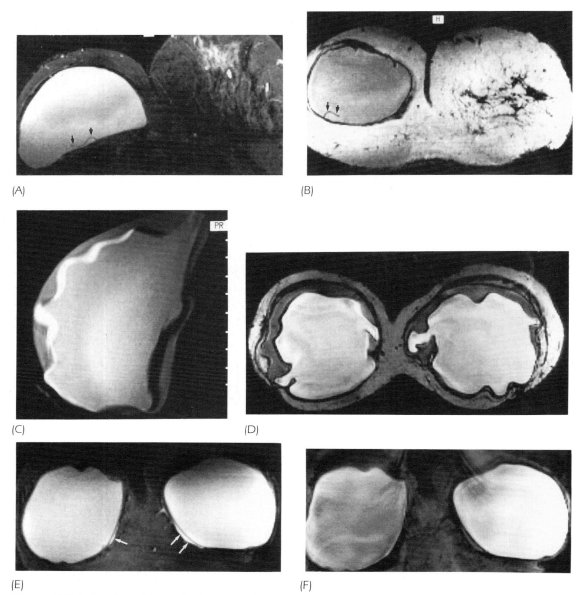

(A)

(B)

(C)

(D)

(E)

(F)

Figure 8.2.   *A variety of breast implants are shown. (A) Axial fat-suppressed STIR scan shows silicone implant in the right breast of this patient who had prior right mastectomy; the left breast has had no surgery. Note the radial folds (arrows) seen in the bright silicone, with the fat having low signal because of the fat suppression effect of the STIR method. (B) Coronal PSIF image of the same patient; note that the silicone is similar in signal intensity to the fat on this GRE T2*-weighted method. Note again the radial folds, which extend from the periphery and end in the implant (arrows). (C) Sagittal STIR image of a double-lumen implant that is not ruptured. (D) Coronal PSIF scan of same patient; note that the central portion of the implant is brighter than fat; this indicates it is saline. This is one of the less common double-lumen implants with saline surrounded by silicone. (E) Coronal STIR scan of patient with saline implant. Note the small amount of fluid around the implant (arrows). (F) Coronal PSIF scan of same patient; note that this saline is more evident on PSIF because the implant is brighter than fat (compare with Figure 2B). Note also that the fluid is relatively bright and probably is reactive fluid.*

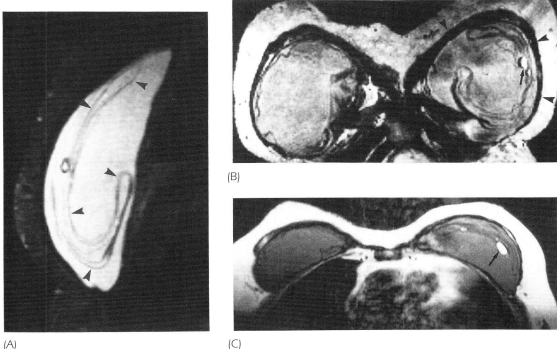

(A)   (C)

Figure 8.3.   This patient with silicone implants has a confined intracapsular rupture of the left implant. On sagittal STIR image (A), there are serpiginous lines (*arrowheads*)—the linguine sign—within the silicone, which remains confined by the fibrous capsule. On the coronal PSIF scan (B), the fibrous capsule is better seen (*arrowheads*). In addition to the linguine sign, there is a small drop of fluid (*arrow*). Axial silicone-suppressed STIR proves this drop (*arrow*) is fluid, because it does not drop in signal intensity like the silicone (C).

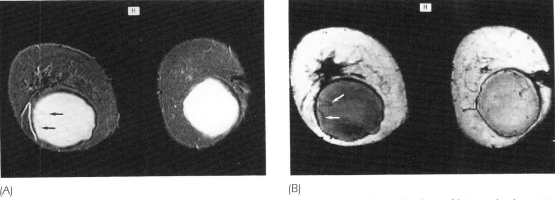

(A)   (B)

Figure 8.4.   A subtle confined rupture is present in this patient with silicone implants. Note on both coronal STIR (A) and PSIF (B) images that there is a wavy line (*arrows*) that is not simply a fold because it does not extend into and end in the silicone.

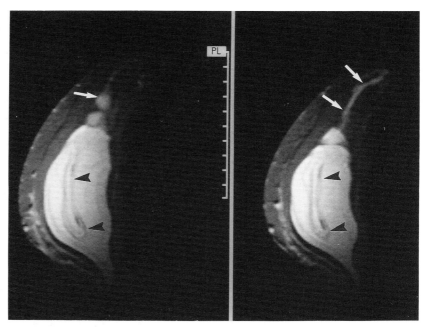

Figure 8.5. An extracapsular rupture occurred in this patient with silicone implants. The sagittal STIR image shows a linguine sign (*arrowheads*). Note in addition that silicone tracks superiorly (*arrows*) through the fibrous capsule.

MRI of silicone implants is directed at detection of rupture. Although only reported as of 1992 (12,13), MRI has rapidly been demonstrated to be very effective for this purpose. One study of 80 patients who had MRI and then surgical removal of the implants revealed a sensitivity of 79% and a specificity of 96%; there were three false-negative results (14). Another study that used better silicone-sensitive technique found a sensitivity of 94% and specificity of 100% with no false-positive results and only one false-negative result (15). In a comparison of several diagnostic imaging methods, MRI has been shown to be the most accurate procedure for diagnosing implant rupture (2). Thirty-two women with 63 silicone implants had x-ray mammography, sonography, computed tomography (CT), and MRI. Readings were correlated with surgical findings: There were 21 intracapsular ruptures and 1 extracapsular rupture. Mammography had only a 23% sensitivity (17 false-negative results) but a 98% specificity; sonography had a sensitivity of 59% and specificity of 79%; CT had a sensitivity of 82% and specificity of 88%. MRI had sensitivity of 95% and specificity of 93% with only one false-negative result. MRI correctly categorized both intracapsular and extracapsular ruptures.

Several findings on MRI have been shown to be reliable evidence of implant rupture. Although extracapsular rupture is uncommon, direct extension of silicone both through the envelope and through the fibrous capsule is definite indication of extracapsular rupture (see

Fig. 8.5). Detection of small bits of apparent silicone distant from the implant is not a diagnostic finding because of the problem of gel bleed.

With the most common form of rupture, the silicone remains confined within the capsule and, in fact, often has the conformation of an implant. The envelope collapses within the silicone gel and may be seen as a collection of wavy lines (see Fig. 8.3). This appearance has been termed the *linguine sign* because the cross-sectional image resembles noodles lying on a plate (12,14). These wavy lines have been documented to be due to the collapsed envelope (16) and are definitive evidence of rupture. Sometimes this sign may be seen with extracapsular rupture, but if there is no extension of silicone beyond the fibrous capsule, the diagnosis is intracapsular rupture.

If the implant envelope has not fully collapsed within the gel, there may not be a true linguine sign but rather irregular linear structures with silicone seen between the lines and the capsule (see Fig. 8.4). There may be only a very small layer of silicone outside the envelope. Sometimes a looped or "whip" appearance may be seen (see Fig. 8.4). These findings must be distinguished from radial folds (see Fig. 8.2). These radial folds are not signs of rupture and are very common. They probably result from some compression of the implant by the fibrous contracture, which produces invagination of the envelope into the gel. If a linear structure is seen that begins at the periphery and ends with a point in the gel, it is a fold. Imaging in all three planes helps in this determination.

Other signs that are not reliable evidence of rupture are deformity of the implant, bulging or irregular contour of the implant, and fluid around the implant (17). Droplets of fluid (water signal) that are clearly inside the implant (see Fig. 8.3), are considered suggestive of rupture but not definitive in the absence of the linguine sign (17). Occasionally, the implant may migrate or be compressed into a pointed shape in some location; if no linear structure is seen separating portions of silicone, this is not a clear-cut rupture. Calcification around the implant, which is a suggestive sign on mammography, cannot be clearly recognized on MRI.

Most experience and publications have emphasized silicone implants. Double-lumen implants can be very difficult to evaluate. There are often complex interdigitations of the two lumens (see Fig. 8.2). Reliable criteria for rupture have not been established. In one report (18), it was noted that rupture of double-lumen implants usually involves the outer, saline-filled layer. This is seen as a smaller than usual saline component and may be clinically unrecognized because the overall volume of the breast is little changed. If all of the saline component has leaked out through a rupture, the implants may have the appearance of silicone-only implants, so correct surgical history is necessary (18). The finding of saline within the silicone component may also be a sign of rupture.

Saline implants usually present less of a clinical concern. Most often, rupture is readily apparent clinically because of change in shape and rapid loss of volume of the breast as the saline is absorbed. On MRI, saline implants often show fibrous capsule and folds. With loss of saline, the implants shrink and have a corrugated surface. When there is a fluid collection around the implant, it is difficult to distinguish reactive fluid from extravasated saline because saline and serous fluid have similar signals. Whether saline implants demonstrate the same findings, such as the linguine sign, has not been documented in the literature.

The focus of MRI performed on implants is to detect implant rupture. The exact anatomic location of the implant, including whether it is subpectoral or subglandular and whether it has migrated, can be readily seen. The presence of a fibrous contracture can be recognized both from the low signal band surrounding the implant that results from the fibrous tissue and from deformity of the implant. Residual breast tissue, if present, can also be seen. However, because the sequences in these studies have been selected to optimize evaluation of the implants, diseases of the breast tissue may not be diagnosed.

MRI of Breast Tumors

The second potential use of MRI of the breast is in the investigation of intrinsic breast disease. Nearly all of the investigations have been directed at the use of MRI in the detection and diagnosis of breast cancer. This interest has been spurred in part by the recognition of breast cancer as a very significant health risk for the female population and by realizing that there are limitations in the diagnostic armamentarium. Even with state-of-the-art x-ray mammography and breast ultrasonography, there are considerable difficulties in early diagnosis of breast cancer. Only 20% to 30% of lesions suspicious for carcinoma on conventional mammography are, in fact, cancer on biopsy (19). Thus, there is room for improvement in noninvasive diagnosis. Many patients could avoid biopsies that are now necessary if there were a more accurate noninvasive diagnostic method. MRI theoretically should be capable of detecting breast tumors because it has been shown in other areas to be highly sensitive to the different tissue characteristics of neoplasms. MRI would also avoid any concern about carcinogenesis because no study has demonstrated any carcinogenic effect of diagnostic MRI in animals or humans.

Even very early studies did show that MRI was capable of depicting breast tumors (1). Several studies have now documented that MRI, particularly contrast-enhanced procedures, are capable of very high detection rates for breast tumors. Nevertheless, MRI is not yet a standard method for evaluation of suspected breast tumors. To a large degree, this is due to the high cost of MRI, which makes it difficult to identify a cost-effective role in competition with the other methods; even biopsy may be less costly than MRI! Technical limitations and controversies about the most useful role for MRI have not been resolved.

Initial studies did show that MRI could depict breast tumors (1,20,21). Large masses can be seen with standard MRI equipment. However, to achieve the high spatial resolution while maintaining high signal-noise ratios needed to detect small tumors (<5 mm), a specialized coil is essential. It was also recognized quite early that standard T1- and T2-weighted images that are commonly useful in other parts of the body were not sufficient for breast tumor diagnosis. Benign masses could not be adequately distinguished from malignant lesions, and malignant masses could be missed; 20% of cases of cancer were not detected in one study (20). This is because the appearance of small cancers is not very dissimilar from that of normal glandular tissue or benign masses. The use of intravenous MRI contrast (gado-pentetate dimeglumine has been most commonly investigated) was found to markedly improve the detection rate for breast tumors (21). Sensitivity of greater than 90% was reported in relatively early studies (22,23). The value of gadolinium contrast agents probably is due to the neovascularity in breast cancer, which results in very early and bright enhancement. Cysts do not enhance; normal breast tissue enhances only slightly (Fig. 8.6).

Although use of contrast markedly improved sensitivity, in early studies specificity was poor. Heywang reported 98% specificity but only 34% specificity. This is because many benign lesions do enhance. Most cases of fibroadenoma, inflammatory lesion, sclerosing adeno-sis, proliferative dysplasia, and some carcinoma in situ will enhance significantly (22). In studies that used standard T1-weighted spin echo scans after contrast, in which data are acquired throughout the

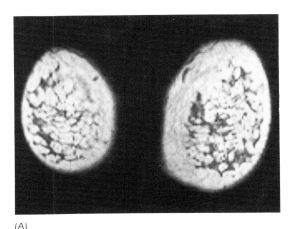
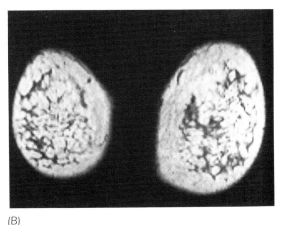

(A)   (B)

Figure 8.6.   Precontrast (A) and postcontrast (B) scans of a normal premenopausal woman shows there is little recognizable enhancement.

entire scan period of 5 minutes or so, no distinct enhancement differences in benign and malignant lesions could be recognized. However, when rapid-sequence studies were performed—in which images were acquired through a lesion in 1 minute or so, with repeated imaging for several minutes—it was discovered that breast cancers typically demonstrated strong early enhancement that peaked by about 90 to 120 seconds after contrast (23). Benign lesions show a slower enhancement profile, with less enhancement in the first 2 minutes after contrast but a gradual rise so that there may be overlap with carcinoma after several minutes. Thus, rapid imaging techniques, usually gradient-recalled echo methods, have become common for investigation of breast tumors.

Because both fat and enhanced cancers are bright on T1-weighted scans, it can be difficult to visually recognize small enhancing areas. Some investigators have used fat suppression methods to make cancers more obvious (24–26). Others have reported subtraction methods that make the areas of enhancement obvious because the precontrast baseline image is subtracted from the postcontrast image; thus, any tissue showing little or no enhancement, including both fat and normal breast tissue, is eliminated (Fig. 8.7) (27).

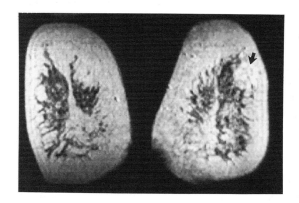

(A)

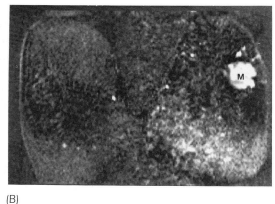

(B)

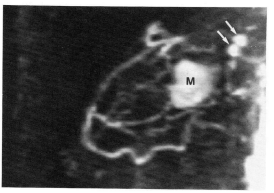

(C)

Figure 8.7. Mammography showed a mass in the upper outer quadrant of the left breast consistent with breast carcinoma in this patient. Coronal FISP scan after gadopentetate dimeglumine (A) shows an enhancing mass (arrow). On subtracted image (B), the mass (M) is much more obvious. Sagittal subtracted image (C) shows pathologic axillary nodes (arrows) in addition to the mass. The tumor was removed and proven to be invasive ductal carcinoma.

It is clear that use of contrast such as gadolinium DTPA is needed to have high sensitivity for detection of breast cancer by MRI. To achieve high specificity, it is necessary to use an imaging sequence with a short time of acquisition to distinguish benign from malignant enhancement patterns. Exactly how short a sequence is needed is unanswered. Most work indicates it must be less than 2 minutes (23,28); sequences providing 8 to 10 slices in 47 to 54 seconds have been reported (27,29); others have reported work with single-slice methods acquired in 30 seconds (30), 20 seconds (4), 14 seconds (31), 12.4 seconds (28), and fewer than 10 seconds (32). Some have suggested that imaging in fewer than 20 seconds is needed to achieve the highest specificity (32).

A dichotomy in current opinions regarding MRI methods for breast tumors has developed, with the division based on limitations of current MRI technology and on philosophy regarding the goals of MRI of patients who may have breast cancer. Current scanners do not allow high-resolution imaging of the entire breast with thin slices in a very short time period (and surely not both breasts). Thus, one must choose whether to perform a rapid-sequence study, which has the best specificity and would be most useful for accurate diagnosis of a breast mass that is known to exist. Good results have been reported with such methods; some investigators have been able to distinguish breast cancer from benign lesions in all cases (30). However, if it is not known where the region of interest lies, it is not possible to select the proper location for a sequential single-slice study! To screen a breast that may or may not be diseased, the entire breast must be scanned, which will require a longer acquisition time, at the cost of specificity. Similarly, if one is searching for multifocal disease in a patient with one known lesion, the entire breast must be imaged (3).

It seems that, at present, true screening for breast cancer with MRI is not feasible or cost effective. Even with relatively high sensitivity—in several studies, all breast cancers were detected by MRI, even several that could not be seen by x-ray mammography (3) and many nonpalpable lesions (27)—the cost of MRI would be prohibitive. MRI may be useful for evaluation of patients at high risk and for difficult mammography patients, such as those with dense breasts (33), those with implants (34), and those who have had surgery or radiotherapy, or both, for breast cancer (35–37). Early detection of local recurrence is difficult by x-ray mammography in those who have had limited surgical resection of cancer. With the high sensitivity of contrast-enhanced MRI that allows distinction of cancer from scar, MRI may be a useful tool. However, it has been shown that there may be enhancement persisting after radiotherapy for as long as 18 months (37).

Another potentially appealing use for MRI is as a noninvasive diagnostic tool to decide which patient with a palpable or mammographic lesion requires biopsy. In this circumstance, one can limit imaging to the region of interest and perform a high-sensitivity and high-specificity rapid-sequence study. In one study of this use, 100% sensitivity was achieved, meaning all breast cancers were correctly detected and sent for biopsy; specificity was 83%. By using MRI, 20 of the 39 biopsies done in 35 women with breast masses on mammography could have been avoided, with no cancers missed (29). One difficulty that can arise is the detection on MRI of a lesion suspicious for cancer that is nonpalpable and not visible on any other imaging method. Localization for biopsy cannot be done using standard methods! Although standard MRI scanners and breast coils cannot be used to direct biopsies, investigational MR biopsy localization methods are being developed (38).

Because of the variable techniques reported, there are not yet any universal criteria of enhancement that can be used clinically. Signal intensity depends on numerous factors, including the pulse sequence, magnetic field strength, contrast dose, and time of imaging, and it can be affected by artifacts such as volume averaging. Little investigation has been done on optimal dose of contrast. One study suggests that contrast doses that are higher than standard doses may be advantageous (39). Further comparative work may be needed to develop generally useful techniques and measurements.

Conclusions

At present, MRI of the female breast remains a diagnostic tool of great promise but limited clinical application. Because of high cost and limited availability (especially because not all imaging centers with MRI units can perform high-quality breast MRI), MRI is still largely investigational.

The most valuable role for MRI at present is in the evaluation of a patient with silicone breast implants. MRI is the most accurate noninvasive diagnostic procedure for these patients and should be used to detect implant rupture. Whether there is any usefulness in searching for gel bleed or whether MRI is needed for detection of saline implant rupture is less clear.

With respect to breast cancer, MRI probably will at some point play a very important role. It can be a high-sensitivity and high-specificity diagnostic tool with minimal adverse effects. It may be most useful at present to help determine which patients should undergo lesion biopsy. However, further investigation probably is needed to establish the accuracy of MRI solidly in large studies. Whether MRI can be cost effective as a screening tool is debatable. It may be possible but likely will require development of a dedicated breast MRI scanner that can be constructed, bought, and operated at low cost.

References

1. Mansfield P, Morris PG, Ordidge R. Cancer of breast imaged by MRI. Br J Radiol 1979;52:242–243.
2. Everson LI, Parantainen H, Detlie T, et al. Diagnosis of breast implant rupture: imaging findings and relative efficacies of imaging techniques. AJR 1994;163:57–60.
3. Harms SE, Flamig DP, Hesley KL, et al. MR imaging of the breast with rotating delivery of excitation off resonance: clinical experience with pathologic correlation. Radiology 1993;187:493–501.
4. Hickman PF, Moore NR, Shepstone BJ. The indeterminate breast mass: assessment using contrast enhanced magnetic resonance imaging. Br J Radiol 1994;67:14–20.
5. D'Orsi CJ, Adler DD, Ikeda DM, et al. RSNA '93 meeting notes—breast imaging. Radiology 1994;190:936–937.
6. Mund DF, Farria DM, Gorczyca DP, et al. MR imaging of the breast in patients with silicone-gel implants: spectrum of findings. AJR 1993;161:773–778.
7. Derby KA, Frankel SD, Kaufman L, et al. Differentiation of silicone gel from water and fat in MR phase imaging of protons at 0.064 T^1. Radiology 1993;189:617–620.
8. Schneider E, Chan TW. Selective MR imaging of silicone with the three-point Dixon technique. Radiology 1993;187:89–93.
9. Gorczyca DP, Schneider E, DeBruhl ND, et al. Silicone breast implant rupture: comparison between three-point Dixon and fast spin-echo MR imaging. AJR 1994;162:305–310.
10. Steinbach BG, Hardt NS, Abbitt PL, et al. Breast implants, common complications, and concurrent breast disease. Radiographics 1993;32:95–118.
11. Park AJ, Black RJ, Watson ACH. Silicone gel breast implants, breast cancer and connective tissue disorders. Br J Surg 1993;80:1097–1100.
12. Gorczyca DP, Shantanu S, Ahn CY, et al. Silicone breast implants in vivo: MR imaging. Radiology 1992;185:407–410.
13. Brem RF, Tempany CMC, Zerhouni EA. MR detection of breast implant rupture. J Comput Assist Tomogr 1992;16:157–159.
14. Ahn CY, Shaw WW, Narayanan K, et al. Definitive diagnosis of breast implant rupture using magnetic resonance imaging. Plast Reconstr Surg 1993;92:681–691.
15. Monticciolo DL, Nelson RC, Dixon WT, et al. MR detection of leakage from silicone breast implants: value of a silicone-selective pulse sequence. AJR 1994;163:51–56.
16. Gorczyca DP, DeBruhl ND, Mund DF, Bassett LW. Linguine sign at MR

imaging: does it represent the collapsed silicone implant shell? Radiology 1994;191:576–577.

17. Berg WA, Caskey CI, Hamper UM, et al. Diagnosing breast implant rupture with MR imaging, US, and mammography. Radiographics 1993; 13:1323–1336.

18. DeAngelis GA, deLange EE, Miller LR, Morgan RF. MR imaging of breast implants. Radiographics 1994;14:783–794.

19. Rosen PP, Braun DW Jr, Kinne DG. The clinical significance of breast carcinoma. Cancer 1980;46:919–925.

20. Dash N, Lupetin AR, Daffner RH, et al. Magnetic resonance imaging in the diagnosis of breast disease. AJR 1986;146:119–125.

21. Heywang SH, Hahn D, Schmidt H, et al. MR imaging of the breast using gadolinium-DTPA. J Comput Assist Tomogr 1986;10:199–204.

22. Heywang SH, Wolf A, Pruss E, et al. MR imaging of the breast with Gd-DTPA: use and limitations. Radiology 1989;171:95–103.

23. Kaiser WA, Zeitler E. MR imaging of the breast: fast imaging sequences with and without Gd-DTPA. Radiology 1989;170:681–686.

24. Pierce WB, Harms SE, Flamig DP, et al. Three-dimensional gadolinium-enhanced MR imaging of the breast: pulse sequence with fat suppression and magnetization transfer contrast. Radiology 1991;181:757–763.

25. Merchant TE, Thelissen GRP, Kievit HCE, et al. Breast disease evaluation with fat-suppressed magnetic resonance imaging. Magn Reson Imaging 1992;10:335–340.

26. Rubens D, Totterman S, Chacko AK, et al. Gadopentetate dimeglumine-enhanced chemical-shift MR imaging of the breast. AJR 1991;157:267–270.

27. Gilles R, Guinebretière J, Lucidarme O, et al. Nonpalpable breast tumors: diagnosis with contrast-enhanced subtraction dynamic MR imaging. Radiology 1994;191:625–631.

28. Stack JP, Redmond OM, Codd MB, et al. Breast disease: tissue characterization with Gd-DTPA enhancement profiles. Radiology 1990;174:491–494.

29. Turkat TJ, Klein BD, Polan RL, Richman RH. Dynamic MR mammography: a technique for potentially reducing the biopsy rate for benign breast disease. J Magn Reson Imaging 1994;4:563–568.

30. Gribbestad IS, Nilsen G, Fjøsne H, et al. Contrast-enhanced magnetic resonance imaging of the breast. Acta Oncol 1992;31:833–842.

31. Flickinger FW, Allison JD, Sherry RM, Wright JC. Differentiation of benign from malignant breast masses by time-intensity evaluation of contrast enhanced MRI. Magn Reson Imaging 1993;11:617–620.

32. Mus RD, Boetes C, Barentsz JO, et al. Characterization of breast lesions with a combination of gadolinium-enhanced dynamic TurboFLASH and MP-RAGE techniques. Presented at the annual meeting of RSNA, Chicago, December 1993.

33. Jackson VP, Hendrick RE, Feig SA, Kopans DB. Imaging of the radiographically dense breast. Radiology 1992;188:297–301.

34. Heywang SH, Hilbertz T, Beck R, et al. Gd-DTPA enhanced MR imaging of the breast in patients with postoperative scarring and silicone implants. J Comput Assist Tomogr 1990;14:348–356.

35. Dao TH, Rahmouni A, Campana F, et al. Tumor recurrence versus fibrosis in the irradiated breast: differentiation with dynamic gadolinium-enhanced MR imaging. Radiology 1993;187:751–755.

36. Gilles R, Guinebretière J, Shapeero LG, et al. Assessment of breast cancer

recurrence with contrast-enhanced subtraction MR imaging: preliminary results in 26 patients. Radiology 1993;188:473–478.

37. Heywang-Köbrunner SH, Schlegel A, Beck R, et al. Contrast-enhanced MRI of the breast after limited surgery and radiation therapy. J Comput Assist Tomogr 1993;17:891–900.

38. Hussman K, Renslo R, Phillips JJ, et al. MR mammographic localization work in progress. Radiology 1993;189:915–917.

39. Heywang-Köbrunner SH, Haustein J, Pohl C, et al. Contrast-enhanced MR imaging of the breast: comparison of two different doses of gadopentetate dimeglumine. Radiology 1994;191:639–646.

Surgical Evaluation and Treatment of Breast Cancer

Charles R. Shumate

Breast cancer has been described since antiquity. Galen noted the importance of accurate planning and precise surgical treatment when he stated, "Make accurate incisions surrounding the whole tumor so as not to leave a single root" (1). The modern application of this concept was the radical mastectomy, but currently a multimodality approach allows a limited surgical resection, maintaining good local tumor control and maximizing cosmetic result. The treatment of breast cancer has, therefore, evolved into a complex interplay among surgeons, radiation oncologists, and medical oncologists. Thus, it is imperative to begin planning treatment at the time of diagnosis to optimize results.

SURGICAL EVALUATION

The purpose of biopsy is to differentiate benign and malignant processes. The pathologist must be provided with a sufficient quantity and quality of tissue to accomplish this task. Multiple methods are available, including fine-needle aspiration, core needle biopsy, and open incisional or excisional biopsy. Each has advantages, disadvantages, and specific clinical applications. The surgeon providing definitive surgical treatment, should malignancy be diagnosed, needs to be involved in the diagnostic evaluation, including biopsy, because properly chosen and oriented biopsy incisions are critical for optimal oncologic and cosmetic outcome.

Fine-needle aspiration is an accurate, minimally invasive diagnostic tool, especially when combined with physical examination and mammography. A positive predictive value of 0.99 has been reported by some authors for fine-needle aspiration, indicating that definitive surgical treatment can be directed by fine-needle aspiration results (2). However, the results of this technique are dependent on a number of factors, especially the expertise of the individuals performing the aspiration and cytologic interpretation. Therefore, the surgeon's confidence in fine-needle aspiration must be individualized according to local expertise.

Typically, fine-needle aspiration is performed on a palpable breast mass. However, with improving mammographic and ultrasonographic techniques, nonpalpable lesions are accessible as well. The mass is stabilized and multiple passes are made with a 23-gauge needle attached to a syringe after induction of local anesthesia (Fig. 9.1). Cells should not be aspirated into the barrel of the syringe because they are then unrecoverable. This is best avoided by releasing the needle vacuum before removal from the lesion. The needle contents are transferred to slides immediately and fixed with either 95% ethanol or spray fixative.

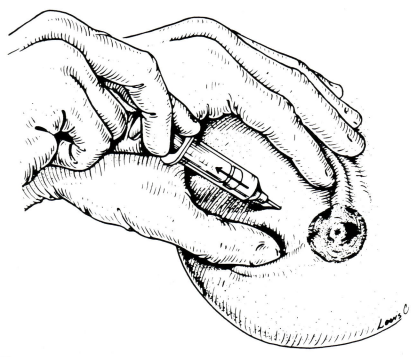

Figure 9.1. Technique of fine-needle aspiration. (Reproduced by permission from Copeland EM, III, Blond, KI. Sabiston's essentials of surgery. Philadelphia: WB Saunders, 1987.)

Despite its accuracy, the fine-needle aspiration technique's Achilles heel is sampling error (i.e., the possibility of missing cancer cells), because a tumor is a heterogeneous accumulation of supporting and malignant tissue. Therefore, if the cytologic results do not correlate with the clinical scenario, an open biopsy is indicated. Thus, patients with clinically and radiographically suspicious masses and negative fine-needle aspiration should not be monitored but should have an open biopsy. Likewise, a clinically benign mass and suspicious fine-needle aspiration need further evaluation with open biopsy before proceeding with a definitive cancer procedure.

The primary indication for fine-needle aspiration is to establish a diagnosis in patients with locally advanced breast cancer and in those who do not desire or who are not candidates for breast conservation. Patients with highly suspicious breast abnormalities wishing to proceed with breast-conservation therapy (i.e., lumpectomy and radiation) will require complete extirpation of the mass. Therefore, fine-needle aspiration can be avoided, unless the patient has an urgent need for diagnosis before excisional biopsy.

The main shortcoming of fine-needle aspiration is sampling error, as noted previously. Additionally, estrogen and progesterone receptor status is more difficult to quantitate with fine-needle aspiration, although it can be established with immunohistochemistry (3). Deoxyribonucleic acid analysis from a fine-needle aspirate is possible but less reliable than if performed on a larger specimen because of intratumoral heterogeneity (4).

Core needle biopsy is less often performed with the increasing availability and confidence of fine-needle aspiration. Core needle biopsy allows a histologic diagnosis compared with a cytologic diagnosis with fine-needle aspiration. More information is, therefore, available, especially for benign lesions, and quantitative estrogen and progesterone receptor data are possible. The larger needle size increases discomfort and postbiopsy ecchymosis and occasionally makes the biopsy of small lesions challenging.

Core needle biopsy's primary role is to establish tissue diagnosis of locally advanced breast cancer before radiation or chemotherapy. Another application is a benign-appearing mass discovered or seen on mammogram or ultrasonogram. Using radiologic guidance, these lesions can undergo biopsy and are proven benign, thereby avoiding open biopsy (5).

Open or surgical biopsy is classified as either incisional (i.e., a subtotal removal of the lesion) or excisional (i.e., complete removal of the lesion). There are several key points to successful biopsy beginning with forethought of possible future operative procedures, should malignancy be diagnosed, and the cosmetic result of the biopsy.

Accurate placement and orientation of incisions optimize cosmesis and assist with further surgical or radiation treatment. Langer's lines or the lines of least tension always lie in a circular direction paralleling

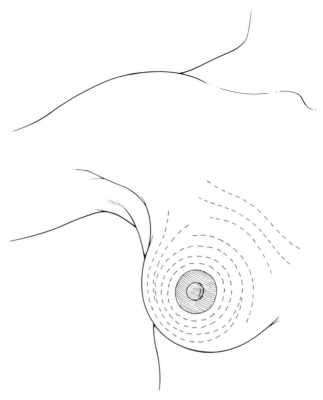

Figure 9.2. Langer's lines of the breast. (Reproduced by permission from Isaacs JH. Breast biopsy and the surgical treatment of early carcinoma of the breast. Obstet Gynecol Clin North Am 1987;14:711.)

the areola (6) (Fig. 9.2). Incisions for open biopsy should be directed in a curvilinear fashion within these lines to optimize cosmesis. Some debate exists over incision orientation in the lower breast. Curvilinear incisions provide better cosmesis if no skin is excised. Radial incisions are indicated in the lower breast if skin excision is required because less downward nipple displacement will occur. Skin is excised for tumor fixation or immediately adjacent to the skin or when re-excision is needed for positive margins and breast conservation therapy is used.

The incision location is as important as its orientation. Temptation to hide the incision immediately adjacent to the areola is avoided unless the mass is located subareolar. Tunneling to a mass through normal breast tissue increases tissue trauma, complicates planning of radiation ports, and boost fields in patients ultimately treated with breast conservation. Additionally, positive margins require re-excision for breast conservative therapy. Re-excision is technically more difficult, and cosmesis impaired, with improperly placed incisions. Dissection should be sharp, performed with scissors, knife, or cautery. Previous reports of heat inactivation of hormone receptors have been refuted and should not deter use of cautery dissection. How-

Table 9.1. *Pathology request*

Ink all margins
Frozen section
  If positive:
     Estrogen and progesterone receptors
     Flow cytometry
Mammographic abnormality
  Specimen radiograph

ever, judicious use of the cautery is recommended to avoid pathologic misinterpretation of margins.

Once the specimen has been removed, the surgeon's job is not complete. Much information is needed to allow consideration of all subsequent treatment options. The surgeon must precisely request the information required and accurately identify specimen margins (Table 9.1). Margins are best interpreted when the specimen is oriented by suture markers, or additional biopsies can be obtained from the wall of the biopsy cavity. The locations of these biopsies is recorded to allow precise re-excision if indicated. Re-excision is indicated when adjacent breast tissue is involved with malignant or premalignant processes. Tissue should also be submitted for estrogen and progesterone receptor status and flow cytometry. This analysis is done on fresh (i.e., nonfixed) tissue. Therefore, all breast biopsy specimens are transported in saline, not formalin. Frozen section is done both for diagnosis and to ensure proper analysis for prognostic factors (i.e., hormone receptors and flow cytometry).

An increasing number of patients are now diagnosed with asymptomatic mammographic abnormalities. The radiologic characteristics of these lesions have been described in a previous chapter. Radiographic identification is only the first step in diagnosis. Depending on the mammographic features, a lesion may have as little as a 1:200 to 1:2 chance of proving malignant (5). Thus, abnormalities that are considered indeterminate or highly suspicious for malignancy must have tissue confirmation by either open or radiographic directed biopsy.

Mammographically detected lesions are usually not palpable; therefore, the surgeon requires an accurate method of lesion localization to allow open biopsy. A reliable method uses a guide wire placed by the radiologist under mammographic or ultrasonogram guidance that permits surgical localization and excision, commonly called needle-localized, or directed, breast biopsy. A strategically located skin incision is chosen that allows optimal exposure and complete removal of the mammographic abnormality with little contamination and disturbance of normal breast tissue (Fig. 9.3). Often the incision is not placed at the site of entry of the guide wire; rather, it is placed at a site that is anatomically superficial to the abnormality. Determination of incision location requires an active dialogue between the surgeon and

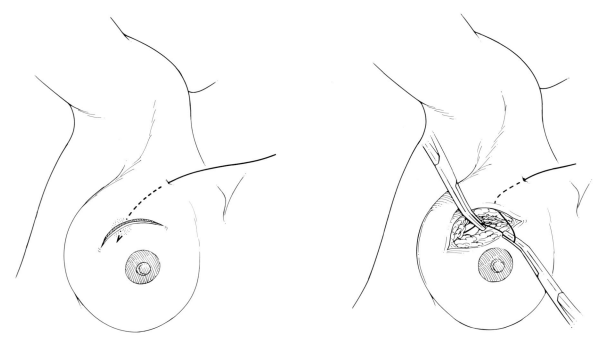

Figure 9.3. Method of needle-directed breast biopsy for nonpalpable mammographic abnormalities. (Reproduced by permission from Bland KI, Copeland EM. The breast. Philadelphia: WB Saunders, 1991.)

the radiologist and an understanding by both that the breast has a different configuration when compressed by the mammogram than when the patient is supine on the operating table. Once the specimen has been removed, a radiograph is taken to ensure that excision of the abnormality has been achieved and then sent to the pathologist for analysis, as noted previously.

Meticulous attention to hemostasis and wound closure is critical to obtain an optimal cosmetic result. Breast hematoma is painful, may delay subsequent therapy, and is potentially disfiguring. The optimal method of closure requires meticulous hemostasis because approximation of breast tissue is avoided to prevent breast deformity (Fig. 9.4). Closure of the subcutaneous tissues and skin only allows the biopsy cavity to fill with fluid and maintain breast contour.

The algorithm in Figure 9.5 illustrates the evaluation of a palpable breast mass. Should the patient's history, physical examination, and appropriate radiographic studies indicate a fibroadenoma or fibrocystic changes, clinical follow-up alone is required. Alternatively, fine-needle aspiration could be performed if the lesion is suggested to be cystic. Return of fluid and resolution of the mass confirm a cyst. The patient is followed up in 3 to 6 months to ensure no recurrence. The aspirated fluid is not sent for cytology because this is an unreliable method of diagnosing carcinoma, unless the fluid is bloody. Multiple recurrent cysts and those that contain bloody fluid should be excised

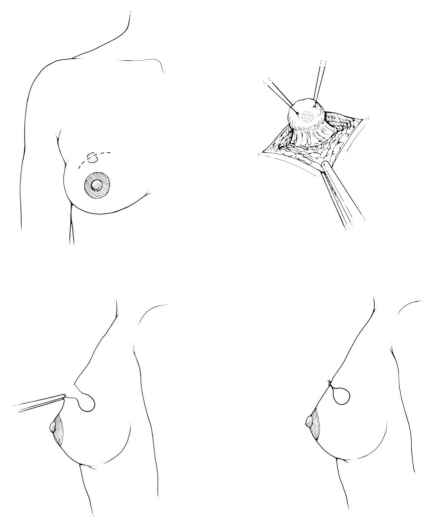

Figure 9.4. Technique of open breast biopsy. (Reproduced by permission from Fisher, B. Reappraisal of breast biopsy prompted by the use of lumpectomy: Surgical strategy. JAMA 1985;253:3587.)

because they may represent neoplasms. Others can be left in situ unless they are painful, are the source of infection, impede satisfactory clinical and radiographic evaluation, or cause patient concern. Fibroadenomas, especially in patients younger than 25 years, need not be excised unless they exhibit enlargement or concerning radiographic features. These situations require excision to exclude a phyllodes tumor.

Patients with suspicious masses by physical or radiographic examination should have a biopsy performed. The choice of biopsy type is dependent on the planned method of treatment and expertise at individual institutions. Those patients with locally advanced malignancies need only tissue confirmation because they will proceed to

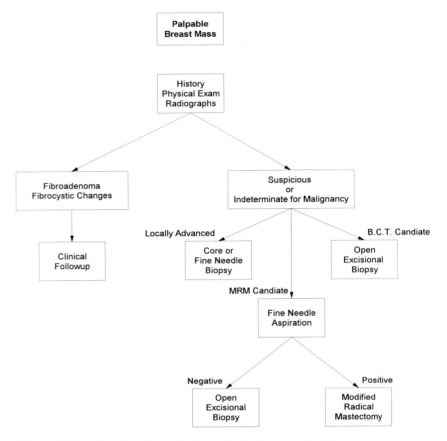

Figure 9.5. *Algorithm for evaluation of palpable breast mass.*

neoadjuvant treatment with radiation or chemotherapy, or both, or mastectomy. Those who believe that breast-conservation therapy is an option should have an excisional biopsy because this is the first step in treatment and the optimal method of determining eligibility for this form of treatment. Candidates for modified radical mastectomy can have a reliable diagnosis with fine-needle aspiration and avoid an open biopsy.

SURGICAL TREATMENT

The surgical management of breast carcinoma has evolved over the last 100 years from a locally radical procedure to less disfiguring operations that preserve normal breast tissue and appearance. However, the goals of surgical treatment remain unchanged. The surgeon's responsibility is to ensure that the entire breast is treated and the malig-

Table 9.2. Summary of survival and recurrence data from randomized, prospective trials of breast-conservation therapy (BCT) versus mastectomy

Study	Overall survival (%)		Disease-free survival (%)		Recurrence (%)	
	BCT	Mastectomy	BCT	Mastectomy	BCT	Mastectomy
NSABP	76	71	59	58	10	8
NCI (Milan)	79	78	77	76	4	2
Institut Gustave-Roussy	78	79	65	56	7	9
Danish Breast Cancer Group	79	82	70	66	4	
NCI (United States)	85	89	66	76	19	6

NSABP = National Surgical Adjuvant Breast & Bowel Project; NCI = National Cancer Institute.

nancy accurately staged with axillary node dissection. An effort is made to balance the goals of tumor control and maintenance of self-image and lifestyle. However, at no time should the primary goal of tumor control be lost.

Radical mastectomy was the mainstay of surgical treatment for breast cancer throughout most of this century (7). Modified radical mastectomy, despite its description in 1932, did not become the standard until the 1970s (8,9). The 1980s brought seven randomized, prospective clinical trials evaluating the efficacy of breast conservative therapy to mastectomy and found them equal for early-stage breast cancer (10–19). Table 9.2 provides survival and recurrence data for five of these trials. As can be seen, overall and disease-free survival and local recurrence are similar in all studies between mastectomy and breast conservation for stage I and stage II breast carcinoma. Currently, the standard of treatment for early breast cancer is to offer modified radical mastectomy or breast-conservation therapy with an explanation of the risks, benefits, and imponderables of both, thus allowing the patient to make an informed decision (20).

Modified radical mastectomy removes the entire breast, sparing the pectoralis major muscle, and involves a partial axillary dissection. The pectoralis major muscle fascia is resected to facilitate complete mastectomy. The pectoralis minor muscle may be excised to improve axillary exposure but is not required because all nodal levels can be visualized with medial retraction of the pectoral muscles. This operation is indicated for women who prefer not to pursue breast-conservation therapy or when breast-conservation therapy is not advised. Skin-sparing procedures are possible, and advised, to facilitate optimal immediate reconstructive results, without compromising the oncologic results, in appropriately selected patients. The oncologic surgeon and reconstructive surgeon must work as a team, having a good understanding of each other's goals and limitations to maximize both the oncologic and cosmetic results.

Incisions are oriented in a transverse or oblique manner, encompassing the nipple-areola complex and any biopsy incisions. An exception is skin-sparing mastectomy, in which the incisions are more limited. Skin flaps are elevated to the clavicle, sternum, superior rectus sheath, and latissimus dorsi muscle to ensure complete breast extirpation. The breast is removed from the chest wall by elevating the pectoralis major muscle fascia from medial to lateral. Dissection parallel to the pectoralis major muscle fibers facilitates dissection and causes less muscle damage. Care is taken at the lateral aspect of the pectoralis minor muscle to expose and protect the medial and lateral pectoral nerves because damage can result in partial atrophy of the pectoralis major.

Axillary dissection is performed in continuity with the mastectomy, removing levels I and II while sparing level III. A complete axillary dissection adds little staging and therapeutic advantage over partial dissection and increases morbidity. The long thoracic and thoracodorsal nerves are identified and protected during the axillary dissection to prevent paralysis of the serratus anterior and latissimus dorsi muscles, respectively.

The indications for axillary lymphadenectomy have changed from the original Halstedian concept of curative resection to the current idea of disease staging (21). Prospective, randomized evaluation has shown that lymphadenectomy does not influence survival; however, nodal metastases are important prognostic variables and often determine the need for adjuvant treatment (20). Controversy exists regarding the need for axillary lymph node dissection, especially in patients with invasive tumors smaller than 5 mm and larger than 2 cm, because nodal metastases are rare with the former and many patients receive chemotherapy on the basis of tumor size alone with the latter. Currently, axillary lymphadenectomy is indicated in all patients with breast carcinoma except those with ductal carcinoma in situ where the incidence of nodal metastases is less than 1% (20).

Seven randomized, prospective clinical trials involving more than 4500 women have proven an equal efficacy between breast-conservation therapy and modified radical mastectomy for stage I and stage II breast carcinoma (10–19). Therefore, approximately 80% of patients presenting with breast cancer are candidates for this form of treatment (20). However, a number of factors will influence treatment choice, including patient preference, tumor and patient physical characteristics, and associated medical factors.

Patient preference is often the most difficult aspect of eligibility determination. The surgeon must honestly discuss the advantages and disadvantages of modified radical mastectomy and breast-conservation therapy without conferring his or her bias. The patient must decide during a period of anxiety and emotional unrest if breast-conservation therapy is important to her self-image and if the treatment requirements will fit into her present lifestyle. The advantages and disadvantages of saving or losing the breast are obvious. Mastectomy is unacceptable to many women, but so is the 6- to 7-week requirement for radiotherapy to others. Many have fears of radiation or lack physical or financial access to radiotherapy units. Therefore, if the patient is an acceptable candidate for breast-conservation therapy, the surgeon should provide the details of treatment, including side effects and time commitments, and allow the patient to choose the treatment method that is best for her.

Tangible, although sometimes controversial, absolute and relative contraindications exist for patient selection (20,22). Figure 9.6 presents the factors most commonly used to direct surgical options for stage I and stage II breast carcinoma. Multiple primary cancers and diffuse malignant-appearing microcalcifications are absolute, and seldom refuted, contraindications for breast-conservation therapy. Prior therapeutic radiation therapy to the breast region is a contraindication if therapeutic doses cannot be delivered. Pregnancy is also a contraindication because the fetus may be exposed to scatter radiation; however, at times the radiotherapy may be delayed to permit breast salvage.

Tumor size is not an absolute contraindication, although few published data exist for tumors larger than 5 cm. The primary problem with tumor size is providing acceptable cosmesis after excision and radiotherapy. Therefore, patients with small breasts may not be candidates,

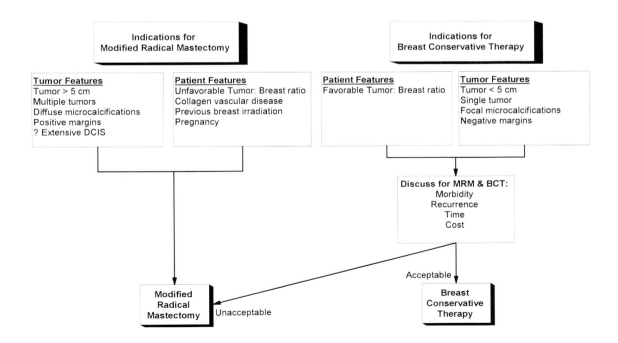

even with small tumors, because a poor cosmetic result may occur. Tumor location likewise should not preclude breast-conservation therapy. Central, or subareolar, tumors may need nipple and areola excision to obtain negative margins, but nipple reconstruction is possible later if desired.

Prior breast augmentation is not an absolute contraindication, and satisfactory cosmetic results occur after breast-conservation therapy. Capsular contraction is a potential concern after therapeutic radiotherapy, and breast-conservation therapy may be best avoided in patients with a history of capsular contraction. Collagen-vascular disease, such as lupus or scleroderma, may cause the development of severe radiotherapy side effects such as moist desquamation and osteoradionecrosis. These patients should have modified radical mastectomy with or without reconstruction.

Extensive intraductal carcinoma is a controversial issue in breast-conservation therapy. Some have reported higher local recurrence rates after breast-conservation therapy, whereas others show no difference if negative margins can be obtained (23,24). Younger patients may also experience a higher local recurrence rate with breast-conservation therapy. However, these patients are the ones most interested in breast preservation and should not be discouraged, but they need an honest appraisal of the risks (25).

The technical aspects of breast-conservation therapy begin with properly placed biopsy incisions. Often the biopsy can be the definitive breast procedure. Skin incisions are oriented along Langer's lines (see Fig. 9.2), and an effort should be made to obtain a 1- to 2-cm rim of normal-appearing breast tissue beyond the tumor. Additional biopsies are taken of the cavity wall to ensure that margins are free of invasive and in situ ductal carcinoma.

Skin is excised only if the tumor approximates the dermis or if re-excision is required for involved margins. Cosmetic closure is facilitated by not developing thin skin flaps and, as with excisional biopsy, not approximating breast tissue. Drains are avoided to allow the cavity to fill with fluid and maintain breast contour.

Should a margin biopsy prove positive, re-excision is warranted to improve local tumor control. This should be limited to the involved margin, thereby limiting the deficit and maintaining cosmesis. During re-excision, a small amount of skin is removed for oncologic and cosmetic indications.

Axillary dissection is performed via a separate axillary incision, thereby avoiding breast deformity. Levels I and II are removed, as with modified radical mastectomy. Closed suction drains are used to prevent seroma and to facilitate wound healing.

In summary, the modern treatment of breast carcinoma is a complex interplay among surgery, radiotherapy, and chemotherapy. Reports are now available that indicate even locally advanced tumors can occasionally be downstaged with preoperative chemotherapy, allowing breast-conservation therapy. The decision regarding breast conservation or mastectomy is complex. Factors to consider include tumor size, number, and the presence or absence of ductal carcinoma in situ, either pathologically or as strongly suggested by malignant-appearing micro-calcifications throughout the breast. Associated diseases such as lupus and scleroderma as well as the patient's body habitus are also included in the decision algorithm. Breast-conservation therapy certainly re-quires a greater time and monetary commitment by the patient, and this is one that some patients are not willing to provide. The most important consideration the clinician can have is to provide the patient with an informed choice so that a thoughtful decision can be reached.

References

1. Lewison EF. The surgical treatment of breast cancer: an historical and collective review. Recent Adv Surg 1953;34:904–953.
2. Ciatto S, Cecchini S, Grazzini G, et al. Positive predictive value of fine needle aspiration cytology of breast lesions. Acta Cytol 1989;33:894–898.
3. Reiner A, Reiner G, Spencer J, et al. Estrogen receptor immunocyto-chemistry for preoperative determination of estrogen receptor status on fine needle aspirates of breast cancer. Am J Clin Pathol 1987;88:399–404.
4. Levack PA, Mullen P, Anderson TJ, et al. DNA analysis of breast tumor fine needle aspirate using flow cytometry. Br J Cancer 1987;56:643–646.
5. Schmidt RA. Stereotactic breast biopsy. CA Cancer J Clin 1994;44:172–191.
6. Isaacs JH. Breast biopsy and the surgical treatment of early carcinoma of the breast. Obstet Gynecol Clin North Am 1987;14:711–732.
7. Halsted WS. The results of radical operations for the cure of carcinoma of the breast. Ann Surg 1907;46:1–9.
8. Patey DH, Dyson WH. The prognosis of carcinoma of the breast in rela-tion to the type of operation performed. Br J Cancer 1948;2:7–13.
9. Maddox WA, Carpenter JT, Laws HT, et al. Does radical mastectomy still have a place in the treatment of primary operable breast cancer. Arch Surg 1987;122:1317–1320.
10. Fisher B, Redmond C, Poisson R, et al. Eight-year results of a randomized clinical trial comparing total mastectomy and lumpectomy with or without irradiation in the treatment of breast cancer. N Engl J Med 1989;320:822–828.
11. Veronesi U, Banfi A, Del Vecchio M, et al. Comparison of Halsted mastec-tomy with quadrantectomy, axillary dissection, and radiotherapy in early breast cancer: long-term results. Eur J Cancer Clin Oncol 1986;22:1085–1089.
12. Sarrazin D, Le MG, Arriagada R, et al. Ten-year results of a randomized trial comparing a conservative treatment to mastectomy in early breast cancer. Radiother Oncol 1989;14:177–184.
13. Blichert-Toft M. A Danish randomized trial comparing breast conserva-tion with mastectomy in mammary carcinoma. Br J Cancer 1990;62(suppl 12):15.

14. Blichert-Toft M, Brincker H, Anderson JA, et al. A Danish randomized trial comparing breast-preserving therapy with mastectomy in mammary carcinoma: preliminary results. Acta Oncol 1988;27:671–677.

15. Bader J, Lippman ME, Swain SM, et al. Preliminary report of the NCI early breast cancer (BC) study: a prospective randomized comparison of lumpectomy (L) and radiation (XRT) to mastectomy (M) for stage I and II BC. Int J Radiat Oncol Biol Phys 1987;13(suppl 1):160. Abstract.

16. Glatstein E, Straus K, Lichter A, et al. Results of the NCI early breast cancer trial. Presented at the conference of NIH Consensus Development, June 1990.

17. Bartelink H, van Dongen JA, Aaronson N, et al. Randomized clinical trial to assess the value of breast conserving therapy (BCT) in stage II breast cancer: EORTC Trial 10801. Presented at the 7th Annual Meeting of the European Society for Therapeutic Radiology and Oncology, Den Haag, the Netherlands, 1988.

18. van Dongen JA, Bartelink H, Aaronson H, et al. Randomized clinical trial to assess the value of breast conserving therapy in stage I and stage II breast cancer: EORTC Trial 10801. Presented at the conference of NIH Consensus Development, June 1990.

19. Habibollahi F, Fentiman IS, Chaudary MA, et al. Conservation treatment of operable breast cancer. Proc Am Soc Clin Oncol 1987;6:A231. Abstract.

20. NIH Consensus Conference. Treatment of early stage breast cancer. JAMA 1991;265:391–395.

21. Wickerham DL, Fisher B. Surgical treatment of primary breast cancer. Semin Surg Oncol 1988;4:226–233.

22. Fisher B, Wolmack N, Fisher ER, et al. Lumpectomy and axillary dissection for breast cancer: surgical, pathologic and radiation considerations. World J Surg 1985;9:692–698.

23. Schnitt SJ, Connolly JL, Harris JR, et al. Pathologic predictors of early local recurrence in stage I and II breast cancer treated by primary radiation therapy. Cancer 1984;53:1049–1057.

24. Boyages J, Recht A, Connally JL. Early breast cancer: predictors of breast recurrence for patients treated with conservation surgery and radiation therapy. Radiother Oncol 1990;19:29–41.

25. Fowble B, Solin LJ, Schultz DJ. Conservative surgery and radiation for early breast cancer. In: Fowble B, Goodman RL, Glick JH, et al, eds. Breast cancer treatment: a comprehensive guide to management. St. Louis: Mosby-Year Book, 1990:105–150.

10

Aesthetic Breast Surgery

Peter H. Grossman and James C. Grotting

Throughout history, the female breast has been the perceived universal symbol of womanhood and fertility. Today we live in a society that has emphasized the well-developed female breast as an important characteristic of femininity. Attention has been focused on this region of the anatomy by the entertainment, advertising, and fashion media, which play a large part in determining the norms and dreams of modern society. Emphasis on youth and vigor, the pressures of physical acceptability on social consciousness, revealing clothing fashions, and more time spent in leisure and social activities all contribute to a woman's consciousness regarding her breasts. The size, shape, consistency, and function of the breast have assumed great importance for the patient and for her admirers. It is thus not difficult to understand how self-perceived breast deviations from the aesthetic ideals of society may lead to diminished body image. Sometimes surgical correction may be desirable to improve a woman's perception of her body or to correct a functional problem (1–3).

HISTORY OF BREAST AUGMENTATION

The earliest operations for breast augmentation involved the insertion or injection of various foreign substances. In the early years of this century, some physicians began devising operations for the enhancement of the female breast. These procedures were invariably fraught with complications. First came the instillation of wax into the breast tissue, often with such disastrous results from infection and foreign body reaction that amputation was necessary. As time went on, some surgeons began removing fat from the buttocks, shaped it, and placed it beneath the breasts to enlarge them. Unfortunately, these free fat grafts usually resorbed or calcified, and the disappointed woman was left with a defect in the donor area and scarred breasts no larger than they had been before surgery (1,4). Sometimes bad ideas resurface over the decades. Recently, there has been a resurgence in the use of free fat grafts for breast augmentation. In general, fat should not be injected into the breasts. Free fat will usually resorb with no substantial long-term benefit to the patient. Furthermore, fat sometimes calcifies within the breast. This can obscure, confuse, or even delay the diagnosis of a breast cancer. The American Society of Plastic and Reconstructive Surgeons has issued statements strongly condemning this procedure.

After World War II, a substance known as Etheron was developed. This was cut and shaped in a globular fashion and inserted behind the breasts. This substance was initially considered nonreactive. However, extremely thick capsules developed around this material, and fibrous tissue invaded the spongy pores of the Etheron, making the breasts extremely hard (4).

In 1963, Dr. Thomas Cronin devised an implant that had a Silastic capsule filled with a silicone gel. This implant did not develop such a thickened capsule as had the former implants. It was the first major breakthrough in augmentation mammaplasty. For the next 25 years, many modifications of this implant were developed (4). Included among the developmental additions to the breast implant market during this period were the "low bleed" silicone implant, the saline inflatable implant, polyurethane and other texturized surfaced implants, and the adjustable implant.

AUGMENTATION MAMMAPLASTY

Goal of Breast Augmentation

Despite society's ambivalence toward cosmetic breast augmentation, a procedure many consider a frivolous and needless risk, thousands of women each year choose to undergo this operation. There are many reasons why a woman chooses to have breast augmentation surgery. Many do so solely because they believe it will make them more attractive to the opposite sex. Some do so because they believe it will be beneficial for specific career choices. Yet certain women feel such a deep, personal need for breast enhancement that even their loved ones and physicians cannot appreciate the impact on their sense of wholeness and self-esteem. Women who share this need can truly understand the significant increase in the quality of life that breast implants can provide (5).

Most women seeking breast augmentation do not want excessively large breasts that attract attention but rather a pleasing, well-proportioned figure. The realistic goals of breast augmentation surgery are to

1. Create an aesthetically more pleasing body contour
2. Look better in clothing
3. Obtain a better self-image

The surgeon's role in helping the patient achieve the first and second goals are obvious. The third goal can only be achieved by the patient herself. While looking better in clothing and having an aesthetically more pleasing body contour might help a patient obtain a better self-image, it is no guarantee.

Regarding the ideal breast shape, the plastic surgeon has long tried to make objective that which is truly subjective. Nonetheless, it is important to have a standard from which to plan an operation, and from there variations are made appropriate for the individual patient. Although it is physically possible to place very large implants in a small-framed woman, it does not appear natural nor is it aesthetically pleasing. The implants should be proportional to the patient's body habitus. When the width of the implant extends beyond the base width of the breast itself, there is a greater incidence of implant palpability and visible rippling, particularly with saline implants.

The aesthetically ideal breast demonstrates prominent anterior projection. The ideal female torso possesses an equilateral triangle between the suprasternal notch and the left and right nipple. The nipple-areola complex lies slightly above the inframammary fold. There is a straight line or slight concavity of the breast above the nipple-areola complex and a convexity below it. The lower pole of the breast is somewhat fuller laterally. The breast is firm enough to remain well proportioned even against the forces of gravity and yet remains soft to the touch. Finally, the dimension of the breasts should be in harmony with the torso.

Development of the Breast Implant

Since the introduction of the silicone implant in the early 1960s, a variety of devices have been developed and marketed to augment the breast so that it will conform to both visual and tactile ideals. The silicone gel smooth-walled implant was by far the most commonly used implant during the 1970s and early 1980s. However, the phenomenon of "silicone bleed," by which microscopic amounts of silicone gel ooze through the pores of the vulcanized Silastic shell of the implant, had long been believed to be the major culprit in the development of capsular contracture. This led to the development of a thicker, less permeable shell, drastically reducing the incidence of silicone bleed. However, whether "gel bleed" truly represents a physical phenomenon or is the result of a "micropuncture" still remains controversial.

Next in the evolution of breast implants was the development of polyurethane implants and surface texturization. Polyurethane-coated implants were developed in the 1970s in an attempt to disrupt the smooth, linear periprosthetic capsule that develops around the implant. It is this capsule that can contract around the implant, resulting in hard, disfigured, and painful breasts. Several authors showed a significant decrease in the rate of capsular contracture around polyurethane implants compared with other gel-filled implants, but because of rising concerns regarding the safety of the polyurethane coat and its breakdown products, these implants were withdrawn from the market in 1991 (6,7) (Fig. 10.1).

Inflatable implants possess a vulcanized silicone shell and are filled with saline instead of silicone gel. With these implants there is no

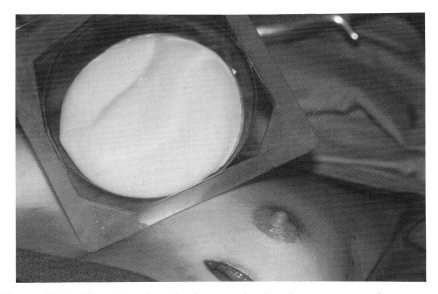

Figure 10.1. The polyurethane implant was developed to prevent capsular contracture. The open-pore polyurethane coating around the silicone gel implant allowed ingrowth of collagen bundles, resulting in a thicker but disarrayed capsule that was less likely to contract.

silicone "bleed"; however, microscopic particulate debris from the implant shell can be found in the wall of the capsule that surrounds the shell (8). In case of implant rupture, only saline escapes from the implant, not silicone gel. Unfortunately, many earlier model implants had been plagued by a high rate of deflation. Recent models have a far lower rate of deflation, but deflation can still occur. In addition, the saline-filled devices have the disadvantage of lacking the natural feel of the gel-filled implants (9) (Figs. 10.2 and 10.3).

Textured silicone envelopes were developed with the hope of achieving the low capsular contracture rate of the polyurethane implants without exposure to the potential health risks of polyurethane (9).

The texturing of the surface of the implant shell disrupts the smooth, linear capsule that develops around the implant, and studies have shown that, with gel implants, the rate of capsular contracture is less with textured implants than with smooth implants (10,11). Studies with saline-filled, inflatable implants have shown similar results with respect to capsular contracture. However, the textured saline implant has a thicker shell with increased palpability. Consequently, many patients prefer the smooth-walled implant despite its higher incidence of capsular contracture (12). The perfect implant has yet to be found (Fig. 10.4).

The ideal implant would be one that, once implanted, looks and feels like a natural breast. The implant would be impervious to tissue fluid, be chemically inert, and cause no inflammatory or foreign body reaction. It should be noncarcinogenic, nonallergenic, resistant to mechanical strains, and capable of being fabricated to the desired form (13).

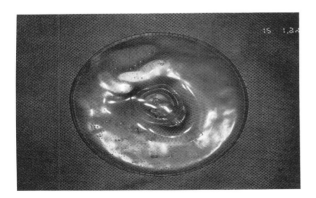

Figure 10.2. Smooth-walled, saline-filled, inflatable implant, the most common implant currently in use for both aesthetic and reconstructive breast surgery.

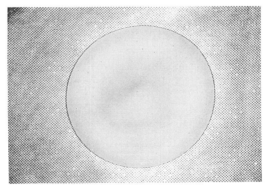

Figure 10.3. Saline-filled, inflatable implant with a textured silicone elastomer shell. This surface was developed to diminish the capsular contracture rate again by affecting the pattern of collagen deposition within the capsule. An irregular capsule with nonparallel collagen bundles will not be as likely to contract as capsules that develop in response to a smooth-walled surface.

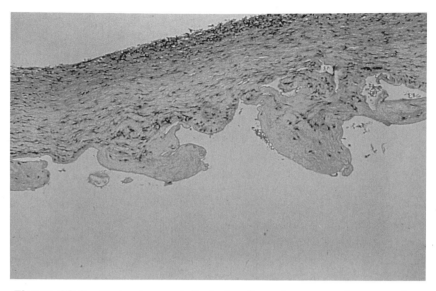

Figure 10.4. *Photomicrograph illustrating the collagen capsule surrounding a textured silicone implant. Note the indentation in the surface of the capsule caused by the textured surface. This disruption of collagen bundles affects its ability to contract, leading to a softer, more natural result.*

IMPORTANT SURGICAL ANATOMY OF THE BREAST

Vascular Supply

Three main arterial routes supply the breast. The internal thoracic (internal mammary) artery lies just lateral to the sternum. It sends perforators through the intercostal spaces and provides 60% of the total breast blood flow, mainly to the medial portion. The lateral thoracic artery from the subclavian artery approaches the breast from the anterolateral thoracic wall. Branches of this artery approach the breast tissue from the upper outer quadrant of the breast, supplying 30% of its blood supply. The blood supply to the lower lateral aspect of the breast is from the branches of the third, fourth, and fifth posterior intercostal arteries (14).

The venous drainage of the breast has a superficial and deep system. The superficial system drains into both the internal mammary veins and the lower neck veins. The deep system is located within the chest wall in the intercostal veins. The intercostal veins drain into the vertebral veins, azygos vein, and the superior vena cava (14) (Fig. 10.5).

Innervation

The breast receives sensory and sympathetic autonomic innervation (Fig. 10.6). The supraclavicular nerves supply the sensory innervation to the upper breast. The small medial branches of the anterior intercostal cutaneous nerves supply the medial and inferior aspects of the breast. The lateral cutaneous nerve branch from the fourth thoracic intercostal nerve is the dominant innervation to the nipple. Sympathetic β-adrenergic stimulation causes contraction of the smooth muscle of the nipple and blood vessels (14).

Lymphatic Drainage

The four main lymphatic routes of the breast are the cutaneous, the internal thoracic, the posterior intercostal, and the axillary areas. The skin lymphatics usually empty into the axillary lymph nodes. The superficial lymphatics of the medial aspect of the breast empty into the internal mammary chain. The inferior portion of the breast may drain to the lymphatics on the rectus abdominis muscle sheath and into the subdiaphragmatic lymphatics and the intra-abdominal nodes (14).

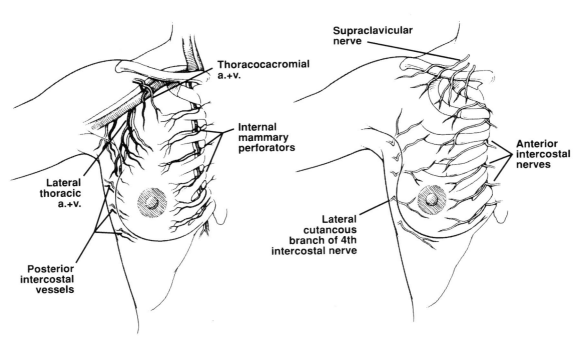

Figure 10.5. Vascular anatomy of the breast.   **Figure 10.6.** Innervation of the breast.

SURGICAL APPROACHES TO AUGMENTATION MAMMAPLASTY

Location of Incisions

The location of the implant incision is variable (Fig. 10.7). The most common incision sites are in the inframammary fold, the periareolar region, and the axilla. Each of these sites has advantages and disadvantages. The inframammary fold allows for good exposure for the development of the pocket into which the implant will be placed. Among the disadvantages of this approach are that it requires a well-defined inframammary crease, and the scars can sometimes be conspicuous on the breast. The periareolar incision usually results in a very inconspicuous scar camouflaged in the junction between the pigmented areolar tissue and the normal breast skin. Among the disadvantages of this incision are the potential for injury to the sensory innervation of the nipple, and, although well camouflaged, there is still a scar directly on the breast. The transaxillary incision avoids placement of the scar on the breast but unfortunately provides limited visibility of the implant pocket. It is also difficult to define and develop the inframammary fold through this incision. The addition of endoscopy to breast surgery may make exposure and development of the inframammary fold easier and again attract surgeons who have abandoned this approach.

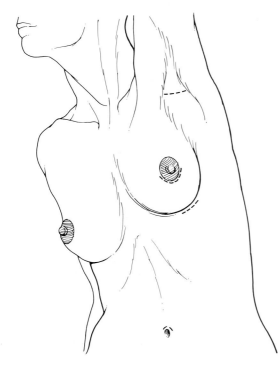

Figure 10.7. Incisions for augmentation mammaplasty: axillary, periareolar, inframammary, periumbilical.

The periumbilical incision has gathered some attention. This approach allows for a small periumbilical incision through which the implant is tunneled subcutaneously via a large cannula to rest under the breast. Placement is checked with an endoscope, and the implant is then inflated by way of long, removable tubing. Although this approach has its appeal in that no scars appear on or near the breast, problems arise with mechanical difficulties and damage to the implant. Development of the pocket can also be difficult through this approach.

Location of Implant Placement

When silicone gel implants were first used, nearly all were placed in the subglandular position. This allowed for excellent projection of the breast. As capsular contracture became more of a problem, many surgeons began to place the implant in the submuscular position. Published reports noted a significantly lower rate of capsular contracture when comparing submuscular versus subglandular placement of smooth-walled silicone implants (15–17). Thus, a trend toward submuscular placement developed. The results of the studies on the formation of capsular contracture have not been repeated, however, when using saline-filled, inflatable, textured implants.

Today, the surgeon and the patient must weigh the advantages and disadvantages of submuscular versus subglandular placement (Fig. 10.8). The advantages of submuscular placement of saline-filled im-

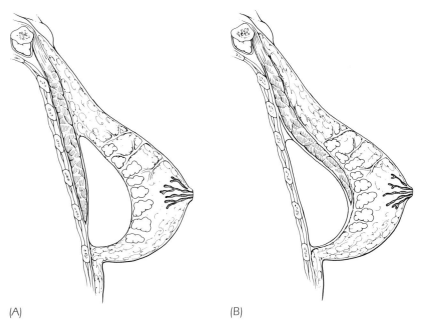

(A)   (B)

Figure 10.8.   *(A) Subglandular position of breast implant. (B) Submusculofascial position of breast implant.*

plants include 1) a theoretically lower incidence of capsular contracture, 2) improved mammographic exposure of the breast gland, 3)
blunting of the palpable edges of the implant by the muscle. The
envelope of the saline-filled, inflatable implant is thicker than the
envelope used for silicone gel. The lower viscosity of saline combined
with the thicker shell often results in visible and palpable ripples and
folds in the implant. These folds and ripples are quite undesirable for
the patient, and placement of the implant below the muscle allows for
an additional layer of tissue for camouflage.

The disadvantage of submuscular placement is that a dynamic tissue lays over the implant, creating the potential for embarrassing
displacement of the implant during active flexion of the pectoralis
major muscle. The advantage of subglandular placement is that, in
the hands of most plastic surgeons, an aesthetically more pleasing
shape of the augmented breast can be achieved. Among the disadvantages is the increased potential risk for capsular contracture. The thick
shell of the saline implant, when placed in the subglandular position,
can usually be palpated, and sometimes folds that develop can be
visualized postoperatively (Fig. 10.9).

COMPLICATIONS

As with any surgical procedure, there are certain risks involved with
augmentation mammaplasty. These risks include hematoma, infection, loss of nipple sensation, extrusion of the implant, and capsular
contracture. The reported incidence of hematoma is 3%. Significant
hematomas that present as painful, disproportionate swelling of the
augmented breast are often associated with high rates of wound infection and capsular contracture. Often this complication is best treated
by surgical evacuation (13).

Wound infections occur in approximately 2.2% of cases. The most
common pathogen is *Staphylococcus aureus.* Treatment consists of
drainage of the implant pocket, removal of the implant in most cases,
and administration of systemic antibiotics (13).

The incidence of decreased nipple sensation probably averages
about 15% overall, but complete lack of nipple sensation is a very rare
complication (13).

Capsular contracture is perhaps the most frustrating complication
of breast augmentation surgery. The exact cause is not fully understood, and its often delayed onset cannot be predicted. The histology
of the fibrous capsule consists of a thin inner membrane layer rich in
fibroblasts surrounded by a thick layer of collagen fiber bundles.

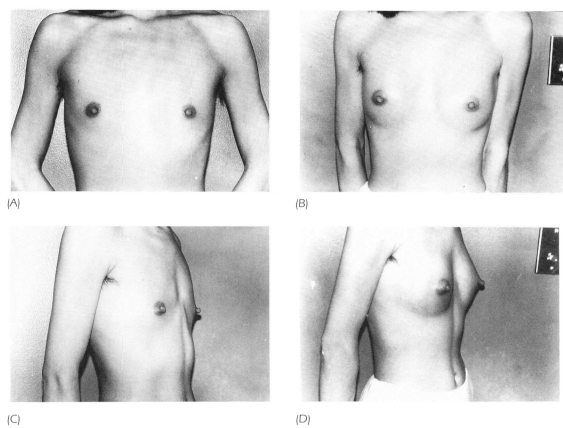

(A)   (B)

(C)   (D)

Figure 10.9.   *Pre- and postoperative views of a young Asian female with essentially agenesis of the breast. Cultural aesthetic values often influence patient requests for ultimate breast size and shape.*

There are hypotheses about why contractures of this membrane develop in some women. Some attribute it to hypertrophic scarring of the capsule, whereas others believe it can be attributed to subclinical infections in the developing capsule (13). The observation of silicone particles in the implant capsule has led yet others to believe that gel bleed was responsible for contracture; however, contracture has continued to be a problem even with low-bleed implants (18). Unfortunately, whatever the true cause, the result is sometimes an unhappy patient and a frustrated surgeon.

The severity of the capsular contracture can range from just minimal firmness of the breast to a breast that is hard, tender, painful, and distorted. Treatment of an established capsular contracture has historically been either by closed or open capsulotomy. The goal of closed capsulotomy is to tear the scar capsule hydraulically without damaging the implant. Closed capsulotomy is done by manually squeezing the breast until there is an audible "rip" or "pop" of the capsule. The long-term success rate of closed capsulotomies has been less than satisfying for most surgeons, and potential complications of this technique include hematoma and deformed or ruptured implants. Most surgeons have abandoned closed capsulotomies and instead perform an open procedure for severe capsular contracture. Once the capsule is surgically entered, it can be scored in several places, partially stripped, or completely excised (13) (Fig. 10.10).

Implant rupture can occur from closed capsulotomy, mammography, or other forms of trauma. Sometimes, however, implant ruptures are noted without any precipitating cause. The rupture can be "silent" and only discovered at the time of routine mammography or at surgery for implant exchange. Physical findings noted with rupture of saline implants simply consist of a decrease in size of the augmented side or sometimes a more prominent rippling of the folds of the implant shell. Findings consistent with rupture of silicone gel implants include nodules, asymmetry, and tenderness. Among the diagnostic studies available to detect rupture of a silicone implant is mammography combined with ultrasonography, interpreted by an experienced mammographer and a plastic surgeon. Magnetic resonance imaging has proven to be more accurate than mammography

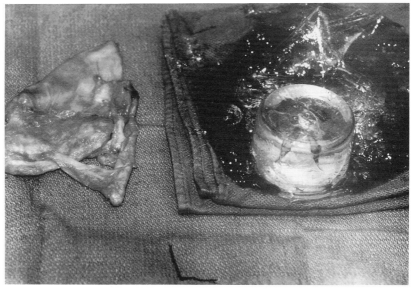

Figure 10.10. The appearance of a ruptured silicone gel implant after removal. Generally, the capsule of scar tissue prevents extrusion of the majority of gel into the breast tissue itself. Removal of the capsule at the time of explantation also facilitates removal of as much implant material as possible. However, excision of the capsule is a more technically difficult procedure usually requiring good exposure and general anesthesia.

(19). The only definitive diagnostic test, however, remains surgical exploration.

DIAGNOSIS OF DISEASE IN THE AUGMENTED BREAST

Silicone is a radiopaque substance and thus has the potential to obscure mammographic visualization of breast tissue. Breast compression and displacement techniques during mammography have improved glandular visualization. However, all implant materials used to date, including saline-filled implants, obscure radiographic visualization of microcalcifications through the prosthesis wall. The search for a radiolucent implant continues (13).

CURRENT STATUS OF BREAST AUGMENTATION

As of this writing, the only implants available for cosmetic augmentation are the saline-filled, inflatable implants. In 1992, the Food and Drug Administration (FDA) placed a moratorium on the use of silicone gel–filled implants for cosmetic breast surgery. The FDA stated that they had continuing concerns regarding the safety of silicone gel implants. These concerns included questions regarding the longevity and durability of the implants; implications of the silicone gel leaking into the body if the shell ruptures; and the possibility of a link between the implants and immune-related disorders and other systemic diseases (20).

The FDA review and the accompanying widespread media coverage have created a considerable amount of anxiety and confusion about the safety of these devices. Concern has arisen about whether silicone breast implants can cause cancer or autoimmune disease. Presently, there is no scientific evidence to show a cause and effect relationship or even a statistical correlation between silicone gel–filled breast prostheses and cancer (21). Furthermore, there is no conclusive evidence now that women with breast implants are at an increased risk for arthritis-like diseases or other autoimmune diseases. Such diseases in women with breast implants may have developed regardless of the implants (22–24).

Silicone is a part of our lives. It is used as a lubricant for intravenous tubing and disposable needles and syringes. In its solid form, silicone is used to coat pacemakers and to make medical tubing, prosthetic joints, hydrocephalus shunts, penile implants, Norplant birth control implants, and similar drug delivery systems. Testicular implants usually consist of a Silastic shell filled with a silicone gel, just the same as breast implants. Further, the methicone found in many drugs is simply medical-grade silicone. Silicone is also used in hair spray, processed foods, skin creams, and cosmetics. Silicone is considered one of the least reactive materials used in medical devices (5).

Despite the lack of scientific evidence, there is a select group of women in whom systemic fibromyalgia-type symptoms have developed after silicone breast implant placement. Although the cause of some of these symptoms may be difficult to diagnose or understand, it would be unfair and probably wrong to dismiss these complaints in all women as unrelated to their breast implants. It is possible that some women experience an adverse response to the presence of implants, and systemic symptoms develop that mimic those of polyarthralgias and fibromyalgia. Further research into this potential problem is under way and certainly warranted (25).

FUTURE OF BREAST AUGMENTATION

Research continues today to find an implant filler material that is as innocuous as saline and creates the same visual and tactile effect as silicone. Any new implant that will be made available to the public will have to be physiologically inert, have long-term durability, and be radiolucent enough so as not to interfere with mammographic oncologic screening.

REDUCTION MAMMAPLASTY

Indications for Breast Reduction

Women seek to reduce the size of their breasts for both physical and psychological reasons. Heavy, pendulous breasts cause physical discomfort. Among the most common complaints of women with large breasts is back pain. The pendulous weight of the breast produces changes in posture, which ultimately may lead to osteoarthrosis and kyphosis, with a compensating lordosis in the vertebral bodies. To support large breasts, heavy bras are needed; these can cut deep, painful grooves into the shoulders. Because of the large size of the breasts, exercise is often difficult and subsequent weight gain becomes a problem. The breasts themselves may be chronically painful, and the skin in the inframammary region is subject to maceration and dermatosis. The inframammary region has a tendency to collect moisture, especially in summer months or in tropical climates. This becomes an ideal environment for fungal infections, which produce intertrigo, which is difficult to treat (26).

From a psychological standpoint, excessively large breasts can be a troublesome focus of embarrassment. Women with macromastia often consider themselves deformed, feel conspicuous and embarrassed, and resent being noted for this aspect of their body, over which they have had no control. They will complain that men fixate on their breasts to the exclusion of their personality or intellect. Many patients openly admit to psychological problems caused by the realization of a serious disfigurement in their body contour. Furthermore, unilateral hypertrophy with asymmetry heightens embarrassment and may prompt undesirable behavioral changes in the teenager (26–28).

HISTORY OF BREAST REDUCTION SURGERY

The earliest written history on the subject of breast surgery deals, for the most part, with mutilation. Hippocrates (c. 460–370 BC) described amputation of the breast among the Scythians by burning the breasts with a hot copper instrument (29).

It is not known who performed the first reduction mammaplasty in a female. Paulas of Aegina, a well-known Byzantine surgeon, described a reduction mammaplasty in the seventh century AD, but this surgery was designed for correction of gynecomastia in the male. Over the centuries, many surgeons were instrumental for refining surgery for the hypertrophied breast, but major contributions to the development of modern reduction mammaplasty did not take place until the twentieth century (2).

Before 1960, most operations for large breast reductions were done in two stages. It was believed that this provided a higher degree of safety for the viability of the nipple-areola complex and also a higher aesthetic standard. By the early 1960s, understanding of the blood supply to the breasts allowed for refinements in techniques, more pleasing aesthetic results, and a higher degree of safety. Most plastic surgeons subsequently began to perform large breast reductions in a single-stage procedure. The key to safety was based on the principles of preserving blood supply and innervation of the nipple-areola complex. This was done by maintaining a parenchymal pedicle to the nipple-areola complex and de-epithelialization of the skin of the pedicle leading toward the nipple-areola complex. The breast tissue is not undermined from the skin.

Despite a century of surgical striving, reduction mammaplasty remains imperfect. Its evolution continues, with emphasis on minimizing cutaneous-glandular interruption, creating a more pleasing form, and reducing incisions to achieve acceptable scars (30,31).

GOALS AND SURGICAL APPROACHES TO BREAST REDUCTION

The surgeon does not necessarily want to recreate a virginal breast in most women but rather a slightly pendulous, gently drooping organ that resembles a mature breast (32).

The vast majority of plastic surgeons perform breast reductions through techniques in which the nipple is transposed and elevated on a parenchymal pedicle. The parenchymal pedicle can be based inferiorly, superiorly, centrally, or a combination of these, so long as the vascular supply and innervation of the nipple-areola complex are preserved. The breast skin flaps are then draped over the remaining parenchymal tissue. The skin incisions are usually planned and marked preoperatively with the patient in the standing position to obtain the most accurate results. The site of the transposed nipple-areola complex is also marked preoperatively to correct associated ptosis.

A superiorly based envelope of skin and breast tissue is elevated and will eventually drape over the remaining reduced breast parenchyma. A portion of the gland and skin is resected while maintaining parenchymal circulation to the nipple-areola complex via the fourth and fifth intercostal vessels. Similarly, preservation of nipple sensation is maintained by leaving intact the cutaneous branches of the fourth and fifth intercostal nerves that enter the breast posterolaterally (32) (Fig. 10.11).

Breast reduction with transplantation of the nipple as a full-thickness graft is an alternative to the parenchymal pedicle technique. It is often indicated for elderly patients to limit anesthesia time, for heavy women who have pronounced ptosis, for women who require massive reductions of more than 1500 to 2000 g per breast, and for women who have had previous breast procedures that have placed in question future viability of the nipple-areola complex (32).

Hypopigmentation of the nipple-areola complex and incomplete graft take are major disadvantages of breast reduction procedures involving free nipple transplantation. Other disadvantages include inability to nurse. Despite the obvious problem of early complete loss of nipple sensation with this procedure, studies have shown that many women eventually have some return of nipple sensation (33) (Figs. 10.12 and 10.13).

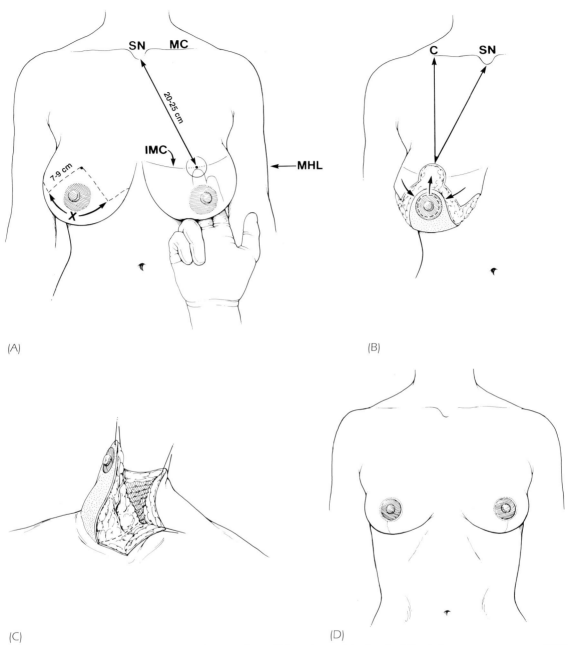

(A)

(B)

(C)

(D)

Figure 10.11. (A) The nipple-areola complex will be elevated to level of the inframammary crease (IMC) reflected to the anterior surface of the breast (approximately 20 to 25 cm from the sternal notch). (B) The nipple-areola complex is pedicled on an inferiorly based dermal parenchymal flap. It is transposed superiorly as the medial and lateral skin flaps are brought together beneath it. (C) From the lateral view, the nipple-areola complex is shown receiving its blood supply through parenchymal pedicle. (D) Final closure results in a periareolar scar and an inverted "T"-shaped scar with the horizontal limb in the inframammary crease.

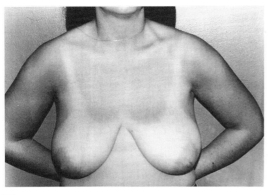

(A)

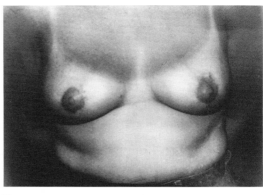

(B)

Figure 10.12. (A) Preoperative view of symptomatic patient with macromastia requesting breast reduction. A short-scar, "L"-shaped technique was used. (B) Postoperative result at 3 months.

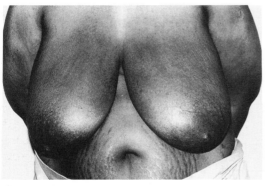

(A)

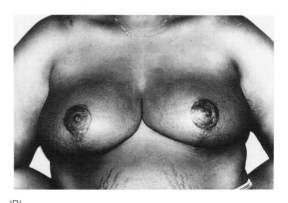

(B)

Figure 10.13. (A) Preoperative view of a patient with true gigantomastia suffering from considerable neck and back discomfort. In this situation, free nipple grafts are often the safest way to transplant the nipple-areola complex despite the propensity for depigmentation of the graft in nonwhite patients. (B) Postoperative view at 6 months.

COMPLICATIONS OF REDUCTION MAMMAPLASTY

Complications of reduction mammaplasty are listed in Table 10.1. Scarring is one of the greatest drawbacks to breast reduction surgery, and the patient should be made aware of this fact preoperatively. The scars resulting from most breast reduction procedures are in the shape of an anchor or inverted "T." The scar encircles the nipple-areola complex, runs in a vertical orientation below this, and proceeds transversely in the inframammary fold. Scar hypertrophy is common

Table 10.1. Complications of
reduction mammaplasty

Infection
Hematoma
Necrosis of the skin flaps
Necrosis of the nipple-areola complex
Nipple inversion
Fat necrosis
Loss of breast sensation
Hypertrophic scarring

Modified by permission from Gupta SC.
A critical review of contemporary procedures for mammary reduction (34).

and usually subsides with time, but the patient must know ahead of time that there will always be some scarring.

Newer techniques of breast reduction and mastopexy aim at reducing the amount of visible scarring. "L," "J," or lateral scar techniques are all aimed at avoiding placement of scars in the medial region of the breast, where hypertrophy can be more of a problem (35). Combining suction lipectomy with short vertical scars has been advocated and in many instances has resulted in more pleasing scars (36,37). Nevertheless, scars continue to be a drawback for this procedure.

Most women have some asymmetry of the breast, some more than others. This holds true for the surgically reduced breast as well. Although every effort is made by the plastic surgeon both preoperatively and intraoperatively to obtain symmetry, a perfect postoperative match is difficult to achieve.

Residual devascularized fat that is not excised may calcify and be visible mammographically, so breast reduction patients should inform their mammographer that reduction mammaplasty has been performed (35).

MASTOPEXY AND CORRECTION OF ASYMMETRY

Indication for Mastopexy

Ptosis or drooping of the breast is an almost universal condition. It may appear in early adulthood, usually following childbirth and protracted periods of breast-feeding, but more commonly it is an inevitable sequela of aging and gravity (1). The physiologic events that result in ptotic changes of the breast include 1) loss of elasticity in the dermis of the skin of the breast and 2) loss of breast bulk (weight loss, postpartum atrophy, aging).

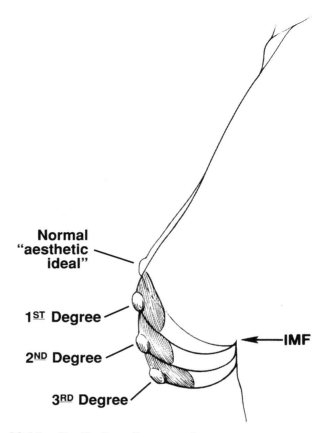

Figure 10.14. *Classification of breast ptosis.*

Mastopexy involves uplift and fixation of the mammary gland with repositioning of the nipple-areola complex. Ptotic deformities of the breast can be classified by the relationship between the nipple and the inframammary fold. First-degree, or minor, ptosis is when the nipple lies at the level of the inframammary fold. In second-degree, or moderate, ptosis, the nipple lies below the level of the fold but remains above the lower contour of the breast. Third-degree, or major, ptosis is when the nipple lies below the fold and at the lower contour of the breast (32) (Fig. 10.14).

GOALS AND SURGICAL APPROACHES TO MASTOPEXY

The goal of mastopexy is to restore a youthful, uplifted contour and to add bulk if necessary (1). In mild cases of ptosis, a simple de-epithelialized ellipse of skin above the areola can elevate the nipple-

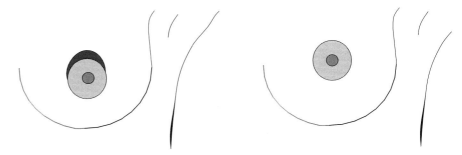

Figure 10.15. *Elliptical excision of skin for correction of minimal ptosis.*

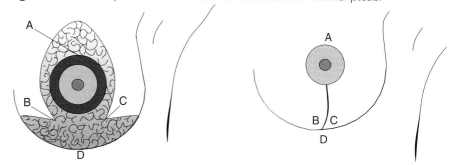

Figure 10.16. *Glandular-based elevation of nipple-areolar complex for moderate to severe ptosis.*

areola complex to a slightly higher position (Fig. 10.15). For a moderate degree of ptosis, a new location for the nipple-areola complex is predetermined. The periareolar tissue is de-epithelialized, the nipple-areola complex placed superiorly, and the redundant inferior skin excess excised. For severe ptosis, the nipple-areola complex may need to be elevated on a parenchymal pedicle, similar to breast reduction surgery but without resection of glandular tissue (Fig. 10.16). Other times it may be better to augment the ptotic skin with an implant to compensate for postpartum or aging breast tissue involution (6).

FUTURE OF BREAST REDUCTION AND MASTOPEXY

The continuing evolution of aesthetic breast surgery is to improve form and minimize scarring. Endoscopic surgery may play a role in this evolution. Surgeons are currently researching endoscopic techniques, and some day endoscopic techniques may be used to augment or reduce breasts with minimal scars. As for now, the art and science of plastic surgery of the breast continue to evolve.

References

1. Weatherly-White RCA. Preface. In: Weatherly-White RCA, ed. Plastic surgery of the female breast. Hagerstown, MD: Harper & Row, 1980:xiii.
2. Aston SJ, Rees TD. Mammary augmentation, correction of asymmetry and gynecomastia. In: Rees TD, ed. Aesthetic plastic surgery, vol. 2. Philadelphia: WB Saunders, 1980:954–965.
3. Pitanguy I. Breast. In: Pitanguy I, ed. Aesthetic surgery of head and body. Berlin: Springer-Verlag, 1981:3–36.
4. Grossman AR. Augmentation mammoplasty. Springfield, IL: Charles C Thomas, 1976.
5. ASPRS Breast Implant Task Force. Overview of silicone gel-filled breast implants. In: American Society of Plastic and Reconstructive Surgeons, eds. Breast implant resource guide. Chicago: ASPRS, 1992.
6. Capozzi A, Pennisi VR. Clinical experience with polyurethane-covered gel filled mammary prostheses. Plast Reconstr Surg 1981;68:512.
7. Hester TR, et al. A 5-year experience with polyurethane-covered mammary prostheses for capsular contracture, primary augmentation mammoplasty, and breast reconstruction. Clin Plast Surg 1988;15:569.
8. Copeland M, Choi M, Bleiweiss IJ. Silicone breakdown and capsular synovial metaplasia in textured-wall saline breast prostheses. Plast Reconstr Surg 1994;94:628.
9. Spear SL, Dawson KL. Augmentation mammoplasty. In: Cohen M, ed. Mastery of plastic and reconstructive surgery, vol. 3. Boston: Little, Brown, 1994:2099–2113.
10. Picha G. Panel discussion—augmentation mammaplasty. Presented at the 52nd Annual Meeting of the American Society of Plastic and Reconstructive Surgeons, Dallas, TX, October 1983.
11. Ersek RA, Glaes KC, Navarro JA. Results of reaugmentation with MISTI prostheses after failure of smooth silicone prostheses. Plast Reconstr Surg 1992;89:83.
12. Burkhardt BR, Demas CD. The effect of siltex texturing and povidone-iodine irrigation on capsular contracture around saline inflatable breast implants. Plast Reconstr Surg 1994;93:123.
13. Burns AJ, Barton FE Jr. Augmentation mammaplasty. Selected Readings Plast Surg 1991;6.
14. Georgiade NG, Georgiade GS, Riefkohl R. Esthetic breast surgery. In: McCarthy JM, ed. Plastic surgery, Vol. 6: the trunk and lower extremity. Philadelphia: WB Saunders, 1990:3839–3896.
15. Mahler D, Hauben DJ. Retromammary versus retropectoral breast augmentation—a comparative study. Ann Plast Surg 1982;8:370.
16. Puckett CL, et al. A critical look at capsule contracture in subglandular versus subpectoral mammary augmentation. Aesthetic Plast Surg 1987; 11:23.
17. Biggs TM, Yarish RS. Augmentation mammaplasty: a comparative analysis. Plast Reconstr Surg 1990;85:368.
18. Grotting JC, Gardner PM, Caffee HH. Reoperative surgery following breast augmentation. In: Grotting JC, ed. Reoperative aesthetic and reconstructive plastic surgery. St. Louis: Quality Medical Publishing, 1994: 963–1007.
19. Ahn CY, et al. Comparative silicone breast evaluation using mammog-

raphy, sonography, and magnetic resonance imaging: experience with 59 implants. Plast Reconstr Surg 1994;94:620.

20. Kessler DA. Statement regarding FDA's decision on distribution and use of silicone gel-filled breast implants. April 16, 1992.

21. Berkel H, Birdsell DC, Jenkins H. Breast reconstruction: a risk factor for breast cancer? N Engl J Med 1992;326:1649.

22. Giltay EJ, et al. Silicone breast prostheses and rheumatic symptoms: a retrospective follow up study. Ann Rheum Dis 1994;57:194.

23. Park AJ, Black RJ, Watson ACH. Silicone gel breast implants, breast cancer and connective tissue disorders. Br J Surg 1993;80:1097.

24. Duffy MJ, Woods JE. Health risks of failed silicone gel breast implants: a 30 year experience. Plast Reconstr Surg 1994;94:295.

25. Bridges AJ, et al. A clinical and immunologic evaluation of women with silicone breast implants and symptoms of rheumatic disease. Ann Intern Med 1993;118:929.

26. Pitanguy I. Reduction mammaplasty: a personal odyssey. In: Goldwyn RM, ed. Reduction mammaplasty. Boston: Little, Brown, 1990:95–129.

27. Goldwyn RM. Reduction mammaplasty: a personal overview. In: Goldwyn RM, ed. Reduction mammaplasty. Boston: Little, Brown, 1990:73–89.

28. Little JW III, Spear SL, Romm S. Reduction mammaplasty and mastopexy. In: Smith JW, Aston SJ, eds. Grabb and Smith's plastic surgery. 4th ed. Boston: Little, Brown, 1991:1157–1202.

29. Letterman G, Schurter MA. A history of mammaplasty with emphasis on correction of ptosis and macromastia. In: Goldwyn RM, ed. Plastic and reconstructive surgery of the breast. Boston: Little, Brown, 1976:1–35.

30. Psillakis JM, Cardoso de Oliveira M. History of reduction mammaplasty. In: Goldwyn RM, ed. Reduction mammaplasty. Boston: Little, Brown, 1990:1–15.

31. Goldwyn RM. Remarks of reduction mammaplasty. In: Goldwyn RM, ed. Plastic and reconstructive surgery of the breast. Boston: Little, Brown, 1976:147–153.

32. Spicer TE. Reduction mammaplasty and mastopexy. Selected Readings Plast Surg 1991;6.

33. Townsend PLG. Nipple sensation following breast reduction and free nipple transplantation. Br J Plast Surg 1974;27:308.

34. Gupta SC. A critical review of contemporary procedures for mammary reduction. Br J Plast Surg 1965;18:328.

35. Grotting JC, Askren CC. Reoperative breast surgery after reduction mammaplasty and mastopexy. In: Grotting JC, ed. Reoperative aesthetic and reconstructive plastic surgery. St. Louis: Quality Medical Publishing, 1995.

36. Lejour M. Vertical mammaplasty and liposuction of the breast. Plast Reconstr Surg 1994;94:100.

37. Lejour M. Vertical mammaplasty and liposuction. St. Louis: Quality Medical Publishing, 1994.

Breast Reconstruction

Brian J. Hasegawa and James C. Grotting

Breast cancer is the most common malignancy affecting women in the Western world. The National Cancer Institute estimates that the lifetime risk of developing breast cancer is now one in eight, increased from the commonly quoted one in nine (1). Despite intensive research on the cause and prevention of breast cancer, it is believed that the incidence will continue to grow (2). Much effort continues to focus on treatment. Although mastectomy has been the standard treatment for almost a century, there is controversy today over what constitutes the "ideal treatment."

Only three decades ago, the radical mastectomy was still considered by many surgeons to be the treatment of choice for resectable breast cancers. Because the primary goal was cure, both surgeon and patient accepted the mutilating defect it produced with varying degrees of indifference. Reconstructive options were few and required three or four stages to create a crude semblance of a breast mound. Thus, the patient was usually instructed to wear an external breast prosthesis. Although this was adequate for the needs of some women, most found the external prosthesis to be hot, heavy, and a nuisance to wear. Fear of displacement and exposure of the prosthesis severely limited the types of clothing that could be worn. More significantly, the prosthesis served as a constant reminder of the breast cancer.

By the early 1980s, numerous studies had documented the tremendous psychosocial morbidity associated with mastectomy (3,4). Mastectomy patients feel disfigured, have poor body image, lowered self-esteem, and diminished feelings of sexual attractiveness and femininity (5). Breast conservation surgery developed as an alternative to mastectomy with goals of leaving a cosmetically acceptable breast and minimizing the psychosocial morbidity without compromising survival. For stage I and stage II breast cancer, survival is equivalent to modified radical mastectomy (6). However, breast conservation surgery is not indicated for large tumors, multiple tumors, or diffuse disease on mammogram. Also the cosmetic outcome is variable depending on factors such as tumor and breast size, the extent of surgical resection, and the technique of irradiation. Radiotherapy has significant adverse effects that can compromise reconstructive options should mastectomy be required later. Ward reported that many women who elect modified radical mastectomy fear the consequences of radiotherapy more than breast loss (7). When given the option of breast conservation, more than 50% of women will still choose mastectomy (8,9).

In the late 1970s, the field of reconstructive surgery was advancing rapidly with the popularization of tissue expanders, myocutaneous flaps, and microsurgery. Application of these techniques to breast reconstruction made it possible to reconstruct the radical mastectomy defect and create a reasonable facsimile of a breast in a single stage. Reconstruction after mastectomy has been shown to significantly decrease psychological morbidity and improve quality of life (10). Today, immediate reconstruction with autogenous tissue can produce superb cosmetic results. Breast reconstruction has thus become increasingly accepted by women and physicians and should be considered an essential component in the total care of the patient with breast cancer.

ROLE OF THE PLASTIC SURGEON

Breast cancer is a multifaceted problem that, in this day and age, deserves a multidisciplinary team approach along with participation of the patient to determine the most appropriate plan of management. The psychological impact of breast cancer is an important aspect in the total care of the patient. Many women begin to mourn the loss of a breast at the time breast cancer is diagnosed. Early consultation with a plastic surgeon can help to alleviate some of the fears and anxieties that accompany the thought of possibly losing a breast. Discussing reconstruction encourages a more positive outlook for the future. It is then important for the plastic surgeon to determine the patient's needs and expectations regarding breast reconstruction. She must be advised on all the reconstructive options, their capabilities and limitations, and whether or not she is a suitable candidate. The goal of reconstruction is to create a breast safely that meets the needs and expectations of the particular patient. Even patients with late-stage tumors and a poor prognosis for survival can benefit from breast reconstruction with an improved quality of life.

Some women will be offered breast-conservation surgery as an alternative to mastectomy and reconstruction. Ultimately, the patient must make this most difficult decision; therefore, she must be fully informed. From a plastic surgery perspective, radiotherapy may damage tissues, which could complicate and limit reconstructive options if required in the future. Moreover, breast-conservation surgery does not always leave a cosmetically acceptable breast.

If treatment is to be mastectomy followed by reconstruction, the plastic surgeon must then determine the timing of the reconstruction. Immediate reconstruction must be planned and coordinated with both oncologic and plastic surgeons.

Before the mastectomy and reconstruction, it is important that both the oncologic surgeon and the plastic surgeon consider the status of the opposite breast because the risk of cancer developing in it is higher than normal. From an oncology standpoint, a total or subcutaneous mastectomy for prophylaxis is a consideration, especially for women considered high risk because of lobular carcinoma, a strong family history of breast cancer, or precancerous disease on biopsy of the breast. The efficacy of subcutaneous mastectomy compared with total mastectomy remains controversial because it removes only 95% of the breast tissue and spares the nipple-areola complex. Some reconstructive surgeons find difficulty in justifying subcutaneous mastectomy because reconstruction is not any easier, and the results of reconstruction are not significantly better than after a total mastectomy. With current methods, bilateral breast reconstruction can be done safely in a single stage with the advantage of excellent symmetry.

For most women, however, a prophylactic mastectomy is not warranted because the opposite breast can be adequately monitored with regular examination and mammography. From a reconstructive standpoint, it may be desirable to alter the opposite breast if it is large or ptotic because matching these features with even the most complex of the current methods of reconstruction is difficult if not impossible.

For large breasts, a breast reduction may be necessary, and if ptosis is the main problem, a skin-tightening mastopexy may be all that is required. Occasionally, the opposite breast requires augmentation. If possible, alterations of the breast parenchyma are kept to a minimum to avoid fat necrosis with subsequent calcification, which might complicate mammography. Some surgeons prefer to perform the opposite breast alterations at the time of mastectomy and reconstruction, finding it easier to achieve symmetry and eliminate the need for another stage, whereas others prefer to delay it to a separate operation, believing that the reconstructed breast needs time to "settle" into a more permanent position and shape.

CURRENT TRENDS IN BREAST RECONSTRUCTION

Immediate Versus Delayed Reconstruction

Immediate breast reconstruction is defined as reconstruction performed at the time of the mastectomy or sometime within the same hospital admission. Not too long ago, it was believed that reconstruction of the breast should be delayed anywhere from 6 months and even up to 5 years after the mastectomy because of oncologic concerns (11). Would immediate reconstruction interfere with the detection and treatment of recurrent cancer or delay and complicate adjuvant therapy if needed? Would the surgeon be more likely to lean toward a suboptimal resection to facilitate the reconstruction? Finally, would there be an adverse affect on overall survival? Numerous studies of patients who have had immediate reconstruction with an implant or expander or myocutaneous flap have shown that 1) diagnosis of local recurrence is not delayed and treatment of the recurrence is not compromised, 2) overall survival is not adversely affected, and 3) adjuvant chemotherapy or radiotherapy are not interfered with, but a delay of 10 days to 2 weeks is preferable for wound healing (12–15).

Over the last decade the trend has been increasingly toward immediate reconstruction for many reasons. First, immediate reconstruction reduces the degree of psychological morbidity experienced by the patient. The reconstructed breast seems to be better integrated into the body image when reconstruction is performed immediately (5). The changes in femininity, self-esteem, body image, feelings of attractiveness, and sexual functioning that occur in women after mastectomy are experienced to a much lesser degree than if reconstruction is delayed. The concept of allowing the patient to live with the mastectomy defect in order that the reconstructed breast will be better appreciated is cruel and unfounded.

Second, at the time of mastectomy, the integrity of the soft tissue that enveloped the breast tissue is intact except for the segment of skin taken as part of the resection. There is no fibrosis, contraction, or radiation damage of the soft tissues with which to contend. The inframammary fold is usually still present and need not be recreated surgically. In essence, to reconstruct the mastectomy defect accurately, one needs only to replace the missing breast tissue and overlying segment of skin with soft tissue and skin of identical volume and shape. This is especially true of immediate reconstruction after a skin-sparing mastectomy, with which perhaps the best possible results in breast reconstruction are achieved.

Third, the design of the mastectomy may be planned in consultation with the plastic surgeon such that the best cosmetic reconstruction can be achieved without compromising the adequacy of the resection. Finally, the patient is subjected to only a single admission, operation, and recovery period. This results in a significant cost savings over delayed reconstruction (16). Occasionally, at the time of mastectomy, the margins of resection are uncertain, and it is prudent to delay reconstruction. Delayed reconstruction should also be considered in obese patients and in patients who reveal some ambivalence about reconstruction.

Implant Versus Autogenous Tissue

The silicone breast implant was developed in the 1960s and was the standard method of breast reconstruction during the 1970s. In 1992, the Food and Drug Administration (FDA) issued a moratorium on silicone gel–filled breast implants, which effectively eliminated their use. Saline-filled implants are still commonly used but are currently under review by the FDA. To date, studies have not shown any association between breast implants and subsequent development of breast cancer, connective tissue disorders, or human adjuvant disease (17–20). Nevertheless, the extensive media coverage and sensationalism concerning the safety of breast implants have had a tremendous impact on women. Although the use of an implant remains the simplest and most expedient option of breast reconstruction, fewer and fewer women are selecting it when given the alternative of "natural tissue" reconstruction.

It is very difficult to obtain ptosis and a well-defined inframammary fold to match the opposite breast with an implant. Moreover, to achieve an acceptable result with minimal complications, implants should be restricted to defects with a stable and supple nonirradiated scar, adequate surrounding skin and pectoralis muscle, and a small minimally or nonptotic opposite breast. Perhaps the most problematic complication specific to implants is capsular contracture. Despite research and improvements in implants, the rate of capsular contracture continues to be in the range of 20% to 30% (21). Thus, it should be understood that the result obtained with an implant is not necessarily permanent and that a revision procedure may be required at some point in the future. Even though saline implants are more reliable today than in the 1970s, most manufacturers state that the device will deflate at some point during the patient's lifetime.

The trend in the 1990s is definitely toward autogenous tissue breast reconstruction (22). The use of autogenous tissue offers a soft, "natural" reconstructed breast without the need for foreign material. Ptosis can be readily achieved. Symmetry and overall aesthetics are superior, and long-term results more predictable compared to implant or expander reconstruction. This is understandable because the mastectomy defect is simply filled with what was removed: skin and soft tissue. Virtually any type of mastectomy defect can be reconstructed with autogenous tissue. It is, however, a complex procedure with greater anesthetic and surgical risk, necessitating certain criteria in selecting candidates. As current techniques continue to be refined and new donor sites described, it is hoped that autogenous tissue reconstruction will become an option for more and more patients.

METHODS OF RECONSTRUCTION

Simple Insertion of an Implant

Breast reconstruction with simple insertion of an implant can yield very acceptable results in a patient with small breasts, minimal or no ptotis, and an abundance of healthy tissue remaining at the mastectomy site. It is also an option to consider for the patient with larger or ptotic breasts if she does not mind having a breast reduction or mastopexy performed on the normal breast to achieve better symmetry. Implants may be used for patients who prefer the simplest most expeditious reconstruction possible, even though a better aesthetic result can be achieved with autogenous tissue or expander reconstruction.

The original mastectomy incision is used to gain access for insertion of the implant. It is preferable to place the implant either completely covered by muscle (pectoralis major, serratus anterior, anterior rectus sheath) or partially covered by muscle (pectoralis major), with the lower pole of the implant in a subcutaneous plane. It is believed that muscle coverage decreases the rate of significant capsular contracture as well as the risk of implant exposure when compared to a purely subcutaneous placement. With the implant in place, it is inflated with saline until the volume approximates that of the opposite breast as closely as possible without causing excessive tension in the overlying tissues.

Timing

The implant may be placed immediately after mastectomy or delayed. In the immediate setting, there is always a degree of uncertainty with regards to the viability of the skin flaps remaining at the mastectomy site. Complete submuscular placement is thought to be even more important in this setting to prevent implant exposure should the skin flaps or wound break down.

Complete muscle coverage of the implant is not essential in the delayed setting because there is usually no concern about the viability of the skin flaps raised at this time. Leaving the lower pole of the implant in a subcutaneous location produces a more natural contour and makes it easier to create a well-defined inframammary fold.

Reconstruction with Tissue Expander

A point is reached when the difference between the amount of skin over the breast to be matched and the amount of skin remaining at the mastectomy site becomes too great for simple insertion of an implant to yield an acceptable result. In these cases, either tissue expansion or autogenous tissue is needed to add skin effectively to the deficient mastectomy site to obtain an aesthetic result. Tissue expansion can usually match an opposite breast of moderate to large size with minimal or no ptosis. Most women who are good candidates for reconstruction with tissue expanders are also good candidates for a transverse rectus abdominis myocutaneous (TRAM) flap.

Gradual expansion of the mastectomy site produces a dividend of additional tissue in both the vertical and transverse dimensions. If the skin is maintained in the expanded state for approximately 6 months, the gain in skin will become a permanent one. As witness to this effect, recall the permanent redundancy of skin in the lower abdomen of women who have had children.

The operative technique is similar to simple insertion of an implant. Whether the implant is completely covered by muscle or only partially covered with the lower pole in the subcutaneous plane is left to the preference of the surgeon. The expander is placed below the level of the previous inframammary fold to compensate for the tendency to rise with any degree of capsular contracture. A separate subcutaneous pocket is then made in the midaxillary area for the injection portal. Just enough saline is injected into the expander to ensure that it remains smooth and flat. Wrinkles in the expander are notorious for causing points of excessive pressure to the overlying skin, leading to exposure of the expander.

Approximately 2 weeks are allowed for the wounds to gain some tensile strength before beginning further expansion. Ideally, both the patient and surgeon would prefer as rapid an expansion phase as possible but realistically, only 50 to 100 mL can be comfortably injected at weekly intervals. Care should be taken that capillary perfusion is maintained in the overlying skin after each injection.

It is generally agreed that, to produce some degree of ptosis and a soft, natural-appearing breast, the expander should be overinflated beyond the desired breast size, maintained in the overexpanded state for 4 to 6 months, and then deflated back to the desired size. The amount of overinflation needed to achieve this is controversial, but we generally anticipate 10% to 15% of the final desired volume (Fig. 11.1).

Latissimus Dorsi Myocutaneous Flap

In the late 1970s, the use of the latissimus dorsi myocutaneous (LDM) flap for mastectomy defects with tight, thin, or radiated skin was a

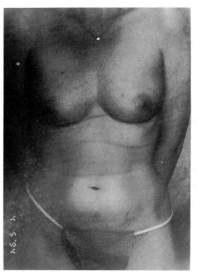 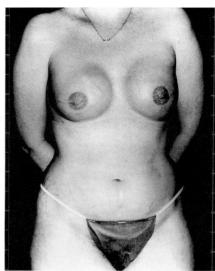

(A)   (B)

Figure 11.1. (A) Preoperative view of patient with a very strong family history of carcinoma of the breast with ductal carcinoma in situ on recent biopsy. She was believed to be a good candidate for prophylactic simple mastectomies. (B) View after placement of tissue expanders followed by permanent implants and nipple-areola reconstruction.

major advance in breast reconstruction (23). It was the standard method of reconstructing the radical mastectomy defect commonly encountered at that time. The latissimus dorsi muscle effectively replaced the missing pectoralis major muscle, thereby restoring the anterior axillary fold, allowed creation of an inframammary fold, and added fill to the subclavicular hollow.

In almost all cases, however, an implant was needed to provide much of the shape and volume of the new breast. It was hoped that the rate of capsular contracture would be significantly less than that observed in reconstructions using implants alone, because the implant would be completely covered by healthy latissimus dorsi muscle. After studies revealed an incidence of significant capsular contracture of at least 20% and with the introduction of tissue expansion and the TRAM flap in the early 1980s, the use of the LDM flap quickly dwindled (24). Today, use of the LDM flap remains exceptionally safe and reliable and has found its niche mainly as a backup for the failed TRAM flap. It is also very useful for improving thin coverage over a saline implant.

Anatomy

The latissimus dorsi originates from the posterior iliac crest, the lumbar fascia, the spines of the lower six thoracic vertebrae, and the lower three ribs. Its tendon inserts on the medial lip of the bicipital groove of the humerus. The thoracodorsal artery, a branch of the subscapular artery, is the dominant arterial supply. Numerous myocutaneous perforators exist, allowing the skin paddle to be designed anywhere over the entire surface of the latissimus.

Technique

The patient is placed in the lateral position. The skin paddle is oriented transversely or obliquely just below the scapula and is designed for maximum width that will still allow primary closure. Ideally, the final scar should be hidden by a bra strap or swimsuit top. Leaving the skin paddle attached to the muscle, a plane is developed between the muscle and overlying fat. The muscle is then freed from the underlying chest wall. The thoracodorsal pedicle is identified and the muscle divided from its origins. The skin paddle is ideally placed low and lateral on the breast rather than into the mastectomy scar. The latissimus muscle is attached to the lower border of the pectoralis major muscle. The free margin of the latissimus muscle is attached to the chest wall 1 to 2 cm below the inframammary line to recreate the fold. The implant is placed so that complete muscle coverage is obtained. An expander may be used if an implant is too tight.

Autogenous Latissimus Flap

The autogenous latissimus flap (ALF) carries additional fat on the surface of the latissimus muscle to achieve a completely autogenous breast reconstruction without the need for an implant. The amount of skin and soft tissue that can be transferred is still less than with the TRAM flap in most patients. There is also less flexibility in positioning and shaping the flap. Thus, when autogenous tissue reconstruction is considered, the TRAM flap remains the first choice. Sometimes the TRAM flap is not an option because of either previous abdominal scars or patient preference for a different donor site. In these cases, the ALF is a reasonable alternative. The best indication for its use is after partial loss of a TRAM flap, when up to a moderate amount of additional skin and soft tissue is needed.

Flap design and technique are very similar to the standard LDM flap already described. A layer of fat, however, is left on the surface of the latissimus muscle, which provides the added volume needed to form a breast mound. Infraclavicular fill is excellent, and ptosis can be obtained. As with the standard LDM flap, vascularity and reliability are excellent. Arguably, the donor site scar and possible contour deformity are disadvantages. If the random skin flaps on the back are dissected too thinly, necrosis at the wound margin is common.

TRAM Flap

Most surgeons would agree that the TRAM flap is by far the flap of choice when considering autogenous reconstruction. The skin and subcutaneous tissue of the lower abdomen is often redundant, especially in women who have borne children, making it an excellent donor site for tissue transfer. The abundance of tissue that this site usually provides allows the surgeon an unparalleled flexibility in positioning, shaping, and achieving volume of the tissue to obtain as close a match of the opposite breast as possible. As an added bonus, abdominal contour is improved and the transverse suprapubic scar is usually well hidden.

Anatomy

The main blood supply to the anterior abdominal wall is via myocutaneous perforators from the deep superior and inferior epigastric systems. The deep superior epigastric artery (DSEA) originates from the internal thoracic artery at the level of the sixth intercostal space. It initially descends along the deep surface of the rectus abdominis muscle and then courses within the muscle, where it begins to arborize. The deep inferior epigastric artery (DIEA) arises from the external iliac artery just proximal to the inguinal ligament and ascends along the deep surface of the rectus abdominis to the level of the arcuate line, where its course becomes intramuscular. The two systems branch extensively within the muscle to form anastomoses at a level superior to the umbilicus (Fig. 11.2). Branches that perforate the muscle to supply the overlying skin and subcutaneous fat are concentrated in the periumbilical area. The DSEA is the main blood supply to the abdominal wall tissue superior to the umbilicus, and the DIEA is the main blood supply to the tissue below the umbilicus. It is preferable to design the flap over the lower abdomen, where there is the most tissue redundancy, so that the scar will lie in the suprapubic location. The flap may be based on either the DSEA (pedicled or "conventional" TRAM flap) or the DIEA (free TRAM flap).

Pedicled TRAM Flap

Because the DIEA is the predominant blood supply to the lower abdomen, perfusion of the flap based on the DSEA occurs only by flow from the DSEA through the anastomoses into the DIEA in a retrograde fashion. It is not surprising that flap necrosis resulting from inadequate perfusion is the major difficulty with this technique. Care-

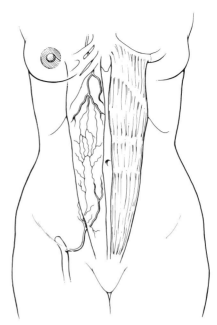

Figure 11.2. *Arterial anatomy of the rectus abdominis muscle. The muscle receives its major blood supply from the deep inferior epigastric artery, a branch from the external iliac artery. The deep superior epigastric artery represents the continuation of the internal mammary. Both of these systems branch into an arteriolar network, which anastomose with each other in the central part of the muscle.*

ful patient selection is, therefore, crucial in obtaining a predictable result with minimal morbidity. The operation is basically reserved for the healthy patient. Contraindications include significant medical problems (severe atherosclerosis, congestive heart failure, diabetes mellitus, chronic obstructive pulmonary disease, previous transection of the DSEA or previous abdominoplasty, smoking, obesity, and psychological instability).

Technique

The flap is usually based on the DSEA pedicle contralateral to the mastectomy for unilateral reconstruction. A transverse elliptical flap is designed over the lower abdomen from just above the umbilicus to the suprapubic level (Figs. 11.3 and 11.4). The upper abdominal skin and subcutaneous fat are then undermined in a plane just superficial to the anterior rectus sheath until the costal margin and xiphoid are reached. Two longitudinal incisions are made in the anterior rectus sheath about 4 cm apart from above the costal margin to the upper edge of the flap. The rectus muscle is then freed within its sheath,

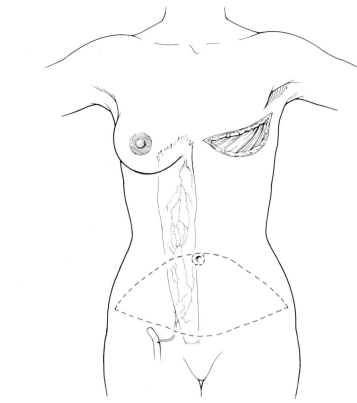

Figure 11.3. The transverse rectus abdominis myocutaneous flap is designed over the lower abdomen much like an aesthetic abdominoplasty. The flap receives its blood supply from perforators through the rectus muscle from the epigastric system.

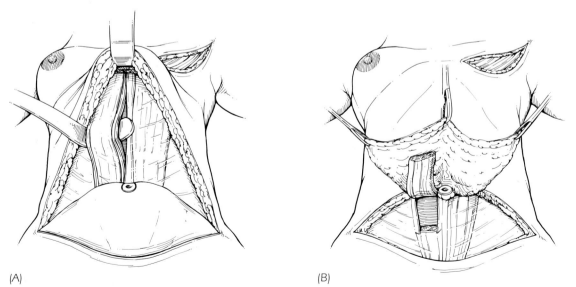

(A)

(B)

Figure 11.4. (A, B). In the conventional transverse rectus abdominis myocutaneous procedure, the flap is isolated on either the ipsilateral or contralateral rectus abdominis muscle. (See text for more detail.)

leaving the anterior strip of fascia adherent to the muscle. The flap on the nonpedicle side is then elevated off the anterior rectus sheath to 1 to 2 cm beyond the midline until the medial row of perforators is encountered. The pedicle side of the flap is elevated until the lateral row of perforators is encountered. The fascia is then incised around the two rows of perforators. The rectus muscle is further freed from its sheath, and the deep inferior epigastic vessels are identified and ligated (Fig. 11.5A, B). The muscle is then divided just below the semicircular line. The flap is now free and attached only to the rectus muscle and DSEA pedicle.

A tunnel is created to connect the abdominal wound to the mastectomy wound. The flap is passed through this tunnel and delivered into the mastectomy wound undergoing a 90-degree rotation in the process (Fig. 11.6). The flap is then shaped and molded to match the opposite breast. The anterior rectus sheath is closed primarily. Marlex mesh can be used to reinforce the closure but is rarely necessary.

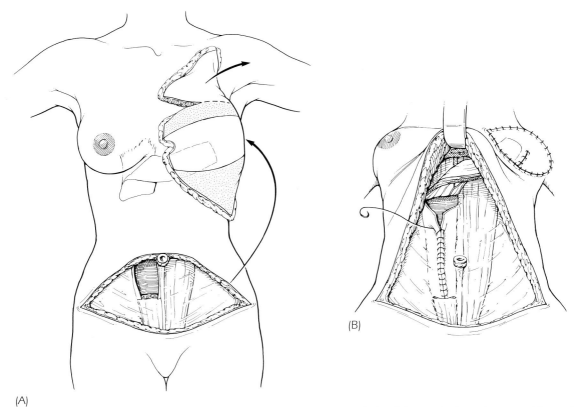

(A)

(B)

Figure 11.5.   (A, B). Once the flap has been isolated on the rectus abdominis muscle, it can be passed through a subcutaneous tunnel into the mastectomy site. The anterior rectus sheath must then be repaired, taking care to include both the internal and external oblique aponeuroses in the repair.

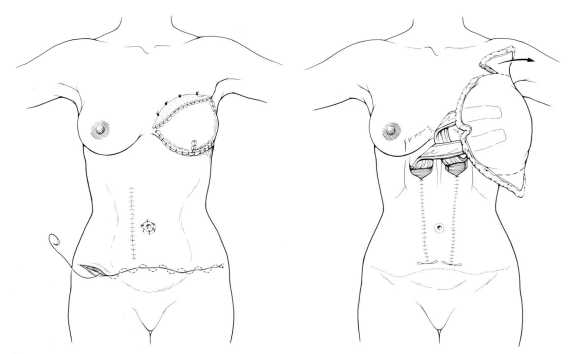

Figure 11.6. The transverse rectus abdominis myocutaneous (TRAM) flap is then inset to attempt to gain symmetry with the opposite side. One rectus abdominis muscle will provide adequate blood supply to carry approximately 50% to 60% of the TRAM flap skin and fat. The remainder must be debrided. The donor site is closed in much the same way as an aesthetic abdominoplasty.

Figure 11.7. Schematic illustration of the bipedicle conventional transverse rectus abdominis myocutaneous (TRAM) flap. This operation is used if more than half of the TRAM flap skin island is required for reconstruction of the breast. This provides a dual source of blood supply through both rectus muscles; therefore, the incidence of fat necrosis in the flap is less. However, more muscle must be sacrificed from the abdominal wall, leaving the abdominal wall strength entirely dependent on the oblique musculature.

Bipedicled TRAM Flap

Because of its somewhat tenuous blood supply, the pedicled TRAM flap (Fig. 11.7) must be restricted to the carefully selected healthy patient. To minimize the risk of partial flap necrosis, it is believed that not more than 60% of the volume of the abdominal ellipse should be carried on a single DSEA pedicle. In many cases the volume of tissue that can be safely carried is not enough to match the opposite breast. In these cases and for patients considered at higher risk for partial flap necrosis, such as smokers, use of the double-pedicled TRAM flap has been advocated to improve the blood supply (25). Essentially, the entire abdominal flap can be carried safely on both DSEA pedicles. Because both rectus muscles are taken with the flap, an obvious disadvantage is increased abdominal wall weakness with an increased need for synthetic mesh to facilitate the abdominal wall closure. The epigastric bulge tends to be quite prominent especially in thinner patients.

Free TRAM Flap

An alternative method of improving the blood supply to the TRAM flap with less abdominal wall disruption is the free TRAM flap. The free TRAM flap is based on the deep inferior epigastric artery and vein, which is the largest set of axial vessels entering the anterior abdominal wall. It represents the primary source of blood supply to the TRAM flap territory. However, because the pedicle clearly cannot reach the mastectomy site, it must be divided and the flap transferred as a microsurgical free flap with subsequent reanastomosis of the inferior epigastric artery and vein to recipient vessels around the mastectomy site. Because the inferior epigastric vessels are considerably larger than the superior epigastric vessels, the free TRAM flap is a better profused flap than the pedicle TRAM. As such, more tissue can be transferred on a single pedicle than with the conventional pedicled TRAM (Fig. 11.8). As depicted in Figure 11.8, the flap is elevated on a small rectangle of rectus abdominis muscle extending from the arcuate line to the umbilicus. This segment of rectus muscle includes the key perforators from the deep inferior epigastric artery into the flap territory. A medial and lateral strip of rectus muscle can be maintained, thereby improving the ultimate strength of the repaired abdominal wall.

For immediate reconstruction, we prefer skin-sparing mastectomies whereby only the nipple-areola complex and the previous biopsy site are included with the mastectomy specimen (Fig. 11.9). For DCIS or other noninfiltrated lesions, the biopsy site may be left alone. For the reconstructive surgeon, the goal, then, is to replace exactly the volume and shape of tissues that are removed at mastectomy. The free TRAM flap offers this capability in that the nipple-areola complex can be replaced by a disk-shaped skin island, with the abdominal fat restoring the breast mound.

A separate axillary incision is convenient to complete the axillary lymphadenectomy as well as to dissect the thoracodorsal artery and vein, which are the most common recipient vessels for microvascular anastomosis. In Figure 11.10 A, the microvascular anastomosis is schematically depicted. Generally, the thoracodorsal artery is a good size match for the deep inferior epigastric artery, which measures between 1.5 and 2 mm. The thoracodorsal vein is anastomosed to the deep inferior epigastric vein, thereby restoring circulation to the flap via a single arterial and venous anastomosis. The flap is then shaped into a cone matching the opposite breast.

Abdominal closure is somewhat simpler in the free TRAM than in the pedicled TRAM. The fascial defect is considerably smaller, al-

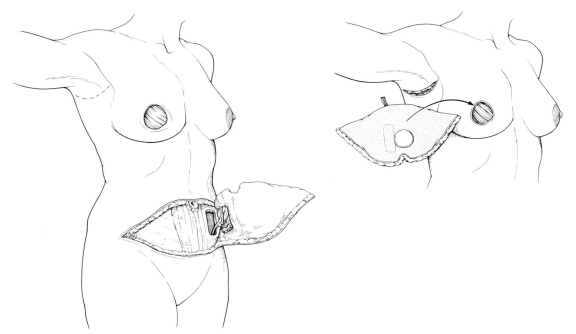

Figure 11.8. Schematic design of the free transverse rectus abdominis myocutaneous procedure. In this operation, the flap is pedicled on the deep inferior epigastric artery and vein. These vessels are then divided, and the flap is transplanted to the mastectomy site.

Figure 11.9. In ideal candidates, the mastectomy can be performed through a periareolar incision only. A separate axillary incision is used to expose the thoracodorsal artery and vein, which is ordinarily selected for recipient microvascular anastomoses.

though it does violate the abdominal wall in its most vulnerable portion (i.e., the area around the arcuate line where there is no posterior sheath); therefore, a very secure closure must be achieved. Plication of the opposite fascia as well as correction of any rectus diastasis and fat contouring is always done to try to achieve the most aesthetic abdominal closure possible.

Overall, the free TRAM flap has been most suitable for immediate reconstruction and, in our opinion, has improved the results of autogenous reconstruction using the TRAM flap to the point at which it has largely replaced the pedicled TRAM in our practice (26, 27) (Figs. 11.11 and 11.12).

Bilateral Reconstruction

Patients who have had cancer in one breast are at increased risk for cancer in the remaining breast. The risk is estimated to be five times greater than that of someone who did not have a first breast cancer. The need for bilateral breast reconstruction may be encountered in patients undergoing a second mastectomy for a second primary breast

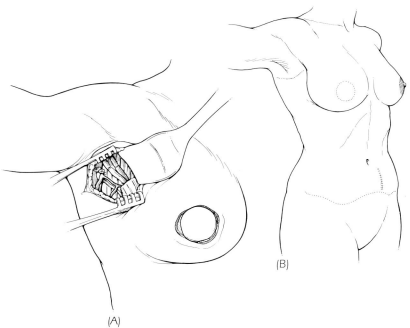

(B)

(A)

Figure 11.10.   (A) The microvascular anastomoses are depicted. The deep inferior epigastric artery is sutured end to end to the thoracodorsal artery just proximal to the serratus branch. The venous anastomosis is similarly done. This single set of microvascular repairs is adequate to supply circulation to the transferred flap at approximately the same level as the bipedicled conventional transverse rectus abdominis myocutaneous (TRAM) flap. It has the advantage of sparing abdominal wall muscle, however. (B) Closure of the free TRAM is simplified because the segment of rectus sheath that has been harvested is quite short. Also no muscle must be tunneled into the mastectomy flap area, so natural breast landmarks are preserved, and no prominence in the superior abdomen is observed.

cancer. Both breasts can be reconstructed in a single stage with either implants and expanders or autogenous tissue. The option of bilateral breast reconstruction is of particular importance to women considering a prophylactic mastectomy of the contralateral breast at the time of modified radical mastectomy.

Symmetry is much more easily obtained in bilateral reconstructions than in unilateral reconstructions for obvious reasons. This is especially true for implants and expanders, although, as with unilateral reconstruction, mature-appearing ptotic breasts are difficult to achieve. The TRAM flap is again the flap of choice when considering autogenous tissue reconstruction. Bilateral free TRAM flaps can be performed safely in a single stage and yield excellent cosmetic results. The superior blood supply to the flaps and decreased abdominal wall disruption may result in lower complication rates and less abdominal wall morbidity compared with bilateral pedicled TRAM flaps (28).

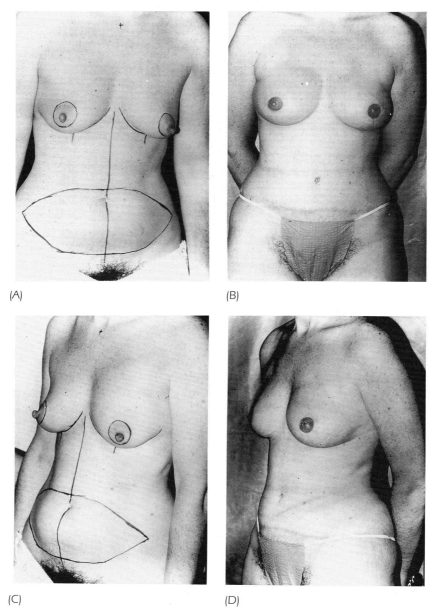

(A)

(B)

(C)

(D)

Figure 11.11. (A) A 44-year-old woman with an early infiltrating lesion in the right breast and a strong family history of breast cancer in first-degree relatives. She elected to undergo bilateral mastectomies through periareolar incisions. Bilateral free transverse rectus abdominis myocutaneous flaps were used. (B) Result after nipple-areola reconstruction and tattooing. (C) Preoperative oblique view. (D) Postoperative oblique view.

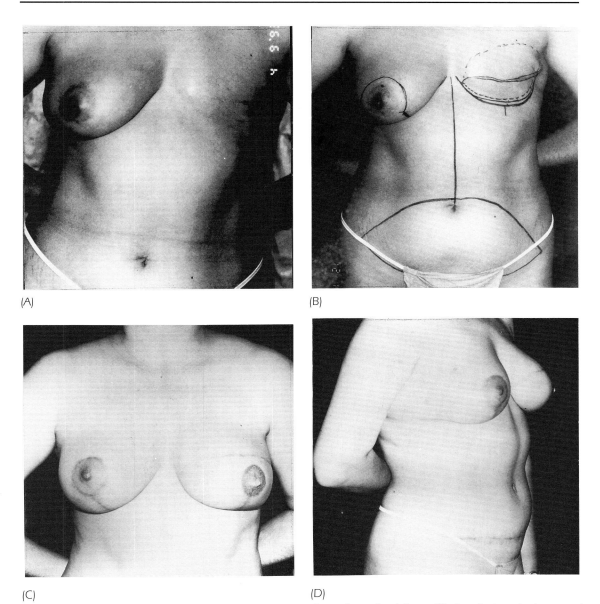

(A)

(B)

(C)

(D)

Figure 11.12.   (A) Preoperative anteroposterior view of a patient after left modified radical mastectomy and adjunctive chemotherapy for a stage I carcinoma of the left breast. (B) The operative plan includes free transverse rectus abdominis myocutaneous (TRAM) flap reconstruction of the left breast and a right mastopexy for ptosis. (C) Result after free TRAM flap reconstruction of the left breast followed by nipple-areola reconstruction. (D) Postoperative oblique view.

Other Donor Sites for Autogenous Tissue Reconstruction

The lateral transverse thigh flap and the gluteal flap have been described as free tissue transfers for breast reconstruction (29,30). Among microsurgeons, however, the free TRAM flap is the flap of choice when considering a free tissue transfer. If conditions preclude the use of a free TRAM flap, such as a previous abdominoplasty, abdominal scars, or patient preference, the lateral transverse thigh (LTT) flap and gluteal flap are useful alternatives.

LTT Flap

The LTT flap is based on the lateral circumflex artery, which supplies the skin over the lateral thigh via myocutaneous perforators from the tensor fascia lata. The flap is designed as a transverse ellipse centered over the greater trochanter. A segment of tensor fascia lata must be included in the flap. It is a well-vascularized, reliable flap that offers a potential improvement of "saddlebag" deformities of the thigh if present. There is negligible functional morbidity. The main problem is that the donor site scar cannot be hidden, and an objectionable contour irregularity may result, especially in a patient without obvious saddlebags.

Inferior Gluteal Flap

The inferior gluteal artery supplies the lower portion of the gluteus maximus muscle and overlying skin by myocutaneous perforators. The flap is designed over the lower buttock such that the resultant scar will lie hidden in the inferior gluteal crease. An inferior portion of the gluteus maximus muscle must be included in the flap. Excellent projection of the reconstructed breast can be achieved because of the inherent characteristics of the buttock tissue. The scar is usually well hidden. The main problem with this flap is that it is technically difficult to perform. Also chronic pain at the donor site is possible as well as buttock asymmetry.

Reconstruction of the Nipple-Areola Complex

The nipple-areola complex is an essential functional and aesthetic component of the female breast. It has unique qualities of form, texture, and pigmentation, which have proven a challenge to the reconstructive surgeon. In the past, a symmetric breast mound was rarely achieved even after multiple stages. The addition of a nipple-areola complex to an asymmetric mound tended to accentuate the asymmetry. Not surprisingly, nipple-areola complex reconstruction was often declined by both patient and surgeon. Today, with much improved methods of achieving breast mound symmetry, nipple-areola complex reconstruction enhances the symmetry and gives the mound a true breast-like appearance. Most women will elect to undergo nipple-areola complex reconstruction if it can be done simply and with little or no morbidity.

The nipple and areola are usually reconstructed as separate components after waiting approximately 3 months to allow settling of the reconstructed breast into its final shape and position. Nipple-areola complex placement is crucial and should be agreed on by both patient and surgeon. The patient may experiment with placement by sticking an electrocardiogram button in various positions on the breast mound until the most aesthetic placement is arrived at. In general, the nipple and areola may be reconstructed using specific tissue (the opposite nipple and areola) or nonspecific tissue (skin grafts, local flaps). The opposite nipple-areola complex represents a sensate, erogenous, and functional component of the only normal breast remaining, and most women prefer that it not be violated.

Nipple Reconstruction

The main difficulty with current methods of nipple reconstruction is obtaining and maintaining adequate nipple projection. The most common method is the use of a local flap. Recently, many ingenious local flaps have been designed to achieve long-term nipple projection (31–33) (Fig. 11.13). The technique can usually be performed under local anesthesia, and complications are rare. As a rule, however, texture and color are not well matched.

A nipple-sharing technique may be a consideration if the opposite nipple is obviously hypertrophic. A portion of the nipple is excised longitudinally, transversely, or in a wedge pattern and transferred to the breast mound as a free composite graft. The donor nipple is closed primarily. Texture and color match is excellent. Adequate nipple projection can be achieved, but symmetry can be difficult. Donor site morbidity must be considered but usually is minimal.

Areola Reconstruction

The main difficulty with reconstruction of the areola is obtaining a good color match. A full-thickness skin graft may be taken in the shape of the opposite areola usually from the pigmented upper inner thigh. An acceptable color match may be initially obtained, but fading of the skin graft to a much paler color is to be expected over time. Donor site wound breakdown and chronic pain over the scar can be a

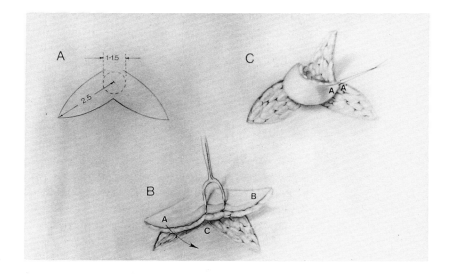

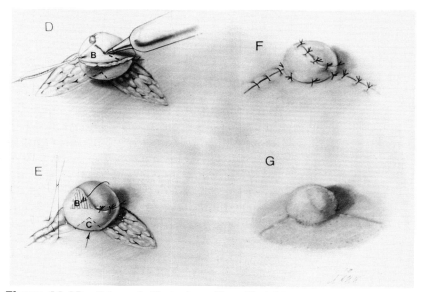

Figure 11.13.   Schematic illustration of "modified fishtail flap" nipple reconstruction. The two flaps are elevated and transposed as shown. Eight weeks later the nipple-areola area is tattoed to match the color of the opposite side.

problem. The more heavily pigmented skin of the labia majora has been used, but donor site morbidity is often unacceptable and the resultant areola may stretch to an unaesthetic size.

If the opposite areola is large and the patient is not averse to a scar around it, areolar sharing may be considered. Numerous techniques have been described, some of which are ingenious but complicated. A simple and effective method is to take a concentric ring of skin from the outer aspect of the opposite areola. The scars surrounding both areolae tend to improve the symmetry. The donor areola may stretch with time, but morbidity is minimal.

Tattooing

The main problem in nipple-areola complex reconstruction using tissue other than the opposite nipple-areola complex is achieving a good color match. This was partly solved, and nipple-areola complex reconstruction was simplified by the popularization of tattooing over the last 5 years. Although a degree of skill and artistry is required to achieve excellent results, the technique itself is easy to learn and can be practiced by any health professional. The challenge is selecting the appropriate pigments to match the opposite nipple-areola complex. Some have advocated tattooing the opposite nipple-areola complex with the same pigment as a means of improving symmetry.

Tattooing is most commonly done after the nipple and areola have been reconstructed. It can be used to "touch up" the shape of the reconstructed areola, which is often distorted or smaller than originally planned because of contraction inherent with skin grafts. The areola can be reconstructed with tattoo alone, thus precluding the need for a skin graft and any associated donor site morbidity. Although areolar texture and projection are not simulated, it is a fair tradeoff for the simplicity of the technique, and excellent results can still be achieved especially with bilateral reconstructions.

Tattooing is usually performed 2 to 3 months after nipple-areola reconstruction is complete. It is generally well tolerated in an office or clinic setting with or without local anesthesia depending on patient preference or comfort. Pigment slightly darker than the opposite areola is chosen to compensate for some degree of fading that all tattoos experience with time. The nipple often requires a slightly darker pigment than the areola.

CONCLUSION

Every woman diagnosed with breast cancer deserves to be informed of all the treatment options so that she may participate in determining the treatment that is best for her. To this end, early consultation with a plastic surgeon is essential. Breast reconstruction is not for all women, and not every woman will choose reconstruction after mastectomy. If reconstruction is an option, then the methods most appropriate for the needs and expectations of the patient can be thoroughly discussed and a sound treatment protocol planned. With current techniques, an excellent match of the opposite breast can be achieved in a single stage. All physicians involved in the care of a patient with breast cancer should be aware that reconstruction after mastectomy has a major impact in terms of minimizing the psychological morbidity, and there is no doubt that quality of life is greatly improved.

References

1. Feuer EJ, Wun L, Boring CC, et al. The lifetime risk of developing breast cancer. J Natl Cancer Inst 1993;85:892–897.
2. Sondik EJ. Breast cancer trends. Cancer 1994;74:995–999.
3. Lewis FM, Bloom JR. Psychosocial adjustment to breast cancer: a review of selected literature. Int J Psychiatry Med 1978;9:1–13.
4. Clifford E. Psychological effects of the mastectomy experience. In: Georgiade NG, ed. Breast reconstruction following mastectomy. St. Louis: CV Mosby, 1979:1–21.
5. Stevens LA, McGrath MH, Druss RG, et al. The psychological impact of immediate breast reconstruction for women with early breast cancer. Plast Reconstr Surg 1984;73:619–626.
6. Fisher B, Redmond C, Poisson R, et al. Eight year results of a randomized clinical trial comparing total mastectomy and lumpectomy with and without irradiation in the treatment of breast cancer. N Engl J Med 1989;320:822–828.
7. Ward S, Heidrich S, Wolberg W. Factors women take into account when deciding upon type of surgery for breast cancer. Cancer Nurs 1989;12:344–351.
8. Wilson RG, Hart A, Dawes PJDK. Mastectomy or conservation: the patient's choice. BMJ 1988;297:1167–1169.
9. Wolberg WH. Surgical options in 424 patients with primary breast cancer without systemic metastases. Arch Surg 1991;126:817–820.
10. Rowland JH, Holland JC, Chaglassian T, et al. Psychological response to breast reconstruction. Psychosomatics 1993;34:241–250.
11. Dowden RV, Yetman RJ. Mastectomy with immediate reconstruction: issues and answers. Cleve Clin J Med 1992;59:499–503.
12. Noone RB, Frazier TG, Noone GC, et al. Recurrence of breast carcinoma following immediate reconstruction: a 13-year review. Plast Reconstr Surg 1994;93:96–106.
13. Slavin SA, Love SM, Goldwyn RM. Recurrent breast cancer following immediate reconstruction with myocutaneous flaps. Plast Reconstr Surg 1994;93:1191–1204.
14. Eberlein TJ, Crespo LD, Smith BL, et al. Prospective evaluation of immediate reconstruction after mastectomy. Ann Surg 1993;218:29–36.
15. Noguchi M, Fukushima W, Ohta N, et al. Oncological aspect of immediate breast reconstruction in mastectomy patients. J Surg Oncol 1992;50:241–246.

16. Elkowitz A, Colen S, Slavin S, et al. Various methods of breast reconstruction after mastectomy: an economic comparison. Plast Reconstr Surg 1993;92:77–83.

17. Berkel H, Birdsell DC, Jenkins H. Breast augmentation: a risk factor for breast cancer? N Engl J Med 1992;326:1649–1653.

18. Park AJ, Black RJ, Watson ACH. Silicone gel breast implants, breast cancer and connective tissue disorders. Br J Surg 1993;80:1097–1100.

19. Gabriel SE, O'Fallon WM, Kurland LT, et al. Risk of connective-tissue diseases and other disorders after breast implantation. N Engl J Med 1994;330:1697–1702.

20. Petit J, Le MG, Mouriesse H, et al. Can breast reconstruction with gel-filled silicone implants increase the risk of death and second primary cancer in patients treated by mastectomy for breast cancer? Plast Reconstr Surg 1994;94:115–119.

21. Holmes JD. Capsular contracture after breast reconstruction with tissue expansion. Br J Plast Surg 1989;42:591–594.

22. Trabulsy PP, Anthony JP, Mathes SJ. Changing trends in postmastectomy breast reconstruction: a 13-year experience. Plast Reconstr Surg 1994;93: 1418–1427.

23. Bostwick J, Nahai F, Wallace JG, Vasconez LO. Sixty latissimus dorsi flaps. Plast Reconstr Surg 1979;63:31–41.

24. McCraw JB, Maxwell GP. Early and late capsular deformation as a cause of unsatisfactory results in the latissimus dorsi breast reconstruction. Clin Plast Surg 1988;15:717–726.

25. Wagner DS, Michelow BJ, Hartrampf CR. Double-pedicle TRAM flap for unilateral breast reconstruction. Plast Reconstr Surg 1991;88:987–997.

26. Grotting JC, Urist MM, Maddox WA, Vasconez LO. Conventional TRAM vs. free microsurgical TRAM flap for immediate breast reconstruction. Plast Reconstr Surg 1989;83:828–841.

27. Grotting JC. Reoperation following free flap breast reconstruction. In: Grotting JC, ed. Reoperative aesthetic and reconstructive plastic surgery, vol. 2. St. Louis: Quality Medical Publishing, 1995:1093–1157.

28. Baldwin BJ, Schusterman MA, Miller MJ, et al. Bilateral breast reconstruction: conventional versus free TRAM. Plast Reconstr Surg 1994;93: 1410–1416.

29. Elliott LF, Beegle PH, Hartrampf CR. The lateral transverse thigh free flap: an alternative for autogenous-tissue breast reconstruction. Plast Reconstr Surg 1990;85:169–178.

30. Paletta CE, Bostwick J, Nahai F. The inferior gluteal free flap in breast reconstruction. Plast Reconstr Surg 1989;84:875–883.

31. Eskenazi L. A one-stage nipple reconstruction with the "modified star" flap and immediate tattoo: a review of 100 cases. Plast Reconstr Surg 1993;92:671–680.

32. Little JW, Spear SL. The finishing touches in nipple-areolar reconstruction. Perspect Plast Surg 1988;2:1–17.

33. Hugo NE, Sultan MR, Hardy SP. Nipple-areolar reconstruction with intradermal tattoo and double-opposing pennant flaps. Ann Plast Surg 1993;30:510–513.

Radiotherapeutic Management of Breast Cancer

Merle M. Salter and Richard L. S. Jennelle

Breast cancer is the most common malignancy in women and the second leading cause of death. It is estimated that in 1996 this disease will develop in 182,000 women, resulting in 46,000 deaths (1). The traditional surgical approach of mastectomy for all stages of this disease has now evolved to add breast-conservation surgery and irradiation as a definitive therapeutic option for many patients with stage I and stage II carcinoma of the breast.

Both large and small randomized trials are now available (2–8) with long-term follow-up that show equivalent survival with breast-preserving surgery versus mastectomy. Retrospective reviews involving breast preservation, some with 10- to 15- and 25-year follow-up (9–13), are also reported and reveal survival rates that are comparable to those for patients who have undergone mastectomy. These studies also show no difference in local recurrence or distant metastases. Low complication rates and good to excellent cosmetic outcomes are well documented.

The studies just cited are the basis of and continue to affirm the June 1990 consensus statement of the National Institutes of Health. A panel of experts concluded that breast-conservation treatment is an appropriate method of primary therapy for a majority of women with stage I and stage II breast cancer. It is preferable because it provided survival rates equivalent to those of total mastectomy and axillary dissection while preserving the breast (14). Despite this, one study revealed that only 5% to 15% of women with early-stage disease undergo conservative surgery (15).

A discussion that involves alternative methods of therapy, the risks, and complications should be offered to all properly selected women with early-stage breast cancer. These issues should be discussed by each discipline involved. Criteria for patient selection should be based on producing the most acceptable cosmesis with the fewest complications and the lowest possible risk of breast recurrence.

PATIENT SELECTION CRITERIA

Tumor Size

Any primary breast tumor up to 4 cm in greatest diameter that can be excised with clear margins may undergo breast preservation. In addition, the tumor must not involve the skin and should be relatively proportional to the size of the breast. Large tumors in small breasts may produce an unacceptable cosmetic result and should be excluded on this basis alone.

Breast Size

Initially patients with large, pendulous breasts were thought to be ineligible for breast preservation because of increased fibrosis and retraction. However, with appropriate radiation technique, this is not a problem, and the result can be more cosmetically pleasing than reconstruction and reduction mammaplasty.

Tumor Location

Tumors in any location in the breast, including the subareolar region, can be treated with breast conservation (16). Subareolar tumor requires excision of the nipple-areola complex, which can impair cosmesis.

Histologic Subtypes

Various histologic subtypes of breast cancer, which include infiltrating ductal carcinoma and infiltrating lobular, medullary, colloid, and tubular carcinoma, have been investigated in regard to being a risk factor in predicting survival and pattern of failure. There is no impact on overall survival, relapse-free survival, or cause-specific survival regardless of histologic subtype (17).

RELATIVE CONTRAINDICATIONS

Multicentricity and Multifocality

It is important to be aware of and understand the differences between these two entities. Mammography is often extremely important in the identification of one or more cancers in the same breast. If the disease is multicentric (one or more totally independent foci of tumor), then mastectomy with reconstruction may well produce the most pleasing cosmetic result as well as a decreased local recurrence rate. Several studies have addressed this specific issue and found actuarial recurrence rates of between 25% and 40% for synchronous ipsilateral breast cancers versus a local recurrence rate of 11% to 12% for single lesions (18,19).

Whether this may apply to multifocal carcinoma of the breast (more than one tumor focus of cancer within the same quadrant) is unclear. Findings from Holland et al (20) suggest that most multiple tumors are multifocal rather than multicentric. We know from the National Surgical Adjuvant Breast Project (NSABP) study B-06 data (21) as well as other series (22,23) that local excision alone gives failure rates of between 25% and 35%, with most local recurrences in close proximity to the primary tumor. It has been proven that the addition of radiation decreases the incidence of local recurrence from 44% to 10% at 10 years (2). Hence, some few selected patients with overt multifocal disease with no more than two lesions may be candidates for breast conservation, if they so desire, knowing that the local recurrence rate is increased.

Age

Patient age has been a controversial issue when one wishes to be treated with radiation for breast preservation. With heightened awareness and an increase in breast education, more and more young patients are asking about breast-conservation surgery. Several published reports examined breast cancer in young women and suggested that they have a lower survival rate than older women (24–31). Several reports also reveal an increased local recurrence rate in women treated with breast conservation who are younger than 30 to 35 years (32–34). However, the most quoted data from this country are from the Joint Center for Radiation Therapy (JCRT) (35). Evaluation of their earlier data found that with pre- and postoperative mammography and careful attention to surgical margins (re-excision in cases with extensive intraductal component [EIC] or uncertain initial margins to obtain negative margins) the local recurrence rate for those patients younger than 35 years was 12%. The recurrence rate for women 35 to 50 years old was 11%; for women aged 51 to 64 years, 3%; and for those older than 65 years, 7% (36). Other articles supported the use of breast-conservation surgery and found no difference in disease-free survival or overall survival with tumorectomy and radiation in this group of younger patients (37–39).

The most recent article by de la Rochefordiere et al (40,41) is the largest reported series examining age as a prognostic factor. Clearly, the younger patients had a significantly lower 5-year survival and higher local and distant relapse rates than did older patients independent of tumor size, nodal status, histologic grade, hormone receptors, locoregional treatment procedure, or adjuvant systemic therapy. This article should put to rest any controversy about young age at diagnosis. Reasons for more aggressive behavior in this subset of patients are unknown.

One should remember also that women who are younger than 30 to 35 years have a longer time to live, are at a greater risk for second primary cancer (42), and may have a disease that in some patients is biologically different.

HISTOPATHOLOGIC FEATURES

Many histopathologic features have been associated with an increase in the local recurrence rate. The presence of EIC as defined by the JCRT is simultaneous invasive carcinoma and an intraductal component of greater than 25% of the primary tumor as well as intraductal carcinoma being present in the surrounding breast tissue. EIC has been said to increase the incidence of local recurrence (43). However, if adequately excised with negative margins, this is not a contraindication to breast preservation (44–47). Other factors such as high nuclear grade (48), vascular invasion (47), lymphatic invasion, and tumor necrosis (49) have been implicated and should be considered along with all the other relative factors that may increase local recurrence.

PSYCHOSOCIAL ISSUES

The psychosocial issues and quality of life studies are also important factors in patient selection. It has been found that when the patient becomes an active participant in the decision-making process with a thorough understanding of all the issues there are no substantial differences in the psychological adjustment favoring either breast preservation or mastectomy. Specifically, there was no difference with regard to changes of life patterns or fear of cancer recurrence and death. However, with respect to body image and sexual functioning, the results favor breast-conserving treatment (50).

CONTRAINDICATIONS

Complications that are unacceptable have been reported in patients with known collagen-vascular disease (51–54). These are exaggerated acute toxicity with increased skin reaction and protracted healing as well as long-term chronic effects of radiation producing fibrosis, scarring, and a painful breast. These patients should not be considered candidates for breast preservation. Patients with a history of Hodgkin's disease or non-Hodgkin's lymphoma who have received irradiation to a supradiaphragmatic mantle and who experience breast cancer are not candidates for conservative treatment. Also patients with chronic obstructive lung disease, myocardial disease with cancer arising in the left breast, and uncontrolled diabetes should be excluded from treatment with radiation. Patients who are uncooperative because of psychiatric disorders or elderly patients with dementia are not candidates. Ongoing pregnancy is also an absolute contraindication to breast irradiation (55).

SURGICAL CONSIDERATIONS

The optimal extent of breast resection before radiation therapy for definitive local control still remains unclear. It seems that the best measure of local control is adequate surgical resection with negative margins and a good to excellent cosmetic outcome. An example is NSABP B-06, in which all patients had negative tumor margins (56). However, what constitutes an adequate surgical margin is still unclear and ranges from quadrantectomy to excisional biopsy of the lesion (57–58) (Table 12.1). Various groups have studied outcome and local recurrence in terms of margin assessment and found no survival or local control difference in selected patients with tumors that had negative margins (defined as >2 mm), close margins (<2 mm), or focally positive margins (59,60). We do know that grossly incomplete removal of the primary tumor results in a significantly higher risk of

Table 12.1. Incidences of local recurrence
related to the extent of breast resection

	Local recurrence (%)	
Series	**Excisional biopsy**	**Quadrantectomy**
Retrospective		
Clarke	369 (5)	43 9.0
Van Limbergen	149 (15)	69 7.0
Chu	110 (10)	18 11.0
Nobler	87 (7)	48 6.0
NSABP	629 (10)	—
Veronesi	—	1232 (3.0)
Prospective		
Veronesi	345 (7)	360 (2.2)

NSABP = National Surgical Adjuvant Breast Project.
Data from Vicini et al (58).

local failure and is generally considered unacceptable in terms of surgical management (61–64).

Patients generally considered for re-excision before radiation are those who initially have unknown margins, EIC without good margins, or residual microcalcification on postexcision mammogram. Patient selection and radiotherapy dose and technique may be contributing factors to the varied outcomes described previously.

Axillary Dissection

An axillary dissection separate from the primary surgery is considered a standard part of breast-conservation surgery (56) at this time. Axillary management by the surgeon may range from a sampling of nodes to a full axillary dissection. It appears that in patients with clinically negative nodes a dissection that includes levels I and II is adequate therapeutically and prognostically (56,65). There is less arm and breast edema associated with the more limited procedure (66,67).

Haffty et al (68) addressed the concept of lumpectomy without axillary dissection followed by irradiation to the breast and regional nodes. Patients outside a protocol setting whose systemic management would not be altered by axillary dissection might be considered candidates for such an approach. Also postmenopausal women whose tumors are estrogen receptor (ER) positive and who will receive tamoxifen as standard adjuvant therapy regardless of microscopic nodal status may also be candidates. There may be some younger patients who, regardless of nodal status, will receive systemic chemotherapy and would be candidates for this approach. These issues should be considered and addressed in randomized trials.

RADIATION TREATMENT TECHNIQUES

Radiotherapy to ensure the best possible results requires a team approach with cooperation among the mammographer, pathologist, surgeon, and radiation oncologist and medical oncologist. This treatment program should be given only in a facility that provides an understanding of the total problem.

Equipment

Low-energy linear accelerators of between 4–6 MeV or a cobalt 60 machine are adequate for treatment. The availability of brachytherapy or electron beam capability is also helpful as is the ability to make compensators or wedge filters.

Patient simulation is mandatory as are dedicated treatment planning computers. Excellent physics and dosimetry support and well-trained technical staff are essential.

Dose and Fractionation

The treatment is delivered 5 days per week, one fraction per day at a dose of 180 to 200 cGy/fraction. A total dose of between 4500 and 5000 cGy is delivered to the entire breast in a 4.5- to 5.5-week interval.

Portals

The entire breast is included using two tangent or oblique fields; each field is treated daily. The margins extend superiorly to the level of the sternoclavicular joint, inferiorly to 1.5 cm below the inframmary fold, medially to the midline of the sternum, and laterally to the mid- to posterior axillary line. The underlying chest wall to include muscle and ribs is included within the tangent volume. Excessive volumes of both lung and heart should be avoided.

CONTROVERSIES IN RADIOTHERAPY

Boost Dose

The administration of additional radiation to the primary area of excision remains controversial. The NSABP B-06 did not give additional treatment to this area with known negative margins, and local recurrence was not increased. However, the use of additional treatment to the site of the primary tumor is routinely given by many institutions in this country as well as in Europe. The added 1000 to 1500 cGy can be administered by photons, electron beam of appropriate energy, or interstitial irradiation. Currently, the validity of adding a boost in patients with negative margins is being investigated in an ongoing trial by the European Organization for Research on Treatment of Cancer (EORTC).

Regional Nodal Irradiation

Regional nodal irradiation postaxillary dissection at levels I and II has also been an ongoing area of controversy. Recht et al (69) retrospectively analyzed 1624 patients treated with breast-conservation surgery and irradiation at the JCRT. They found that the incidence of axillary failure for patients who underwent an axillary dissection and breast irradiation was only 2.7% for patients with negative nodes and 2.1% for patients with one to three positive nodes. The incidence of supraclavicular failure was 1.9% and 0.0%, respectively, for these two groups. They believe that regional nodal irradiation for negative nodes or one to three positive nodes is not routinely indicated. For patients with four or more positive nodes, there are insufficient data to make a recommendation regarding axillary and supraclavicular irradiation, but this is discussed in greater detail in the section on advanced breast cancer. Patients with more than 50% of the nodes positive or with extracapsular extension are a subgroup of patients who may benefit the most from such treatment.

Patients who did not have an axillary dissection, who had clinically negative nodes, and who were treated with nodal irradiation had an 0.8% incidence of axillary recurrence and a 0.3% recurrence in the supraclavicular area region. These patients can be treated effectively for local control, and these areas should be treated if for some reason axillary dissection is not performed.

Fowble et al (70) found that only 27 (3%) of 914 patients developed regional node failure as their first site of failure; axillary failure was the most common. In a subset analysis of the 50.0% node-negative patients who received treatment to the breast, only 2.9% developed nodal recurrence and, among the N1 patients only 2.4% developed local nodal recurrence.

Nodal relapse correlated only with the number of axillary nodes removed and the patient's age and was unrelated to primary tumor size, tumor location, histology, axillary nodal status, and region irradiated. Fowble and others believe that nodal irradiation may be omitted in the node-negative patient. However, they still advocate regional nodal irradiation in patients with positive axillary nodes. There are many other articles both for and against treatment to the regional nodal areas, and this topic remains controversial.

SEQUENCING OF CHEMORADIOTHERAPY

Adjuvant chemotherapy in selected node-negative patients as well as node-positive patients has become the standard of care. Its use in combination with radiation appears to decrease the incidence of breast recurrence. This was seen in NSABP B-06 (71) in node-positive patients. Rose et al (72) also reported on a group of premenopausal node-positive patients in whom chemotherapy appeared to increase the local control rate. In a prospective, randomized trial carried out in NSABP B-13, Fisher reported on a group of node-negative estrogen receptor-progesterone receptor (ER-PR)–negative women in whom the local control rate tended toward improvement with the addition of chemotherapy (73).

The mechanism of action of enhancing the effectiveness of radiotherapy in preventing local recurrence is unknown; hence, the optimum sequencing of these modalities is still unclear. There are results that favor radiotherapy being initiated before chemotherapy; some investigators indicated that the delay of radiation treatment increases local recurrence (74), whereas others have found no difference in local control rates by delaying radiotherapy after lumpectomy until after adjuvant chemotherapy was delivered. Some studies reported on the "sandwich technique," giving one or several courses of chemotherapy immediately after surgery and then radiation followed by further chemotherapy (75,76). Still others have used concurrent chemoradiotherapy (74).

The use of concurrent chemoradiotherapy is generally thought to produce a worse cosmetic result when compared with sequential use of chemotherapy and radiation (77). Other institutions indicated that the impact of concurrent treatment on cosmesis was small or nonexistent when compared with radiotherapy alone (78). The University of Pennsylvania showed fewer excellent cosmetic results with an increase in the fair to poor results when using concurrent treatment (79). Concurrent treatment has also been shown to produce worsened acute skin reactions (80,81) as well as more severe chronic subcutaneous fibrosis (82).

Other complications such as symptomatic pneumonitis, brachial plexopathy, arm edema, and myositis may be increased by the use of concurrent chemoradiotherapy, but the effect of sequential treatment is not clear. The radiotherapeutic technique also plays an important part in producing the best result.

The use of adjuvant tamoxifen during radiotherapy has been widely discussed, and there is some concern that tamoxifen produces a growth-arresting effect, which may make the tumor cells less sensitive to radiation. This datum is from laboratory research and remains to be proven. There is no clinical evidence to support this adverse effect. The NSABP B-14 trial reported a decrease in local failure in patients who were ER-PR positive and node negative who received concurrent tamoxifen (83).

Complications

Long-term complications in conservatively managed patients are and will be ongoing. The final result of the combination of the varying surgical approaches and the sequencing of the chemotherapy as well as radiotherapy technique is yet to be seen. According to a report from the JCRT (84) the risk of significant complications is low. Patients with primary breast cancer have a two- to fivefold increased risk for the development of cancer in the opposite breast. With the increasing use of radiation therapy for definitive control of the initial cancer, the role of radiation in increasing the risk has been assessed. A study by Storm et al (85) provides evidence that there is little, if any, risk of radiation-induced breast cancer associated with the low radiation dose to the opposite breast.

Local Recurrence

The risk of local recurrence is inherent in any patient who chooses breast preservation. The 5-, 10-, 15-, and 20-year results are available from large retrospective studies. A 5% to 10% recurrence rate is seen at 5 years, and a 10% to 20% local recurrence rate is seen at 10 years with a leveling at 15 to 20 years. The local recurrence rate for the patients with mastectomy is no different than local recurrence with breast preservation: approximately 10% to 20% at 10 years (37–39).

Breast recurrence is important to detect early because tumors 2 cm or smaller are associated with the best prognosis. Screening mammography is not as helpful as in the untreated breast, and some series (86,87) reported a rate of lesion detection by mammography alone ranging from 29% to 42%. In other series, mammogram alone detects roughly 35% of lesions; physical examination, 39%; and both methods, 26% (88). Noninvasive recurrences are more commonly detected by mammography (87). It is believed that mammographic follow-up is necessary and complementary to physical examination in the detection of local recurrence.

True or malignant recurrences must be at the site of the original tumor or within the vicinity; and new tumors are those occurring a distance away from the primary site or in a different quadrant of the breast. Time to recurrence is related to the location of the recurrence. True or marginal recurrences occur earlier than elsewhere. Median times to local failure for true recurrence range from 29 months (89) to 48 months (90). For failure in a separate site, the median time to recurrence ranges from 46 months (87) to 68.5 months (91).

A majority of recurrences occur within the vicinity of the primary tumor (91–99). The location of the recurrence has been related to histology in some series, with invasive lobular carcinoma more likely to recur at the primary site. Recurrence may be ductal carcinoma in situ (DCIS), infiltrating duct carcinoma (IDC), lobular carcinoma, or a mixture of any of these. IDC is the most common histology. Approximately 10% of the patients will present with simultaneous distant metastasis. Eighty-five percent to 95% of isolated breast recurrences are operable (100), and the patient can be rendered disease free by salvage mastectomy. Local control is typically 90% to 95%.

Factors able to predict for survival after an operable recurrence are not significantly affected by initial age, pathologic nodal status initially, or, at the time of recurrence, interval to recurrence, location, method of detection, or the use of adjuvant chemotherapy. A trend toward improved survival was noted 1) in patients older than 35 years at initial presentation, 2) in patients with negative nodes initially, 3) when there was a longer time to recurrence, 4) when there was no residual tumor at the time of mastectomy, and 5) in the absence of skin dermal lymphatic, vascular lymphatic, or muscle invasion (87). Others have found the most important prognostic factor to be disease-free intervals from initial biopsy (95). JCRT studied 1593 patients, 166 of whom experienced local recurrence (101). They found that the histology of the recurrent tumor was the most significant prognostic factor, and those patients with predominately invasive tumors fared worse than those with purely noninvasive or focally invasive tumors. Haffty et al (102) examined prognostic factors after local recurrence with a median follow-up of 5 years after recurrence. Patients with tumors smaller than 3 cm without dermal involvement, prolonged time to recurrence, and failure outside the initial area of management did better. Many other investigators have shown better survival for those patients experiencing a recurrence after 3 to 5 years (103–105).

There is no decreased survival in those patients who experience an isolated local recurrence. Forty-five percent to 75% of the patients in whom recurrence develops are alive at 5 years and about 50% are disease free (106–109). Only 30% of the patients are disease free at 5 years; chest wall recurrences have occurred after mastectomy (110). The standard management for local recurrence in the breast is mastectomy.

DCIS

DCIS was reported in only 3% to 5% of the patients before the advent of screening mammography, and most were palpable masses (111). With the spread of mammography, about 15% to 20% (112) of new diagnoses are DCIS, many of which are without a palpable mass.

DCIS is defined as carcinoma confined to the preexisting duct system of the breast without penetration of the basement membrane seen by light microscopy. There are four subtypes of DCIS: micropapillary, comedo, cribriform with necrosis, and cribriform with anaplasia.

The historic management of this disease has been mastectomy. However, the successful use of breast-conserving surgery for invasive cancer has led to the use of breast conservation as an alternative for this group of patients. A large, randomized study (NSABP B-17) (111) examined patients treated with lumpectomy alone versus lumpectomy and irradiation. Initially, this study included axillary dissection, but early on this requirement was dropped from the study because the incidence of axillary nodal involvement was so infrequent (113). With a mean follow-up of 43 months, the 5-year event-free survival was significantly better (84.4% vs. 73.8%) for women receiving radiotherapy (111). Among the women treated by lumpectomy alone, 16.4% developed an ipsilateral recurrence; of these recurrences 50% were invasive cancer. In contrast, only 7% of the women treated with irradiation developed an ipsilateral recurrence; 8 of 20 patients had invasive cancer. Hence, the benefit of radiation treatment was related to its ability to decrease the cumulative incidence of second ipsilateral breast tumors (invasive as well as noninvasive), and radiation is a more appropriate treatment than lumpectomy alone.

One retrospective analysis of combined data from nine institutions (112) studied 10-year results using definitive radiation after lumpectomy for DCIS. The 10-year overall survival rate was 94%, with cause-specific survival of 97%. The local failure rate was 16%; the median time to local recurrence was 50 months. Again, 50% of the recurrences were invasive cancer. This investigation supports high overall survival, cause-specific survival, and freedom from distant metastases. The effectiveness of salvage treatment remains uncertain at this time because of the long, natural history of this disease.

To confuse the issue, Lagios et al (114) reported on 79 patients treated with excision alone; only 10.1%, or 8 patients, experienced local recurrence. However, these patients all met specific criteria for entry into this prospective study. These were DCIS detected by mammographic microcalcification, a maximum tumor focus of 25 mm or less, and adequate excision confirmed histologically as well as mammographically. A majority of the recurrences were detected mammographically and 50% proved to be invasive cancer. Most recurrences were seen in the comedo type and cribriform with necrosis histologic pattern. The pathologic risk factors for increased local recurrence have also been studied by Solin et al (115), and comedo carcinoma as well as nuclear grade 3 resulted in an increased risk of local recurrence. Salvage mastectomy is the treatment of choice for those patients who experience recurrence locally, and to date local recurrence has not been associated with altered survival.

With many retrospective and nonrandomized reports in the literature that are not comparable to one another, the issue of DCIS is still confusing and decisions are difficult.

Advanced Breast Cancer

Advanced breast cancer is fortunately becoming less common in the developed world. The less developed countries are not as fortunate and still struggle with advanced disease. Because of the relative scarcity of advanced disease in the United States, the number of large trials concerning advanced disease is small. We must, therefore, look to Europe for guidance.

This problem is compounded by the growing popularity of the conservative approach to breast cancer in the United States and elsewhere. This is commendable for the improvements obtained in organ preservation but can make analysis of the role of radiation in advanced cancer more difficult. Adjuvant radiation given for organ preservation may have subtle effects beyond its role as the preserver of a woman's intact breast. For example, portions of the axillary lymphatics unavoidably receive therapeutic doses of radiation in any irradiated breast. The results of this and other factors may be difficult to detect unless specifically sought by a study designed to detect them.

Postmastectomy Adjuvant Radiotherapy

The routine use of postmastectomy radiotherapy is controversial at best. Studies supporting and refuting its usefulness have appeared in the literature. Since the appearance of multiagent chemotherapy, routine adjuvant radiotherapy has been largely abandoned. The true value of postmastectomy radiotherapy is difficult to glean from the studies done to date. Many of them have suffered from inadequate technique and study design.

The American experience is most influenced by the results of the NSABP B-04 study (116). The results of this study failed to demonstrate any advantage for extended-field radiotherapy, especially concerning distant metastasis. Specifically, no survival or disease-free survival advantage was detected with the addition of radiotherapy.

Unfortunately, because the study included all patients with breast cancer whatever their prognostic category, its power in subset analysis is somewhat decreased. The initial article dealing with NSABP B-04 describes in detail the techniques used in the study (117). The patients were randomized on the basis of clinical nodal involvement, which is known to be inaccurate. In addition, the patients who underwent a total mastectomy had no sampling of the axillary contents. This was encouraged at the time because there was some thought that leaving the axillary contents intact might bolster the immune defense. It is impossible to separate patients with histologically positive nodes when proceeding with subset analysis. Because of this difficulty in the study design, a more proper conclusion is that there is no advantage to postmastectomy radiotherapy in an unselected patient population within the limits of this study.

Subsequent NSABP studies were based on the results of this study and so do not include extended-field radiotherapy. The most proper conclusion for the subsequent studies would include the disclaimer that the radiotherapy was limited to the chest wall only. In any event, on the basis of these results adjuvant radiotherapy after radical surgery fell into a period of disfavor in the United States.

One analysis of the world literature incorporating radiotherapy without chemotherapy suggests that there is no benefit and perhaps an increase in mortality (118). Other authors suggest that there is a difference favoring radiotherapy (119) in certain subgroups of patients (120). The M.D. Anderson group also published their results that, when compared retrospectively with an older NSABP surgery-only series, may show a benefit (121).

Notably, it has been suggested that extended-field radiotherapy may potentially affect the rate of distant metastasis (122). Only node-positive patients demonstrated this effect, but it was of statistical significance and seen in two studies. This would lead one to consider the possibility that increased local control of breast cancer may decrease the rate of distant metastasis. This theory is more in keeping with the classic school of thought rather than that championed by the NSABP. The NSABP views breast cancer as a systemic disease almost from the outset. In that model, lymph nodes serve as biologic markers of aggressiveness rather than as the first stage in a stepwise progression from local to systemic disease.

The question of radiotherapy alone after mastectomy is largely moot. Patients with bad prognostic findings will almost uniformly receive chemotherapy. In the modern era, the question is whether local radiotherapy can contribute to the management of the postmastectomy patient who is to receive chemotherapy. The best support for adding radiotherapy is the ongoing results of the Danish Breast Cancer Cooperative Group (DBCG) (123). In contrast to the NSABP B-04, the DBCG limited their study to high-risk patients. In Protocol 82, 1473 premenopausal patients were randomized between radiation plus a combination of cyclophosphamide, methotrexate, and 5-fluorouracil (CMF) and CMF alone. The 1202 postmenopausal patients received radiation plus tamoxifen or tamoxifen alone. This large study found a small but significant absolute survival advantage in the premenopausal group as well as a significant increase in disease-free survival and local control in all groups. The group with the most benefit appeared to be women younger than 45 years with four or more positive lymph nodes. The data continue to mature, and further updates are eagerly expected. It is interesting as well that chemotherapy alone was unable to prevent local recurrence adequately unless combined with radiotherapy.

High-risk postmenopausal patients also demonstrated similar results. In a randomized study of radiotherapy, radiotherapy plus tamoxifen, chemotherapy (CMF), or chemotherapy plus tamoxifen, improved local control and recurrence-free survival was seen in the groups receiving radiotherapy. There was also a trend toward improved survival with radiotherapy, but this did not achieve statistical significance (124).

Analysis of the Eastern Cooperative Oncology Group's studies of patients receiving adjuvant chemotherapy also suggests there is a subgroup of patients who could benefit from adjuvant radiation (125). Overall, the available evidence supports adding radiotherapy to mastectomy and chemotherapy when the tumor is larger than 5 cm or when four or more lymph nodes are involved.

Radiation Technique

The optimal fields of radiotherapy remain undefined. The studies that establish the utility of radiation in the postmastectomy population use extended-field radiotherapy for the supraclavicular, axillary, and internal mammary nodal regions as well as the chest wall. Figure 12.1 shows the regions that typically are included. Although the detailed radiotherapeutic technique is beyond the scope of this chapter, a brief overview of the options is certainly warranted.

The two major techniques used in the treatment of postmastectomy patients are the tangent field technique (Fig. 12.2) and the electron

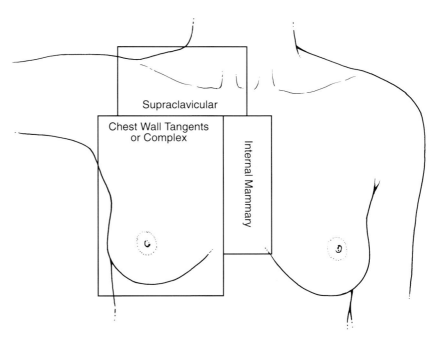

Figure 12.1. Separate radiation fields used in the extended-field technique.

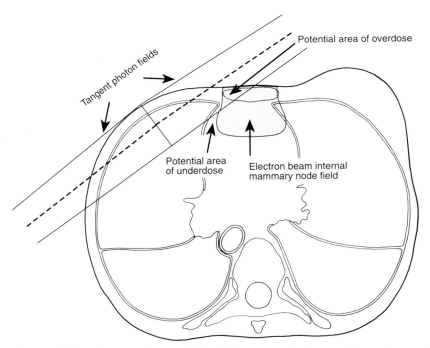

Figure 12.2. *Tangent photon field technique matched to an electron internal mammary node field.*

beam technique (Fig. 12.3). The goal of each technique is to optimally irradiate the target volume while sparing normal tissue. Each technique has its proponents and certain advantages. A review of techniques has been published (126).

The electron beam technique has the advantage of geometric simplicity. The geometric problems of beam divergence are simplified by the use of the anterior electron port. The technique suffers from the uncertainties of dosimetry in the match lines (sites of adjoining fields). Electron dosimetry in lung is also poorly understood. Some authors indicate that there might be differences in the pulmonary function of these patients (127). However, many confounding factors prevent a conclusion regarding this technique. Despite these concerns, the technique is of proven clinical utility.

The alternate method, utilized in most institutions, uses tangent photon fields to treat the chest wall (see Fig. 12.2). These are matched to a supraclavicular field and an internal mammary node field. The resulting complex geometric arrangement is less intuitive. One must then trust in the calculations that govern the match (128) or in a semiempiric method of determination (129).

The match line of the supraclavicular field is adequately controlled, but the internal mammary field still runs the risk of a potential underdose or overdose if an anterior port is used. Most institutions do not use a separate internal mammary field but state that it is included

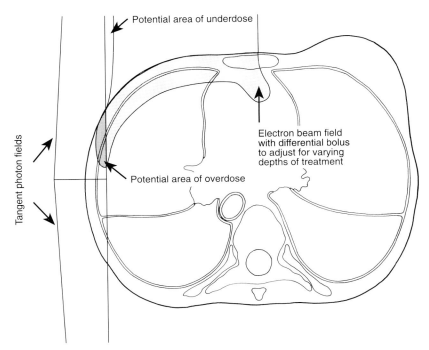

Potential area of underdose

Tangent photon fields

Electron beam field
with differential bolus
to adjust for varying
depths of treatment

Potential area of overdose

Figure 12.3. *Electron beam chest wall field matched to tangent photon beams on the side wall.*

in the tangents. Unfortunately, individual anatomy varies too much to rely on this technique (130).

Studies of pulmonary function indicate that the tangent technique has little or no significant pulmonary toxicity compared with the electron technique (127,131). On the basis of the limited studies, it is impossible to state with certainty that the tangent technique is superior. However, the available evidence supports caution when the electron technique is used.

Lesser radiotherapy (chest wall or chest wall plus supraclavicular) has not been adequately evaluated. The studies that support a survival advantage use extended-field radiotherapy, including an internal mammary node field. It remains unclear whether lesser radiotherapy will be as effective. American radiation oncologists rarely treat the internal mammary nodes and supraclavicular fields. Many are guided by the reasoning of the NSABP, which is based on a single study (NSABP B-04). Further evaluation is clearly warranted.

Radiotherapy in Unresectable Disease

Unresectable disease encompasses many different situations. Patients can be medically unresectable because of their inability to tolerate anesthesia or surgically unresectable because of tumor factors. Usually such factors as chest wall fixation, skin infiltration, axillary nodal fixation, satellite nodules, inflammatory carcinoma, or supraclavicular nodal involvement imply disease that is classically outside the domain of surgery.

The treatment used most often in the past has been primary radiotherapy. This technique can provide local management of the cancer with acceptable morbidity. Most typically, the radiation technique is that described previously and shown in Figure 12.2.

Therapy for locally advanced disease requires doses greater than those typically given for adjuvant treatment. Doses larger than 60 Gy are required to achieve local control, and there is a dose-response relationship. Dose increments of 15 Gy can decrease the chance of local failure by a factor of two (132).

As expected, the risk of complications is related to the total dose, the area treated, and the technical aspects of administration. The patients who often receive the highest doses to the most extensive area are those treated with primary radiotherapy alone. The addition of surgery allows less dose to be given. An analysis of treatment-related complications in the previously cited study was performed regarding treatment and tumor characteristics (133). The improved local control achieved with high-dose radiotherapy must be carefully balanced with the increased complications seen, but the treatment is well tolerated and can prevent the complications associated with uncontrolled local disease.

Recently, combination chemotherapy along with local treatment has been advocated in the management of unresectable disease. Patients with locally advanced disease have a high rate of distant failure that is theoretically addressed by chemotherapy. In addition, there is evidence from the studies cited in the previous section that chemotherapy may contribute to improving local control.

Two randomized, prospective trials, which contained a control arm, have been conducted to address these theories. Both studies use extended-field therapy as described previously. The first is a series reporting on 118 patients randomized between radiotherapy, radiotherapy plus 12 cycles of chemotherapy (CMF) and tamoxifen, and radiotherapy sandwiched between eight cycles of chemotherapy (CMF alternating with doxorubicin and vincristine [AV]) (134). The results of this study failed to demonstrate any advantage over radiotherapy alone for survival, complete response, local control, and relapse-free survival.

In the second study, conducted by the EORTC, 363 assessable patients with locally advanced disease received radiotherapy and then were randomized between observation, chemotherapy (CMF for 12 cycles), endocrine therapy, or chemotherapy combined with endocrine therapy (135). Combined therapy demonstrated an advantage in local control but not in survival or metastatic rate. The local effects were seen in both pre- and postmenopausal women but were most pronounced for the latter. They concluded that present cytotoxic and hormonal manipulation remained of only marginal value in this patient population and that the benefits were limited to improved local control. They believed that increasing the radiation dose may be able to increase local control in the radiotherapy-alone arm without the need to add chemotherapy.

Despite the lack of firm support, it seems reasonable to consider the use of up-front chemotherapy in this patient group. The large tumor mass can serve as an objective measure of response, and the decrease in tumor volume would theoretically improve the efficacy of local therapy. In those cases in which the tumor fails to respond, a different chemotherapy regimen can be tried or further chemotherapy avoided. This spares the patient unnecessary toxicity from useless drugs. These theoretic advantages should be weighed against the very real increase in morbidity from chemotherapy when deciding a course of therapy. Further evaluation is warranted before any conclusion can be reached.

Inflammatory Breast Cancer

Inflammatory cancer is a special case both in diagnosis and management. Radiotherapy has largely been the treatment of choice, but the results have been suboptimal. Local and regional recurrence rates are between 49% and 69% with conventional radiotherapy (136,137). The adoption of twice-daily radiotherapy can improve the local control rates so that local or regional failure is seen in 27% of cases (137).

Given the unacceptable local control rates and the risk of distant metastasis, many have tried more aggressive therapy (138–140). The results have been a decided improvement over the historic experience with this disease but not necessarily better than more aggressive local therapy. A modern series using more standard therapy suggests that some of the benefit implied may not be real (141).

Current strategies that incorporate aggressive local therapy (usually combined surgery and radiation) with aggressive systemic therapy have become increasingly popular. The technique is promising, but it lacks the support of randomized, prospective trials. Given the nature of the disease, it is unlikely that these trials will ever be done. The author routinely recommends such treatment with these realizations.

Radiotherapy of Chest Wall Recurrence

Modern aggressive therapy of breast cancer is quite effective in preventing local recurrence. The risk of local recurrence is very dependent on the nature of the original treatment, most notably, the inclusion of local radiotherapy as discussed previously.

In the patient who has not received prior radiotherapy, the current recommendation would be to proceed with radiotherapy (142). Whether or not to proceed with surgery or chemotherapy is less clear. The role of cytotoxic chemotherapy in assisting radiation in local control of recurrent disease is not established (143). However, there may be benefits in control of systemic disease. Certainly, the role that surgery can play depends to a great extent on the nature of the chest wall failure. Diffuse lesions are often not amenable to resection and can be adequately addressed with radiation (142,144). Even in those patients who present with metastatic disease at the time of local failure, radiation in adequate doses (>45 Gy) is needed to provide optimal palliation of local symptoms (145).

Those patients who have previously undergone radiotherapy to the chest wall can benefit from further treatment (146,147). The technique is similar to the previously described techniques. Some more inventive approaches have been used. Mold therapy, in which brachytherapy sources are placed at a specified distance from the skin, can be used to achieve the benefits of both previously described techniques while avoiding some of their weaknesses (148). The addition of hyperthermia (therapeutic heat) to radiation has demonstrated some promise in helping improve local control of this disease (149,150).

Complications of High-Dose Radiotherapy

The complications of high-dose radiotherapy are similar to those of the lower doses used in adjuvant radiation. Those have been covered elsewhere and are not repeated here. Along with an increased risk of fibrosis of the soft tissues and rib fractures, there is a very real danger of cardiac toxicity from the internal mammary field. The Oslo data demonstrate an increased morbidity from cardiac events that may be due to the hormonal manipulation, the internal mammary nodal radiation, or some combination of the two (151).

Another area of concern is damage to the brachial plexus. As the total dose is increased, the often disabling complication of brachial plexopathy becomes more prominent. The rate of brachial plexopathy was analyzed in a subset of patients from the DBCG study cited previously (152). The findings indicated that the rate of disabling plexopathy was 5% with a rate of 9% for mild symptoms. The addition of chemotherapy increased the risk of damage to the brachial plexus. The most common signs and symptoms were paresthesia (100%), hypoesthesia (74%), weakness (58%), decreased muscle stretch reflexes (47%), and pain (47%). Unfortunately, no effective therapy exists to treat this complication.

CONCLUSION

This chapter has briefly touched on some of the aspects of radiation treatment for breast cancer. Because of space constraints, it is impossible to evaluate this treatment modality exhaustively here. Undoubtedly, the base of knowledge will continue to expand. It is essential for all physicians dealing with this disease to understand the contributions that radiation can make. The participation of a properly trained radiation oncologist in formulating a treatment plan is mandatory.

References

1. Cancer statistics: 1994. CA Cancer J Clin 1995;44:18–19.
2. Fisher B, Redmond C, Others for the National Surgical Adjuvant Breast and Bowel Project. Lumpectomy for breast cancer: an update of the NSABP experience. J Natl Cancer Inst Monogr 1992;11:7–13.
3. Clark RM, McCulloch PB, Levine MN, et al. Randomized clinical trial to assess the effectiveness of breast irradiation following lumpectomy and axillary dissection for node-negative breast cancer. J Natl Cancer Inst 1992;84:683–689.
4. Sarrazin D, Le MG, Arriagada R, et al. Ten-year results of a randomized trial comparing a conservative treatment to mastectomy in early breast cancer. Radiother Oncol 1989;14:177–184.
5. Veronesi U, Banfi A, Salvadori B, et al. Breast conservation is the treatment of choice in small breast cancer: long-term results of a randomized trial. Eur J Cancer 1990;26:668–670.
6. Straus K, Lichter A, Lippman M, et al. Results of the National Cancer Institute early breast cancer trial. J Natl Cancer Inst Monogr 1992;11:27–32.
7. van Dongen J, Bartelink H, Fentiman IS, et al. Randomized clinical trial to assess the value of breast-conserving therapy in stage I and II breast cancer, EORTC 10801 trial. J Natl Cancer Inst Monogr 1992;11:15–18.
8. Blichert-Toft M, Rose C, Andersen JA, et al. Danish randomized trial comparing breast conservation therapy with mastectomy: six years of life-table analysis. J Natl Cancer Inst Monogr 1991;11:19–25.
9. Pierquin B, Huart J, Raynal M, et al. Conservative treatment for breast cancer: long-term results (15 years). Radiother Oncol 1991;20:16–23.
10. Veronesi U, Salvadori B, Luini A, et al. Conservative treatment of early breast cancer. Ann Surg 1990;211:250–259.
11. Spitalier JM, Bambarelli J, Brandone H, et al. Breast-conserving surgery with radiation therapy for operable mammary carcinoma: a 25-year experience. World J Surg 1986;10:1014–1020.
12. Clark RM, Wilkinson RH, Mahoney LJ, et al. Breast cancer: a 21 year

experience with conservative surgery and radiation. Int J Radiat Oncol Biol Phys 1982;8:967–975.

13. Fowble BL, Solin LJ, Schultz DJ, Goodman RL. Ten year results of conservative surgery and irradiation for stage I and II breast cancer. JAMA 1991;21:269–277.

14. NIH Consensus Conference. Treatment of early-stage breast cancer. JAMA 1991;265:391–395.

15. Nattinger AB, Gottlieb MS, Veum J, et al. Geographic variation in the use of breast-conserving treatment for breast cancer. N Engl J Med 1992;326:1102–1107.

16. Fowble B, Solin LJ, Schultz DJ, Weiss M. Breast recurrence and survival related to primary tumor location in patients undergoing conservative surgery and radiation for early-stage breast cancer. Int J Radiat Oncol Biol Phys 1992;23:933–939.

17. Weiss MC, Fowble BL, Solin LJ, et al. Outcome of conservative therapy for invasive breast cancer by histologic subtype. Int J Radiat Oncol Biol Phys 1992;23:941–947.

18. Leopold KA, Recht A, Schnitt ST, et al. Results of conservative surgery and radiation therapy for multiple synchronous cancers of one breast. Int J Radiat Oncol Biol Phys 1989;16:11–16.

19. Fowble B, Yeh IT, Schultz DJ, et al. The role of mastectomy in patients with stage I–II breast cancer presenting with gross multifocal or multicentric disease or diffuse microcalcifications. Int J Radiat Oncol Biol Phys 1993;27:566–573.

20. Holland R, Veling S, Mravunac M, Hendricks J. Histologic multifocality of Tis, T1–2 breast carcinomas: implications for clinical trials of breast-conserving surgery. CA Cancer J Clin 1985;56:979–990.

21. Fisher B, Redmond C, Poisson R, et al. Eight year results of a randomized clinical trial comparing total mastectomy and lumpectomy with or without irradiation in the treatment of breast cancer. N Engl J Med 1989;320:822–828.

22. Clark R, Wilkinson R, Mahoney L. Breast cancer: a 21-year experience with conservative surgery and radiation. Int J Radiat Oncol Biol Phys 1982;8:967–978.

23. Freeman C, Belliveau N, Kim T. Limited surgery with or without radiotherapy for early breast carcinoma. J Can Assoc Radiol 1981;32:125–128.

24. Nixon AJ, Neuberg D, Hayes DF, et al. Relationship of patient age to pathologic features of the tumor and prognosis for patients with stage I or II breast cancer. J Clin Oncol 1994;12:888–894.

25. Adami H-O, Malker B, Holmberg L, et al. The relation between survival and age at diagnosis in breast cancer. N Engl J Med 1986;315:559–563.

26. Host H, Lund E. Age as a prognostic factor in breast cancer. Cancer 1986;57:2217–2221.

27. Vicini FA, Eberlein TJ, Connolly JL, et al. The optimal extent of resection for patients with stages I or II breast cancer treated with conservative surgery and radiotherapy. Ann Surg 1991;214:200–204.

28. Svensson GK, Bjarngard BE, Larson RD, et al. A modified three-field technique for breast treatment. Int J Radiat Oncol Biol Phys 1980;6:689–694.

29. SAS Institute. SAS. Cary, NC: SAS Institute, 1990.

30. Rosner B. Fundamentals of biostatistics. 3rd ed. Boston: PWS-Kent, 1990.

31. Kaplan EL, Meier P. Nonparametric estimation from incomplete observations. J Am Stat Assoc 1958;53:457–481.

32. Fourquet A, Campana F, Zafrani B, et al. Prognostic factors of breast recurrence in the conservative management of early breast cancer: a 25 year follow-up. Int J Radiat Oncol Biol Phys 1989;17:719–725.

33. Recht A, Connolly JL, Schnitt SJ, et al. The effect of young age on tumor recurrence in the treated breast after conservative surgery and radiotherapy. 1988;14:3–10.

34. Viloq JR, Calle R, Stacey P, Ghossein N. The outcome of treatment by tumorectomy and radiotherapy of patients with operable breast cancer. Int J Radiat Oncol Biol Phys 1981;7:1327–1332.

35. Harris JR, Connolly JL, Schnitt SJ, et al. The use of pathologic features in selecting the extent of surgical resection necessary for breast cancer patients treated by primary radiation therapy. Ann Surg 1985;201:164–169.

36. Vicini F, Recht A, Abner A, et al. The association between very young age and recurrence in the breast in patients treated with conservative surgery (CS) and radiation therapy (RT). Int J Radiat Oncol Biol Phys 1990; 19(suppl):132.

37. Solin LJ, Fowble B, Schultz DJ, Goodman RL. Age as a prognostic factor for patients treated with definitive irradiation for early stage breast cancer. Int J Radiat Oncol Biol Phys 1989;16:373–381.

38. Matthews RH, McNeese MD, Montague ED, Oswald MJ. Prognostic implications of age in breast cancer patients treated with tumorectomy and irradiation or with mastectomy. Int J Radiat Oncol Biol Phys 1988;14:659–663.

39. van Dongen JA, Bartelink H, Fentiman IS, et al. Factors influencing local relapse and survival and results of salvage treatment after breast-conserving therapy in operable breast cancer: EORTC trials 10801, breast conservation compared with mastectomy in TNM stage I and II breast cancer. Eur J Cancer 1992;28:805–810.

40. de la Rochefordiere A, Asselain B, Campana F, et al. Age as prognostic factor in premenopausal breast carcinoma. Lancet 1993;341:1039–1043.

41. Solin LJ, Yeh I-T, Kurtz J, et al. Ductal carcinoma in situ (intraductal carcinoma) of the breast treated with breast-conserving surgery and definitive irradiation: correlation of pathologic parameters with outcome of treatment. CA Cancer J Clin 1993;71:2532–2542.

42. Lee CG, McCormick B, Mzaumdar M, et al. Infiltrating breast carcinoma in patients age 30 years and younger: long term outcome for life, relapse, and second primary tumors. Int J Radiat Oncol Biol Phys 1992;23:969–975.

43. Amalric R, Santamaria F, Robert F, et al. Radiation therapy with or without primary limited surgery for operable breast cancers: a 20-year experience at the Marseilles Cancer Institute. CA Cancer J Clin 1982;49:30–34.

44. Abner A, Recht A, Connolly J, et al. The relationship between microscopic margins of resection and the risk of local recurrence in patients treated with breast-conserving therapy. Presented at the 34th Annual Meeting of the American Society of Therapeutic Radiology and Oncology. 1992.

45. Schnitt S, Abner A, Gelman R, et al. The relationship between microscopic margins of resection and the risk of local recurrence in breast cancer patients treated with breast-conserving surgery and radiation therapy. Cancer 1995 (in press).

46. Fisher E, Anderson S, Redmond C, et al. Ipsilateral breast tumor recurrence and survival following lumpectomy and irradiation: pathologic findings from NSABP protocol B-06. Semin Surg Oncol 1992;8:161–166.

47. Borger J, Kemperman H, Hart A, et al. Risk factors in breast-conservation therapy. J Clin Oncol 1994;12:653–660.

48. Fisher ER, Anderson S, Redmond C, Fisher B, for NSABP collaborating investigators: pathologic findings from the national surgical adjuvant breast project protocol B-06. Cancer 1993;71:2507–2514.

49. Gilchrist K, Gray R, Fowble B, et al. Tumor necrosis is a prognostic predictor for early recurrence and death in lymph node-positive breast cancer: a 10-year follow-up study of 728 eastern cooperative oncology group patients. J Clin Oncol 1993;11:1929–1935.

50. Kiebert GM, De Haes JCJM, van de Velde CJH. The impact of breast-conserving treatment and mastectomy on the quality of life of early-stage breast cancer patients: a review. J Clin Oncol 1991;9:1059–1070.

51. Ransom DT, Cameron FG. Scleroderma: a possible contraindication to lumpectomy and radiotherapy in breast carcinoma. Australas Radiol 1987;31:317–318.

52. Robertson JM, Clarke DH, Pevzner MM, Matter RC. Breast conservation therapy: severe breast fibrosis after radiation therapy in patients with collagen vascular disease. Cancer 1991;68:502–508.

53. Varga J, Haustein JF, Creech RH, et al. Exaggerated radiation-induced fibrosis in patients with systemic sclerosis. JAMA 1991;265:3292–3295.

54. Fleck R, McNeese MD, Ellerbroek NA, et al. Consequences of breast irradiation in patients with pre-existing collagen vascular diseases. Int J Radiat Oncol Biol Phys 1989;17:829–833.

55. Harris JR, Morrow M, Bonadonna G. In: DeVita VT Jr, Hellman S, Rosenberg SA, eds. Cancer: principles & practice of oncology. 4th ed. Philadelphia: JB Lippincott, 1993:1286.

56. Margolese R. Surgical considerations in selecting local therapy. J Natl Cancer Inst Monogr 1992;11:41–48.

57. Fagundes MA, Fagundes HM, Brito CS, et al. Breast-conserving surgery and definitive radiation: a comparison between quadrantectomy and local excision with special focus on local-regional control and cosmesis. Int J Radiat Oncol Biol Phys 1993;27:553–560.

58. Vicini FA, Eberlein TJ, Connolly JL, et al. The optimal extent of resection for patients with stages I or II breast cancer treated with conservative surgery and radiotherapy. Ann Surg 1991;214:200–205.

59. Solin LJ, Fowble BL, Schultz DJ, Goodman RL. The significance of the pathology margins of the tumor excision on the outcome of patients treated with definitive irradiation for early stage breast cancer. Int J Radiat Oncol Biol Phys 1991;21:279–287.

60. Schmidt-Ullrich R, Wazer DE, Tercilla O, et al. Tumor margin assessment as a guide to optimal conservation surgery and irradiation in early stage breast carcinoma. Int J Radiat Oncol Biol Phys 1989;17:733–738.

61. Bedwinek JM, Perez CA, Kramer S, et al. Irradiation as the primary management of stage I and II adenocarcinoma of the breast: analysis of the RTOG breast registry. Cancer Clin Trials 1980;3:11–18.

62. Chu AM, Cope O, Russo R, Lew R. Patterns of local regional recurrence and results in stages I and II breast cancer treated by irradiation following limited surgery: an update. Am J Clin Oncol 1984;7:221–229.

63. Harris JR, Botnick L, Bloomer WD, et al. Primary radiation therapy for early breast cancer: the experience at the Joint Center for Radiation Therapy. Int J Radiat Oncol Biol Phys 1981;7:1549–1552.

64. Van Limbergen E, van den Bogaert W, van der Schueren E, Rijnders A. Tumor excision and radiotherapy as primary treatment of breast cancer:

analysis of patient and treatment parameters and local control. Radiother Oncol 1987;8:1–9.

65. Danforth DV, Findlay PA, McDonald HD, et al. Complete axillary lymph node dissection for stage I–II carcinoma of the breast. J Clin Oncol 1986;4:655–662.

66. Larson D, Weinstein M, Goldberg I, et al. Edema of the arm as a function of the extent of axillary surgery in patients with stage I–II carcinoma of the breast treated with primary radiotherapy. Int J Radiat Oncol Biol Phys 1986;12:1575–1582.

67. Clarke D, Martinex A, Cos RS, Goffinet DR. Breast edema following staging axillary node dissection in patients with breast carcinoma treated by radical radiotherapy. Cancer 1982;49:2295–2299.

68. Haffty BG, McKhann C, Beinfield M, et al. Breast conservation therapy without axillary dissection. Arch Surg 1993;128:1315–1319.

69. Recht A, Pierce SM, Abner A, et al. Regional nodal failure after conservative surgery and radiotherapy for early-stage breast carcinoma. J Clin Oncol 1991;9:988–996.

70. Fowble B, Solin LJ, Schultz DJ, Goodman RL. Frequency, sites of relapse, and outcome of regional node failures following conservative surgery and radiation for early breast cancer. Int J Radiat Oncol Biol Phys 1989;17:703–710.

71. Fisher B, Redmond C, Poisson R, et al. Eight-year results of a randomized clinical trial comparing total mastectomy and lumpectomy with or without irradiation in the treatment of breast cancer. N Engl J Med 1989;320:822–828.

72. Rose MA, Henderson IC, Gelman R, et al. Premenopausal breast cancer patients treated with conservative surgery, radiotherapy and adjuvant chemotherapy have a low risk of local failure. Int J Radiat Oncol Biol Phys 1989;17:711–717.

73. Fisher B, Redmond C, Dimitrov NV, et al. A randomized clinical trial evaluating sequential methotrexate and fluorouracil in the treatment of patients with node-negative breast cancer who have estrogen-receptor-negative tumors. N Engl J Med 1989;320:473–478.

74. Recht A, Come SE, Gelman RS, et al. Integration of conservative surgery, radiotherapy, and chemotherapy for the treatment of early-stage node-positive breast cancer: sequencing, timing, and outcome. J Clin Oncol 1991;9:1662–1667.

75. Ludwig Breast Cancer Study Group. Combination adjuvant chemotherapy for node-positive breast cancer: inadequacy of a single perioperative cycle. N Engl J Med 1988;319:677–683.

76. Ludwig Breast Cancer Study Group. Prolonged disease-free survival after one course of perioperative adjuvant chemotherapy for node-negative breast cancer. N Engl J Med 1989;320:491–496.

77. Abner AL, Recht A, Vicini FA, et al. Cosmetic results after surgery, chemotherapy, and radiation therapy for early breast cancer. Int J Radiat Oncol Biol Phys 1991;21:331–338.

78. Bader JL, Lippman ME, Swain S, et al. Cosmetic evaluation (CE) following lumpectomy and radiation (XRT) for early breast cancer (BC) is similar with and without adjuvant adriamycin/cytoxan (AC). Proc Am Soc Clin Oncol 1987;6:62.

79. Glick JH, Fowble BL, Haller DG, et al. Integration of full-dose adjuvant chemotherapy with definitive radiotherapy for primary breast cancer: four-year update. Natl Cancer Inst Monogr 1988;6:297–301.

80. Gore SM, Come SE, Griem K, et al. Influence of the sequencing of chemotherapy and radiation therapy in node-positive breast cancer patients treated by conservative surgery and radiation therapy. In: Salmon SE, ed. Adjuvant therapy of cancer V. Orlando, FL: Grune & Stratton, 1987:365–373.

81. Hahn P, Hallbert O, Vikterlof K-J. Acute skin reactions in postoperative breast cancer patients receiving radiotherapy plus adjuvant chemotherapy. AJR 1978;130:137–139.

82. Bentzen SO, Overgaard M, Thames HD, et al. Early and late normal-tissue injury after postmastectomy radiotherapy alone or combined with chemotherapy. Int J Radiat Biol Phys 1989;56:711–715.

83. Fisher B, Constantino J, Redmond C, et al. A randomized clinical trial evaluating tamoxifen in the treatment of patients with node-negative breast cancer who have estrogen-receptor positive tumors. N Engl J Med 1989;320:479–484.

84. Pierce SM, Recht A, Lingos TI, et al. Long-term radiation complications following conservative surgery (CS) and radiation therapy (RT) in patients with early stage breast cancer. Int J Radiat Oncol Biol Phys 1992;23:915–923.

85. Storm HH, Andersson M, Boice JD, et al. Adjuvant radiotherapy and risk of contralateral breast cancer. J Natl Cancer Inst 1992;84:1245–1250.

86. Dershaw DD, McCormick B, Osborne MP. Detection of local recurrence after conservative therapy for breast carcinoma. Cancer 1992;70:493–496.

87. Fowble B, Solin L, Schultz DJ, et al. Breast recurrence following conservative surgery and radiation: patterns of failure, prognosis, and pathologic findings from mastectomy specimens with implications for treatment. Int J Radiat Oncol Biol Phys 1990;19:833–842.

88. Stomper PC, Recht A, Berenberg AL, et al. Mammographic detection of recurrent cancer in the irradiated breast. AJR 1987;148:39–43.

89. Bartelink H, Border JH, van Dongen JA, Peterse JL. The impact of tumor size and histology on local control after breast-conserving therapy. Radiother Oncol 1988;11:297–303.

90. Veronesi U, Banfi A, DelVecchio M, et al. Comparison of Halsted mastectomy vs quadrantectomy, axillary dissection and radiotherapy in early breast cancer: long-term results. Eur J Cancer Clin Oncol 1986;22:1085–1089.

91. Recht A, Silver B, Schnitt S, et al. Time course of local recurrence following conservative surgery and radiotherapy for early stage breast cancer. Int J Radiat Oncol Biol Phys 1988;15:255–261.

92. Clark RM, Wilkinson RH, Mahoney LJ, et al. Breast cancer: a 21-year experience with conservative surgery and radiation. Int J Radiat Oncol Biol Phys 1982;8:967–975.

93. Clark RM, Wilkinson RH, Miceli PN, MacDonald WD. Breast cancer: experiences with conservation therapy. Am J Clin Oncol 1987;10:461–468.

94. Haffty BG, Goldberg NB, Fischer D, et al. Conservative surgery and radiation therapy in breast carcinoma: local recurrence and prognostic implications. Int J Radiat Oncol Biol Phys 1989;17:727–732.

95. Kurtz JM, Amalric R, Brandone H, et al. Local recurrence after breast-conserving surgery and radiotherapy: frequency, time course and prognosis. Cancer 1989;63:1912–1917.

96. Leung S, Otmezguine Y, Calitchi E, et al. Local regional recurrences following radical external beam irradiation and interstitial implantation for operable breast cancer-a 23-year. Radiother Oncol 1986;5:1–10.

97. Nobler MP, Venet L. Prognostic factors in patients undergoing curative irradiation for breast cancer. Int J Radiat Oncol Biol Phys 1985;11:1123–1331.

 98. Ray GR, Fish BJ, Lee RH, et al. Biopsy and definitive radiation therapy in stages I and II carcinoma of the female breast. Int J Radiat Oncol Biol Phys 1983;9:23–28.

 99. Schnitt SJ, Connolly JL, Recht A, et al. Breast relapse following primary radiation therapy for early breast cancer: II. Detection, pathologic features and prognostic significance. Int J Radiat Oncol Biol Phys 1985;11:1277–1284.

100. Solin LJ, Fowble B, Schultz DJ, Goodman RL. A prognostic factor for patients treated with definitive irradiation for early stage breast cancer. Int J Radiat Oncol Biol Phys 1989;16:373–381.

101. Abner AL, Recht A, Eberlein T, et al. Prognosis following salvage mastectomy for recurrence in the breast after conservative surgery and radiation therapy for early-stage breast cancer. J Clin Oncol 1993;11:44–48.

102. Haffty B, Fischer D, Beinfield M, McKhann C. Prognosis following local recurrence in the conservatively treated breast cancer patient. Int J Radiat Oncol Biol Phys 1991;21:293–298.

103. Fourquet A, Campana F, Zafrani B, et al. Prognostic factors in the conservative management of early breast cancer: a 25-year follow-up at the Institut Curie. Int J Radiat Oncol Biol Phys 1989;17:719–725.

104. Kurtz JM, Amalric R, Brandone H, et al. Local recurrence after breast conserving surgery and radiotherapy. Cancer 1989;63:1912–1917.

105. Kurtz JM, Spitalier JM, Amalric R, et al. The prognostic significance of late local recurrence after breast-conserving therapy. Int J Radiat Oncol Biol Phys 1990;18:87–93.

106. Calle R, Vilcoq JR, Zafrani B, et al. Local control and survival of breast cancer treated by limited surgery followed by irradiation. Int J Radiat Oncol Biol Phys 1986;12:873–878.

107. Stotter A, Atkinson EN, Fairston BA, et al. Survival following locoregional recurrence after breast conservation therapy for cancer. Ann Surg 1990;212:166–172.

108. Kurtz JM, Amalric R, Brandone H, et al. Results of salvage surgery for mammary recurrence following breast-conserving therapy. Ann Surg 1988;207:347–351.

109. Vicini FA, Recht A, Abner A, et al. Recurrence in the breast following conservative surgery and radiation therapy for early-stage breast cancer. J Natl Cancer Inst Monogr 1992;11:33–39.

110. Aberizk WJ, Silver B, Henderson IC, et al. The results of radiotherapy in patients with isolated local-regional recurrence of breast carcinoma after mastectomy. Cancer 1986;58:1214–1218.

111. Fisher B, Costantino J, Redmond C, et al. Lumpectomy compared with lumpectomy and radiation therapy for the treatment of intraductal breast cancer. N Engl J Med 1993;328:1581–1586.

112. Solin LJ, Recht A, Fourquet A, et al. Ten-year results of breast-conserving surgery and definitive irradiation for intraductal carcinoma (ductal carcinoma in situ) of the breast. Cancer 1991;68:2337–2344.

113. Silverstein MJ, Rosser RJ, Gierson ED, et al. Axillary lymph node dissection for intraductal breast carcinoma—is it indicated? Cancer 1987;59:1819–1824.

114. Lagios MD, Margolin FR, Westhahl PR, Rose MR. Mammographically detected duct carcinoma in situ. Cancer 1989;63:618–624.

115. Solin LJ, Fowble BL, Schultz DJ, et al. Definitive irradiation for intraductal carcinoma of the breast. Int J Radiat Oncol Biol Phys 1990;19:843–850.

116. Fisher B, Wolmark N, Redmond C, et al. Findings from NSABP Protocol No. B-04: comparison of radical mastectomy with alternative treatments: II. The clinical and biological significance of medial-central breast cancers. Cancer 1981;48:1863–1872.

117. Fisher B, Montague E, Redmond C, et al. Comparison of radical mastectomy with alternative treatments for primary breast cancer: a first report of results from a prospective randomized clinical trial. Cancer 1977;39:2827–2839.

118. Cuzick J, Stewart H, Peto R, et al. Overview of randomized trials of postoperative adjuvant radiotherapy in breast cancer. Cancer Treat Rep 1987;71:15–29.

119. Strom EA, McNeese MD, Fletcher GH, et al. Results of mastectomy and postoperative irradiation in the management of locoregionally advanced carcinoma of the breast. Int J Radiat Oncol Biol Phys 1991;21:319–323.

120. Edland RW. Does adjuvant radiotherapy have a role in the postmastectomy management of patients with operable breast cancer—revisited. Int J Radiat Oncol Biol Phys 1988;15:519–535.

121. Tapley ND, Spanos WJJ, Fletcher GH, et al. Results in patients with breast cancer treated by radical mastectomy and postoperative irradiation with no adjuvant chemotherapy. Cancer 1982;49:1316–1319.

122. Auquier A, Rutqvist LE, Host H, et al. Post-mastectomy megavoltage radiotherapy: the Oslo and Stockholm trials. Eur J Cancer 1992;28:433–437.

123. Overgaard M, Christensen JJ, Johansen H, et al. Evaluation of radiotherapy in high-risk breast cancer patients: report from the Danish Breast Cancer Cooperative Group (DBCG 82) Trial. Int J Radiat Oncol Biol Phys 1990;19:1121–1124.

124. Rutqvist LE, Cedermark B, Glas U, et al. Randomized trial of adjuvant tamoxifen combined with postoperative radiation therapy or adjuvant chemotherapy in postmenopausal breast cancer. Cancer 1990;66:89–96.

125. Fowble B, Gray R, Gilchrist K, et al. Identification of a subgroup of patients with breast cancer and histologically positive axillary nodes receiving adjuvant chemotherapy who may benefit from postoperative radiotherapy. J Clin Oncol 1988;6:1107–1117.

126. Mansfield CM, Ayyangar K, Suntharalingam N. Comparison of various radiation techniques in treatment of the breast and chest wall. Acta Radiol Oncol Radiat Phys Biol 1979;18:17–24.

127. Groth S, Zaric A, Sorensen PB, et al. Regional lung function impairment following post-operative radiotherapy for breast cancer using direct or tangential field techniques. Br J Radiol 1986;59:445–451.

128. Lichter AS, Fraass BA, van de Geijn J, Padikal TN. A technique for field matching in primary breast irradiation. Int J Radiat Oncol Biol Phys 1983;9:263–270.

129. Chu JC, Solin LJ, Hwang CC, et al. A nondivergent three field matching technique for breast irradiation. Int J Radiat Oncol Biol Phys 1990;19:1037–1040.

130. van der Giessen PH. Parasternal lymphoscintigraphy as an aid in radiation treatment planning. Strahlentherapie 1983;159:422–426.

131. Lund MB, Myhre KI, Melsom H, Johansen B. The effect on pulmonary

function of tangential field technique in radiotherapy for carcinoma of the breast. Br J Radiol 1991;64:520–523.

132. Arriagada R, Mouriesse H, Sarrazin D, et al. Radiotherapy alone in breast cancer: I. Analysis of tumor parameters, tumor dose and local control: the experience of the Gustave-Roussy Institute and the Princess Margaret Hospital. Int J Radiat Oncol Biol Phys 1985;11:1751–1757.

133. Arriagada R, Mouriesse H, Rezvani A, et al. Radiotherapy alone in breast cancer: analysis of tumor and lymph node radiation doses and treatment-related complications. The experience of the Gustave-Roussy Institute and the Princess Margaret Hospital. Radiother Oncol 1993;27: 1–6.

134. Schaake-Koning C, Hamersma van der Linden E, Hart G, Engelsman E. Adjuvant chemo- and hormonal therapy in locally advanced breast cancer: a randomized clinical study. Int J Radiat Oncol Biol Phys 1985; 11:1759–1763.

135. Rubens RD, Bartelink H, Engelsman E, et al. Locally advanced breast cancer: the contribution of cytotoxic and endocrine treatment to radiotherapy. An EORTC Breast Cancer Co-operative Group Trial (10792). Eur J Cancer Clin Oncol 1989;25:667–678.

136. Barker JL, Montague ED, Peters LJ. Clinical experience with irradiation of inflammatory carcinoma of the breast with and without elective chemotherapy. Cancer 1980;45:625–629.

137. Chu AM, Wood WC, Doucette JA. Inflammatory breast carcinoma treated by radical radiotherapy. Cancer 1980;45:2730–2737.

138. Fields JN, Perez CA, Kuske RR, et al. Inflammatory carcinoma of the breast: treatment results on 107 patients. Int J Radiat Oncol Biol Phys 1989;17:249–255.

139. Arriagada R, Mouriesse H, Spielmann M, et al. Alternating radiotherapy and chemotherapy in non-metastatic inflammatory breast cancer. Int J Radiat Oncol Biol Phys 1990;19:1207–1210.

140. Chevallier B, Roche H, Olivier JP, et al. Inflammatory breast cancer: pilot study of intensive induction chemotherapy (FEC-HD) results in a high histologic response rate. Am J Clin Oncol 1993;16:223–228.

141. Frank JL, McClish DK, Dawson KS, Bear HD. Stage III breast cancer: is neoadjuvant chemotherapy always necessary? J Surg Oncol 1992;49: 220–225.

142. Rodger A, Stewart HJ, White GK. The efficacy of delayed radiotherapy for locoregionally recurrent postmastectomy breast cancer. Int J Radiat Oncol Biol Phys 1988;14:665–667.

143. Halverson KJ, Perez CA, Kuske RR, et al. Locoregional recurrence of breast cancer: a retrospective comparison of irradiation alone versus irradiation and systemic therapy. Am J Clin Oncol 1992;15:93–101.

144. Deutsch M, Parsons JA, Mittal BB. Radiation therapy for local-regional recurrent breast carcinoma. Int J Radiat Oncol Biol Phys 1986;12:2061–2065.

145. Bedwinek JM, Munro D, Fineberg B. Local-regional treatment of patients with simultaneous local-regional recurrence and distant metastases following mastectomy. Am J Clin Oncol 1983;6:295–300.

146. Laramore GE, Griffin TW, Parker RG, Gerdes AJ. The use of electron beams in treating local recurrence of breast cancer in previously irradiated fields. Cancer 1978;41:991–995.

147. Lo TC, Salzman FA, Wright KA, Costey GE. Megavolt electron irradia-

tion in the treatment of recurrent carcinoma of the breast on the chest wall. Acta Radiol 1983;22:97–99.

148. Delanian S, Housset M, Brunel P, et al. Iridium 192 plesiocurietherapy using silicone elastomer plates for extensive locally recurrent breast cancer following chest wall irradiation. Int J Radiat Oncol Biol Phys 1992;22:1099–1104.

149. Engin K, Tupchong L, Waterman FM, et al. "Patchwork" fields in thermoradiotherapy for extensive chest wall recurrences of breast carcinoma. Breast Cancer Res Treat 1993;27:263–270.

150. Phromratanapongse P, Steeves RA, Severson SB, Paliwal BR. Hyperthermia and irradiation for locally recurrent previously irradiated breast cancer. Strahlenther Onkol 1991;167:93–97.

151. Host H, Brennhovd IO, Loeb M. Postoperative radiotherapy in breast cancer—long-term results from the Oslo study. Int J Radiat Oncol Biol Phys 1986;12:727–732.

152. Olsen NK, Pfeiffer P, Johannsen L, et al. Radiation-induced brachial plexopathy: neurological follow-up in 161 recurrence-free breast cancer patients. Int J Radiat Oncol Biol Phys 1993;26:43–49.

Medical Therapy of Invasive Breast Cancer

John T. Carpenter, Jr.

Breast cancer remains one of the most frequent malignant diseases seen in women. The incidence has increased substantially since the early 1980s at least in part because of more widespread mammographic screening and perhaps other factors as well. Survival is long compared with that of other common malignancies in women; currently, the median survival is more than 10 years. In virtually every type of medical practice, then, particularly any type of primary care practice, it is inevitable that women who have or have had breast cancer will be encountered. This section provides an overview of the medical aspects of breast cancer management, both specific medical therapy for the disease itself as well as other aspects of medical treatment that should be considered in overall management of the patient. Treatment of disease within the breast by mastectomy or by breast conservation therapy (i.e., tumor removal and radiotherapy to the breast) produces long-term local control of the tumor in more than 90% of patients. Survival, however, is related to the stage of disease and not to the type of local therapy used. When patients die from breast cancer, it is from compromise of other vital organs from metastases, particularly liver, lung, and brain, rather than from uncontrolled local disease. It follows, then, that improvement in survival depends on control of systemic disease. Systemic therapy with hormonal or cytotoxic therapy regularly produces tumor shrinkage in patients with advanced breast cancer. In recent years similar treatment used as part of initial therapy—adjuvant systemic therapy—has produced modest improvement in survival for most patients as well.

EARLY BREAST CANCER

The goal of local therapy with mastectomy or breast conservation therapy is control of disease in the breast and surrounding tissues. In the past, most patients with breast cancer died from systemic recurrence after a period of years despite local control of the tumor. Early detection has altered the situation to some extent. Almost all patients with clinically or mammographically detected tumors 1 cm or smaller that have not spread to regional lymph nodes remain well 5 to 15 years or longer after local treatment only. This group still comprises a rather small minority of the breast cancer population at present. If any patients can reasonably be said to be cured by current therapy, this is the group. Most patients with clinically detected (a lump in the breast is found) or larger mammographically detected tumors continue to be at risk for death from their cancer. In general, that risk is related to the stage of disease—the tumor burden—at the time of diagnosis as well as to the biologic characteristics of the tumor (i.e., its aggressiveness or rate of growth). It has been demonstrated conclusively that administration of hormonal or cytotoxic chemotherapy after local treatment reduces the odds of recurrence and of death in the 10-year period after operation. The observed reduction in the odds of death during that period was about 25% in the overview analysis (1). No group of patients was identified who appear to be cured by the addition of systemic therapy, but the extension in survival observed was unequivocal, although of a modest magnitude (e.g., several years for those with involved axillary nodes). A realistic goal of present studies of adjuvant systemic therapy is to increase the magnitude of extension of survival while improving quality of life.

Early studies by the National Surgical Adjuvant Breast and Bowel Project (NSABP) in the United States (2) and the group at the National Tumor Institute in Milan, Italy (3), showed that adjuvant chemotherapy after mastectomy decreased relapse rates and improved survival in women at high risk for systemic relapse (i.e., those with involved axillary lymph nodes at mastectomy). Later adjuvant tamoxifen, a hormonal agent, was also shown to be effective (4). A representative summary of the results of early studies of adjuvant systemic therapy is found in the overview published by the Early Breast Cancer Trialists' Collaborative Group in 1993 (1). This summation of the results of all known prospective, randomized studies of systemic therapy in early breast cancer found a reduction in the annual odds of death of approximately 25% in the 10 years after mastectomy from the use of adjuvant combination chemotherapy for 6 or more months, tamoxifen for 1 to 2 years, or ovarian ablation. The reduction in mortality is almost certainly somewhat greater in patients who actually receive and complete treatment because the overview data were analyzed using an intention-to-treat methodology. The reduction in the odds of death was of a similar proportion across all subgroups. The absolute reduction in the odds of death for any individual, then, was related to that person's risk from the cancer. A woman whose risk of death from cancer was 15% in 10 years would have that risk reduced to 10% to 12%, whereas a woman whose risk of death was 60% in 10 years would have that risk reduced to 40% to 45% by adjuvant systemic therapy. Adjuvant systemic therapy probably reduces the risk of death for every woman who takes it after local therapy for invasive breast cancer. The decision as to whether an individual should take it should be based on 1) a careful estimation of that person's risk of recurrence and death in the 5- to 10-year period after diagnosis, 2) estimation of the proportional and absolute benefit to be expected from adjuvant therapy as well as the anticipated risks and side effects, and 3) discussion between the woman and her physician as to what is medically advisable and personally acceptable, given the information just discussed. It is certainly not indicated in every situation.

An individual's chance of recurrence or death in the 5 to 10 years after local treatment is ordinarily estimated on the basis of clinical or pathologic prognostic factors related to the cancer. Those with advanced local disease all have greater than a 50% chance of recurrence within 5 years (5). For those with positive axillary lymph nodes, the chance of recurrence within 5 to 10 years ranges from about 30% to 90%, depending on the number of nodes involved (6). The most dependable prognostic factor in those tumors with negative axillary nodes is size: 10-year relapse rates are about 10% or less for tumors 1 cm or smaller, 25% for those 1 to 3 cm in size, and 45% for those 3 to 5 cm in size (7). Tumors of similar size with some special histologic types have lower relapse rates (7). Other factors such as extent of differentiation, nuclear grade, hormone receptor status, proliferative index, and so on may be helpful in borderline situations but are not needed in most situations.

Once an individual's baseline risk of recurrence has been determined, then the decision about adjuvant systemic therapy can reasonably be discussed, knowing that available adjuvant therapies can reduce that risk by 25% to 35%. Most oncologists do not recommend any adjuvant systemic therapy for those whose risk of recurrence is 10% or less, such as those with tumors 1 cm or smaller and negative axillary lymph nodes. It usually is recommended for those with a risk of recurrence of 20% to 25% and higher. For those in between, a frank discussion of the magnitude of improvement and side effects expected as well as the individual's desires and preferences is appropriate.

Current recommendations for adjuvant systemic therapy are certain to evolve as the results of ongoing studies become available. At present (mid-1995), several general approaches are well established. For women of any age and menopausal status whose tumors lack hormone receptors, an established combination chemotherapy regimen of 4 to 6 months' duration should be used. For those whose tumors contain hormone receptors, the choice is more complicated. Postmenopausal women at increased risk with estrogen or progesterone receptor–positive tumors should receive tamoxifen for at least 2 years. In the United States, combination chemotherapy is frequently also recommended in addition, although most available studies do not show any advantage from the addition of chemotherapy to tamoxifen alone for these women (8,9). Premenopausal women with hormone receptor–positive tumors usually receive a combination chemotherapy regimen in the United States; limited data suggest that ovarian ablation or tamoxifen are probably comparably effective (1).

There are several caveats. 1) In no subset of women has combined or sequential endocrine and cytotoxic chemotherapy been shown to be superior to either alone despite their widespread use. 2) Durations of chemotherapy longer than 6 months are not more effective than durations of about 6 months (1), and they may increase long-term toxicity. 3) Low-dose regimens have been demonstrated to be inferior to standard doses of chemotherapy and are not recommended (10). 4) Higher doses of cytotoxic therapy than conventional or standard doses (including myeloablative therapy [bone marrow transplant]) are not known to be superior for any subset of patients; several prospective studies comparing these directly are in progress. 5) Most commonly used combination chemotherapy regimens have been shown to be similarly effective when compared directly in the same patient population; a regimen of doxorubicin followed by the combination of cyclophosphamide, methotrexate, and fluorouracil may be somewhat more effective (11) but unfortunately has not been compared directly to any other conventional regimen in a prospective study. 6) The optimal duration of therapy with tamoxifen is not known; extrapolations from early data suggest that it is 2 to 5 years in postmenopausal women and 5 years in premenopausal women. The usual recommendation in the United States is 5 years. Although experimental data have suggested that longer durations may be superior, preliminary results of two prospective studies indicate no advantage for 10 years over 5 years of tamoxifin treatment in premenopausal or postmenopausal women. 7) No data exist from prospective comparisons to indicate that any particular sequence of modalities is superior to any other despite the strong feelings of some therapists; thus, local custom and oncologists' preferences usually determine the sequencing of multimodality therapy; prospective data on sequential versus simultaneous combined modality therapies are similarly lacking.

It is worth noting that many current recommendations about adjuvant systemic therapy are based on the results of older studies that used what would currently be thought to be flawed designs. These have included suboptimal dosing of chemotherapy, age-related arbitrary dose reductions or excessive dose reductions for numerical toxicities in the absence of clinical toxicity (bleeding or infection), use of oral drugs without any monitoring of compliance or of drug absorption, and use of study designs with patient numbers too small to detect or to exclude moderate sized but clinically important differences in the therapies compared. Important points that should be clarified by ongoing studies include the extent of the benefit of higher doses of conventional outpatient chemotherapy and of myeloablative therapy (i.e., autologous transplantation) compared with conventional chemotherapy and the extent of the benefit of combined endocrine and chemotherapy to chemotherapy alone in premenopausal women or to endocrine therapy alone in postmenopausal women.

Despite increased public awareness and more widespread use of screening mammography, a minority of patients still present with large lesions, with lesions fixed to the chest wall, with skin invasion or edema, or with relatively large palpable axillary lymph nodes, which is locally advanced disease. Survival in this group of patients is inferior overall to that of patients with earlier stages of disease (5). Management nearly always consists of multimodality therapy but differs somewhat from that of earlier stage disease. Most of the caveats listed previously also apply here. The combination of local and systemic therapies used ordinarily includes local or locoregional radiotherapy because control of locoregional disease is more problematic in this group of patients. For the group who presents simply with large, nonfixed lesions, primary chemotherapy followed by breast conservation therapy produces excellent local control rates and survival at least comparable to that seen with other approaches (12).

ADVANCED BREAST CANCER

Although patients with very small tumors fare very well with current therapy, the great majority of patients with clinically detected breast cancer die from their disease sooner or later. This may occur within several years after diagnosis for those with a poorer prognosis or after one or more decades for those with better prognosis. For all groups the range is wide, however. A series from the nineteenth century in which no treatment was used (none was known to be helpful) showed a median survival of about 3 years, but a long gradual decline in the group followed with a few surviving 20 years (13). In the modern era, median survival after systemic recurrence has been of a similar magnitude (i.e., about 3 years). At this point, long-term eradication of disease is not ordinarily a feasible or realistic goal. Available therapy may shrink or eliminate metastatic disease temporarily and may improve quality of life, but the effect on survival is modest. Appropriate goals of treatment in patients with advanced breast cancer are palliation of symptoms and improvement in quality of life. Here the price (i.e., toxicity and side effects) of any treatment should be weighed carefully against the benefits to be obtained. "Doing something" is frequently not the best approach.

Although a detailed guide to the management of advanced breast cancer would constitute an appropriate topic for a book or several chapters, some overall guidelines may be helpful. First, if the goals of treatment are improvement of symptoms and quality of life, then no intervention is needed or helpful for the patient with advanced breast cancer who has normal or near-normal function and no symptoms of disease. For some it may be days or weeks before symptomatic metastatic disease develops, but for others it may be years. Careful observation alone may suffice for this variable period. Once symptomatic metastatic disease appears, treatment may be helpful. Local modalities (radiotherapy) may suffice when symptoms are well localized. Hormonal therapy will frequently be helpful when symptoms are generalized or multifocal, but its effects occur gradually (i.e., over weeks to a few months). It is not an appropriate choice for rapidly progressive, life-threatening situations. Cytotoxic chemotherapy produces improvement in half or more of patients and acts relatively rapidly—days to a few weeks—but at the cost of considerably more toxicity and distressing side effects. It is the correct choice for rapidly progressive or life-threatening situations. Every systemic therapy has a failure rate; optimal usage requires a specific goal for the therapy, some parameter to assess the success of the treatment (such as shrinkage of an index lesion), and a basis for continuing or terminating the therapy.

Initial systemic therapy should start with a hormonal modality such as tamoxifen for all except those with rapidly progressive or life-threatening metastases. Side effects are not usually severe; the chance of tumor shrinkage, that is response, is higher when hormone receptor assays are positive. The treatment should be continued for at least several months to assess response unless there is objective evidence of disease progression. The median duration of response to initial hormonal therapy is about 1 year, although it may be quite long in a few, more than 10 years. Those who experience initial response to hormonal therapy are good candidates for other hormonal modalities when the disease later progresses (e.g., progestins, estrogens, medical or surgical oophorectomy, androgens, aromatase inhibitors). Those who are not good candidates for hormonal therapy or whose tumors later become resistant to it should receive cytotoxic chemotherapy. Although drug combinations have been widely recommended and used in the past, full doses of effective single agents are at least as effective as most drug combinations. Doxorubicin, paclitaxel, cyclophosphamide, methotrexate, and fluorouracil are usually effective either alone or in various combinations. Once symptoms of metastatic disease have been controlled after 4 to 6 months of any given systemic therapy, it is frequently helpful to withhold further systemic treatment until symptoms reappear, a "vacation" from both drug side effects and symptoms of disease.

Other supportive measures may prove extremely helpful for specific situations. The majority of patients will experience pain of at least moderate severity at some point; careful attention to pain relief is essential for satisfactory quality of life. Repetitive doses of oral opiates titrated to the individual's need are usually most satisfactory. The risk of addiction is minimal in this situation; doses should not be withheld or attenuated to avoid a nonexistent risk of addiction. Depression is not an infrequent accompaniment to the situation, which may minimize pain tolerance and lead to disturbed sleep patterns, among other effects. Use of antidepressant medications frequently helps patients to enjoy and make the most of a limited remaining life span. The pain and morbidity of bone metastases may be ameliorated by biphosphonate therapy (14). Pain on weight bearing may portend impending hip or femur fracture from bone destruction. Surgical fixation or repair frequently helps to maintain mobility and independence. Severe or new back pain may be due to spinal cord compression by metastatic disease. Early use of magnetic resonance scanning is critically important to detect cord compression early and allow for control by radiotherapy. Once neurologic function is lost, it cannot usually be regained. Brain metastases can usually be palliated with radiotherapy; removal of single lesions surgically and treatment of limited brain metastases by radiosurgery represent newer approaches that may be helpful in some situations. Pleural effusions resulting from pleural metastases may cause major distress from dyspnea. These may be controlled using systemic therapy, but pleurodesis and sclerosis may be helpful in selected situations. Finally, ongoing support and concern from a physician may be invaluable in dealing with a difficult and trying medical and personal dilemma.

OTHER ASPECTS OF THERAPY

Use of Imaging and Other Diagnostic Studies in Initial Staging and Follow-up

As a general observation, radiographic studies are overused and frequently used inappropriately in patients with breast cancer. For the patient who presents with a breast mass smaller than 5 cm and with no symptoms suggestive of metastasis, initial staging should include physical examination with particular attention to the breasts, regional lymph node–bearing areas, and liver size as well as a complete blood cell count and chemistry survey; radiographic studies should include a chest x-ray film and mammograms of both breasts. Liver imaging with computed tomography or ultrasonography is not needed if liver size and biochemical studies are normal (15). The rate of true positivity for bone scans in this group is 1% to 2%, with a false-positive rate in the same range; in the absence of symptoms or unexplained elevation of alkaline phosphatase, bone scans are not needed and are expensive. For patients with breast masses 5 cm or larger or with locally advanced disease, the rate of positive bone scans approaches 25% (15); here they should be obtained routinely in initial staging. Areas of abnormal uptake on bone scan should always be evaluated with plain x-ray films to distinguish benign from malignant causes. Because bone scintigraphy is quite sensitive, changes resulting from arthritis, osteoporosis, old trauma, and other benign processes are detected frequently; these should be distinguished from malignant bone destruction with bone x-ray films.

For follow-up of patients after initial treatment for breast cancer, a minimalist approach is suggested. Routine history and physical examination should be done several times yearly for 5 years or so and annually thereafter. Annual mammograms are recommended. Other studies (i.e., blood tests, chest x-ray films, and scans) should not be done routinely but performed only if symptoms or abnormal findings dictate. Several studies have shown no improvement in disease outcome or in quality of life from the use of routine imaging studies in follow-up (16,17).

Toxicities of Systemic Therapy

The immediate toxicities of commonly used chemotherapy regimens are well known and largely temporary: nausea and vomiting, hair loss, blood count depression, menstrual irregularity, and so on. Cardiac failure is seen in 1% or less of patients who receive adjuvant doxorubicin. There does not appear to be any increase in second tumors. Of concern, however, are reports of secondary myelodysplasia and acute leukemia after adjuvant chemotherapy (18). Earlier reports described patients who had received melphalan, an oral alkylating agent no longer used for this indication. Recent reports include two distinct syndromes, one occurring within the first few years after topoisomerase II inhibitors (such as doxorubicin or etoposide) with a high proportion of 11q23 translocations, and a second delayed type seen 3 to 7 years after treatment with alkylating agents (such as cyclophosphamide), which frequently has deletion or abnormalities of chromosomes 5 and 7. These syndromes have been seen only occasionally in the past but have been reported more often in recent years after the use of more dose-intensive regimens. It remains to be seen whether more intensive and myeloablative treatment regimens will be sufficiently more effective than conventional regimens to justify this additional major late toxicity.

For women who receive adjuvant tamoxifen, immediate toxicities include hot flashes, changes in vaginal secretions, and hepatic enzyme abnormalities as well as vaginal thinning or atrophy in a few; only a few discontinue the therapy because of side effects. In recent years an increased incidence of endometrial cancer has been reported in a large North American study (19) (and others) of about 2.0 per 1000 per year, up from the baseline U.S. rate of 0.7 per 1000 per year. A few patients have died from these secondary malignancies. Current recommendations for patients who receive adjuvant tamoxifen are that they undergo routine annual pelvic examination as well as definitive evaluation at any time for any other symptoms or signs suggestive of endometrial cancer such as postmenopausal bleeding or new pelvic discomfort or fullness. Transvaginal ultrasonography and endometrial aspiration cytology may be helpful. Endometrial biopsy or dilation and curettage should be performed if needed. Even more recent information suggests that at least some of this apparent increase may be due to exacerbation by tamoxifen of preexisting subclinical endometrial cancers (20). For patients who receive tamoxifen as treatment for breast cancer, the benefit still outweighs this risk by a considerable margin. Further studies are needed and will be forthcoming to clarify the nature and extent of the risk of secondary endometrial cancer.

Early Menopause

One common consequence of treatment with combination chemotherapy in younger women is permanent cessation of menses with early onset of menopause. The likelihood of amenorrhea is strongly related to age; it is usually reversible in women in their 20s but is permanent in about half of women in their 30s and in the majority of women in their 40s. Two major resulting problems are 1) the earlier risk of cardiovascular disease, the principal cause of death in postmenopausal women, and 2) menopausal symptoms, particularly hot flashes, vaginal dryness, and emotional changes, which are superimposed on the emotional changes related to the development of a malignancy. Replacement estrogen is effective in relieving menopausal symptoms but is not widely used in women with previous breast cancer and is thought to be contraindicated by some (21). In fact, no definitive study has been performed to evaluate the safety of hormone replacement therapy in women with a previous breast cancer.

Common symptoms may be ameliorated by other available options. Low doses of progestins are effective in relieving hot flashes; they are not widely used but are thought to be safe in this situation. Definitive studies are again lacking. Low doses of clonidine or vitamin E may also be helpful. Vaginal dryness may be relieved effectively with over-the-counter lubricating preparations (Replens and others). Vaginal atrophy occurs in some, with resultant discomfort and sexual difficulty; topical estrogen preparations provide relief, but this must be balanced against the possible risk of exacerbation of their malignancy.

No studies are available to help with advice about reducing the risk of cardiovascular disease after early menopause in women with breast cancer. Certainly, attention to other known cardiovascular risk factors is advisable: smoking cessation, blood pressure control, and so on. Encouragement of a healthy diet (high in fiber and fresh fruits, vegetables, and grains, and low in fat) and avoidance of obesity are advisable, but adoption of neither of these in midlife is known to affect the course of breast cancer. Tamoxifen lowers both total and low-density lipoprotein cholesterol, and it stabilizes bone mineral density, but it has not been prospectively evaluated as a hormone replacement treatment either alone or combined with estrogen or estrogen-progestin preparations.

Pregnancy After Breast Cancer

In women with a previous breast cancer pregnancy does not appear to change the risk of recurrence (22). Women with a previous breast cancer who inquire about the advisability of having a child may reasonably be told that 1) the risk of recurrence will be unchanged by the pregnancy, 2) it is reasonable to wait several years after primary treatment of the breast cancer, the period of highest risk of recurrence, before considering pregnancy, 3) the decision to bear a child should be based on the woman's desires in light of her overall health situation (i.e., the chance that she will survive to be able to raise the child). The decision is best based on careful consideration of the child's as well as the mother's needs. The physician's responsibility should be to help the woman make her decision with accurate information about her own prognosis and how it will be affected by subsequent childbearing.

References

1. Early Breast Cancer Trialists' Collaborative Group. Systemic treatment of early breast cancer by hormonal, cytotoxic, or immune therapy. Lancet 1992;1–15, 71–85.
2. Fisher B, Fisher ER, Redmond C, and Participating NSABP Investigators.

Ten-year results from the National Surgical Adjuvant Breast and Bowel Project (NSABP) clinical trial evaluating the use of L-phenylalanine mustard (L-PAM) in the management of primary breast cancer. J Clin Oncol 1986;4:929–941.

3. Bonadonna G, Valagussa P, Moliterni A, et al. Adjuvant cyclophosphamide, methotrexate, and fluorouracil in node-positive breast cancer: the results of 20 years of followup. N Engl J Med 1995;332:901–906.

4. Nolvadex Adjuvant Trial Organization. Controlled trial of tamoxifen as a single adjuvant agent in management of early breast cancer: analysis at eight years by the Nolvadex Adjuvant Trial Organization. Br J Cancer 1988;57:608–611.

5. Wood WC. Neoadjuvant chemotherapy. In: Henderson IC, ed. Adjuvant therapy of breast cancer. Boston: Kluwer Academic Publishers, 1992: 279–291.

6. Nemoto T, Vana J, Bedwani R, et al. Management and survival of female breast cancer: results of a national survey by the American College of Surgeons. Cancer 1980;45:2917–2924.

7. Rosen PP, Groshen S, Kinne DW, Norton L. Factors influencing prognosis in node-negative breast carcinoma: analysis of 767 T1N0M0/T2N0M0 patients with long-term follow-up. J Clin Oncol 1994;11:2090–2100.

8. Rivkin SE, Green S, Metch B, et al. Adjuvant CMFVP versus tamoxifen versus concurrent CMFVP and tamoxifen for postmenopausal, node-positive, and estrogen receptor-positive breast cancer patients: a Southwest Oncology Group study. J Clin Oncol 1994;12:2078–2085.

9. Boccardo F, Rubagotti A, Bruzzi P, et al. Chemotherapy versus tamoxifen versus chemotherapy plus tamoxifen in node-positive, estrogen receptor-positive breast cancer patients: results of a multicentric Italian study. J Clin Oncol 1990;8:1310–1320.

10. Wood WC, Budman DR, Korzun AH, et al. Dose and dose intensity of adjuvant chemotherapy for stage II, node-positive breast carcinoma. N Engl J Med 1994;330:1253–1259.

11. Bonadonna G, Zambetti M, Valagussa P. Sequential or alternating doxorubicin and CMF regimens in breast cancer with more than three positive nodes: ten year results. JAMA 1995;273:542–547.

12. Bonadonna G, Veronesi U, Brambilla C, et al. Primary chemotherapy to avoid mastectomy in tumors with diameters of three centimeters or more. J Natl Cancer Inst 1990;82:1539–1545.

13. Bloom HJG, Richardson WW, Harries EJ. Natural history of untreated breast cancer (1805–1933): comparison of untreated and treated cases according to histological grade of malignancy. BMJ 1962;2:213–221.

14. Paterson AHG, Powles J, Kanis JA, et al. Double-blind controlled trial of oral clodronate in patients with bone metastases from breast cancer. J Clin Oncol 1993;11:59–65.

15. Harris JR, Morrow M, Bonadonna G. Cancer of the breast. In: DeVita VT, Hellman S, Rosenberg SA, eds. Cancer principles and practice of oncology. Philadelphia: JB Lippincott, 1993:1278.

16. The GIVIO Investigators. Impact of follow-up testing on survival and health-related quality of life in breast cancer patients: a multicenter randomized controlled trial. JAMA 1994;271:1587–1592.

17. Roselli Del Turco M, Palli D, Cariddi A, et al. Intensive diagnostic follow-up after treatment of primary breast cancer: a randomized trial. JAMA 1994;271:1593–1597.

18. DeCillis A, Anderson S, Wickerham DL, et al. Acute myeloid leukemia (AML) in NSABP B-25. Proc American Society of Clinical Oncology 1995;14:98.

19. Fisher B, Costantino JP, Redmond CK, et al. Endometrial cancer in tamoxifen-treated breast cancer patients: findings from the National Surgical Adjuvant Breast and Bowel Project (NSABP) B-14. J Natl Cancer Inst 1994;86:527–537.

20. Jordan VC, Assikis VJ. Tamoxifen and endometrial cancer: clearing up a controversy. Clin Cancer Res 1995;1:467–472.

21. Cobleigh MA, Berris RF, Bush T, et al. Estrogen replacement therapy in breast cancer survivors: a time for change. JAMA 1994;272:540–545.

22. von Schoultz E, Johansson H, Wilking N, Rutqvist L-E. Influence of prior and subsequent pregnancy on breast cancer prognosis. J Clin Oncol 1995;139:430–434.

INDEX